THE SERPENT'S TALE

THE SERPENT'S TALE

KUṆḌALINĪ, YOGA, AND THE HISTORY OF AN EXPERIENCE

SRAVANA BORKATAKY-VARMA AND ANYA FOXEN

Columbia University Press *New York*

Columbia University Press
Publishers Since 1893
New York Chichester, West Sussex

Library of Congress Cataloging-in-Publication Data
Names: Borkataky-Varma, Sravana author | Foxen, Anya P., 1986– author
Title: The serpent's tale : Kuṇḍalinī yoga and the history of an experience / Sravana Borkataky-Varma and Anya Foxen.
Description: New York : Columbia University Press, [2025] | Includes bibliographical references and index.
Identifiers: LCCN 2025003267 (print) | LCCN 2025003268 (ebook) | ISBN 9780231212526 hardback | ISBN 9780231212533 trade paperback | ISBN 9780231559430 ebook
Subjects: LCSH: Kuṇḍalinī—History
Classification: LCC BL1238.56.K86 B67 2025 (print) | LCC BL1238.56.K86 (ebook) | DDC 294.5/436—dc23/eng/20250411

Cover design: Julia Kushnirsky
Cover image: gettyimages

GPSR Authorized Representative: Easy Access System Europe, Mustamäe tee 50, 10621 Tallinn, Estonia, gpsr.requests@easproject.com

CONTENTS

Prologue 1

1 South Asian Roots: Serpents, Fire, and the Ascent of Kuṇḍalinī 29

2 Western Roots: Subtle Bodies, Mystical Ascents, and Assorted Serpents 55

3 West Meets East: Kuṇḍalinī and the Serpent Power 81

4 East Meets West: Kuṇḍalinī and the Evolution of Modern Yoga 121

5 When the Serpent Rises: What Happened to Gopi Krishna? 163

6 The Serpent in the Marketplace: Global Gurus Make Their Mark 205

7 The Serpent in the Melting Pot: Kuṇḍalinī in North American Counterculture 247

8 The Serpent in the Web: Contemporary Interweavings 285

Notes *327*

Bibliography *363*

Index *377*

PROLOGUE

Turning and turning in the widening gyre

—WILLIAM BUTLER YEATS, "THE SECOND COMING"

She is the dragon in the deep. The primordial force at the foundation. She coils low down in the gut—the reptilian brain, wound tight with the potential energy of our evolution. She is the time-scorching heat of the Sun, the fire that smolders in the heart of the Earth. She is Power. She is Śakti. She is Devī. Maybe She is All.

And above all, perhaps, She is transmutation. In the words of one semi-reluctant mystic, who happened to encounter Her around Christmastime in 1937:

> Little did I realize that from that day onwards I was never to be my old normal self again, that I had unwittingly and without preparation or even adequate knowledge of it roused to activity the most wonderful and stern power in man, that I had stepped unknowingly upon the key to the most guarded secret of the ancients, and that thenceforth for a long time I had to live suspended by a thread, swinging between life on the one hand and

> death on the other, between sanity and insanity, between light and darkness, between heaven and earth.[1]

Kuṇḍalinī is everywhere and nowhere. As scholars of religion, we mean this quite literally: passing references to Kuṇḍalinī consistently show up in the vast majority of scholarly works on tantra, yoga, and the like. It's striking how frequently Kuṇḍalinī appears as a footnote. And yet, to date, there exists no sustained academic study of Kuṇḍalinī. The closest we have come to a scholarly book devoted exclusively to the topic is Lilian Silburn's *Kuṇḍalinī: The Energy of the Depths* (1983). But, excepting a few thematic diversions, Silburn (understandably) treats only the medieval nondual Śaiva texts where Kuṇḍalinī receives Her fullest development.

Things look different, of course, if we step outside the walled gardens of academia. In the popular sphere, there is no shortage of material on Kuṇḍalinī, including book-length treatments that purport to give a holistic account of what Kuṇḍalinī is, does, and means. Perusing this material, it does not take long to arrive at a standard shorthand model: Kuṇḍalinī is the Serpent Power. She rests coiled at the base of the spine. If awakened, She rises, weaving like a fiery snake along the spine and up to the crown of the head. Sometimes *cakras* are mentioned.

This notion of a serpentine Kuṇḍalinī rising up through a sequence of seven(ish) *cakras* certainly has precedents in premodern South Asian sources. Historically speaking, however, this model represents only one specific strand of the Indian material, and its modern character is colored substantially (and often in all seven hues of the rainbow) by fusion with Western systems of symbols, concepts, and practices. Though both the South Asian and Western models in question have ancient and complex roots—roots that have probably been interweaving here and there for centuries if not millennia—the Serpent Power, as we know "it" today, rises out of a particularly tenacious tangle created by colonial-era conversations between Indian and Western esotericists, who reinterpreted Kuṇḍalinī not only in light of intersections between their respective worldviews but also evolving understandings of popular science, especially physiology and evolutionary theory.

A couple of notes, before we proceed. This book is about Kuṇḍalinī. At this point you, the reader, might reasonably expect us to tell you what Kuṇḍalinī *actually is*.

We will not do this.

Apologies, dear reader. If you picked up this book looking for an easy answer, we regret to inform you that you will not find it within these pages. The term itself comes from the Sanskrit root (originally borrowed from Dravidian languages) √kuṇḍ, which can be rendered as something like "to burn." As a basic noun (*kuṇḍa*), it refers to a container—a pot, a bowl, or a basin. In this form, it can also signify both a sacred body of water and the brick pit used as an altar for a Vedic fire sacrifice. Add a suffix (*kuṇḍala*), and it means something that curves in upon itself, like an earring, ring, or bracelet. This is probably the level of meaning from which the Kuṇḍalinī we are concerned with derives. At the most basic level, Kuṇḍalinī is simply "the coiled one" (sometimes also rendered as Kuṇḍalī). But of course one can easily read into its significance, stemming from all of the previously mentioned levels of meaning. And so, this is why there are no easy answers to be found here. If even the word itself is so complex, things are unlikely to become simpler once we begin to layer on century upon century of philosophical concepts, religious rituals, and cultural narratives.

At the same time, though this is an academic book, we do not intend it as a book solely for academics. Rather, this is a book that ultimately hopes to bridge the gap between the rigors of history, ethnography, and textual analysis (all of which are scholarly methods we have drawn upon here) and the inherent ambiguities of human experience.

This book is about experience. Kuṇḍalinī is about experience. This is something to which we will return again and again.

But, to begin with, it may be easier to tell you what this book is *not* about. At least, not entirely. We will start with the most straightforward and then come full circle to the more complex aspects.

THIS BOOK IS NOT ABOUT YOGI BHAJAN'S KUNDALINI YOGA

Many if not most, especially in North America, who have ever heard the term "Kuṇḍalinī" will have likely heard it in the context of "Kundalini Yoga as taught by Yogi Bhajan." The method is so common, especially in the world of modern yoga, that this phrase may as well be trademarked. We will look at Yogi Bhajan's teachings in chapter 6, along with the broader question of how Kuṇḍalinī became inextricably attached to and packaged as "yoga" more generally. For the time being, however, let us simply say that this is only one small, and relatively late, aspect of our story.

THIS BOOK IS NOT ABOUT SEX

Which is to say, this book is not about Neo-Tantra.

Sacred eroticism and transcendent sex have become central to what Hugh Urban has called "neo-Tantra" and Jeffrey J. Kripal has named, perhaps somewhat more pointedly, "American Tantra."[2] (Kripal, to be clear, does not think that American Tantra is a bad thing—but it is *American.*) Common to both of these arguments is the notion that what most Americans, and indeed many across the globe, refer to as "tantra" today is a new (that's the "Neo-") cultural synthesis that should not be conflated, much less equated, with historical South Asian tantric philosophies and practices. The same goes for Kuṇḍalinī.

In Neo-Tantra, Kuṇḍalinī becomes, above all else, a *sexual* energy. As we will see, this has some precedent in South Asian tradition. In nondual tantric traditions, especially, the polarity, relationship, and ultimate identity of masculine and feminine are part and parcel of the fundamental nature of the cosmos. Sexual union is not only a metaphor for cosmic creation, but a tool that can be used—especially in a carefully structured ritual context—to tap into these mechanisms for the purpose of self-realization. To the extent that this basic framing can be found in many Neo-Tantric frameworks, they do share something with their South Asian counterparts. However, Neo-Tantra tends to lean less on ritual and more on spontaneity, less on authority and more on self-empowerment. Depending on the context, Kuṇḍalinī may be equated exclusively with sexual awakening, or even simply with orgasm.

This is not to say that Neo-Tantric understandings of Kuṇḍalinī are somehow invalid, or even inauthentic. Approached ethically and with proper framing, Neo-Tantric sexual practices can be sites of profound healing, discovery, and growth. They are capable of being profoundly spiritual experiences in their own right. But their assumptions as well as their goals—to say nothing of their techniques—are simply not the same as those of their South Asian counterparts. Insofar as they often see sexuality as something to be reclaimed and redeemed, they are steeped in a very particular Western, and even more specifically Christian, heritage. It was the serpent, after all, that promised to lead Adam and Eve to immortality. Neo-Tantric traditions take the notion of forbidden fruit and turn it on its head.

We will turn to some of these tensions between historical roots, culture, and framing when it comes to Kuṇḍalinī and sex in the latter chapters of this book. But this is only one aspect, and a relatively minor one, of the overall sweep—both cross-historical and cross-cultural—of Kuṇḍalinī traditions. And it's important to keep in mind, even in Neo-Tantric contexts where sexuality may come to the forefront, that, in the end, it's never quite about the sex itself. We are, after all, dealing with practices that purport to put us into conversation with the divine nature of ultimate reality.

Within the context of sex and gender, it feels appropriate to remark on an aspect of this book that may strike the reader as somewhat of a peculiarity: namely, that we have chosen to refer to Kuṇḍalinī throughout this text not as "it" (except for where we speak more tangibly of the "Kuṇḍalinī force," the "Kuṇḍalinī experience," and so on) but as "She." We do this both to honor the concept's deep roots in the traditions of Goddess tantra and also as a nod to what seems to be a fundamental aspect of the experience as it is described by those familiar with it—whatever it is, it has a mind of its own. In other words, even as a human bodily experience, Kuṇḍalinī is autonomous. And yet, this gendered pronoun should not be taken literally, in the same way that most Abrahamic traditions that refer to God as "He" do not simply mean that God is male in the ordinary human sense. In the case of Kuṇḍalinī, even in traditional ritual spaces where sexual practices may be employed, biological sex and conventional notions of gender mean very little. Indeed, the Śākta (that is, Goddess-oriented) traditions where Kuṇḍalinī is most prominent take an *advaita* or nondual approach to reality. "Enlightenment" means collapsing and moving beyond *all* binaries—pure/impure, good/bad, masculine/feminine—and so, as the ultimate "She," Kuṇḍalinī is perhaps best understood as "nonbinary."

THIS BOOK IS NOT ABOUT THE ONE "TRUE" KUṆḌALINĪ

Though "Kuṇḍalinī" as a term originated in South Asian, and particularly Hindu, sources, we should not endow these with any sort of ultimate authority. Firstly, the medieval Hindu tantric texts where we find the earliest mentions of Kuṇḍalinī are tapestries woven out of many pre-existing concepts, including not only Hindu but also Jain and Buddhist understandings of both the body and the cosmos at large. And then, the Sanskrit sources on Kuṇḍalinī are miniscule relative to the body of literature that begins to coalesce even by the early twentieth century. Most of the texts responsible for modern global understandings of Kuṇḍalinī are written in English.

Of course, this elides the reality that, for most of Kuṇḍalinī's history, texts would have been precisely the wrong place to look if one wished for anything but a cursory understanding. For one, texts are not always direct. Arguably, our number of sources might expand dramatically if we were willing to read between the lines. Take, for instance, the *Yoga Vāsiṣṭha*, a medieval Sanskrit text that is tricky to date—scholars generally place it anywhere between the tenth and thirteenth century, depending on the version—and even trickier to interpret. The *Yoga Vāsiṣṭha* has not generally been treated as having much to say about Kuṇḍalinī, that is, until you look at a very specific episode narrating the diverging paths the king Śikhidhvaja and his queen, Cūḍālā, take towards enlightenment. The story of Śikhidhvaja and Cūḍālā may also be one of the very few explicit mentions of Kuṇḍalinī rising in a female body.[3] But really—especially given the nature of the topic and the practices with which we are dealing—it is likely that most of the actual premodern transmission of Kuṇḍalinī occurred through vernacular, and especially oral, traditions. Looking at the readily available Sanskrit literature means we encounter Kuṇḍalinī only in the forms that catch the attention of a certain class of cultural elites.[4] Some of this is a matter of historical distance—if only we could hop in a time machine—but some of it, as we will come to see, reflects the way things still work today. As our story winds its way into the final chapter, we will invite you to consider whether the Kuṇḍalinī that occupies Western scholars, the Kuṇḍalinī that swirls within social media, and the Kuṇḍalinī that still dwells on the charnel grounds of West Bengal are indeed the same Kuṇḍalinī.

So, with this more modern and global lens in mind, our goal here is to explore how the shape and meaning of Kuṇḍalinī has evolved through conversation between Indian and Western traditions. The second half of that pair deserves some extra qualification, not only because of its vagueness but because of the loaded nature of referring to "Western tradition," especially in a context that inherently involves colonialism. Since the period of exchange we mean to address here begins during British colonialism in India, we will have an occasion to talk about the realities of this situation in later chapters. For the time being, we want to make clear that we are using the term "Western" not as some kind of objective and absolute geographic or ideological marker, but as shorthand for a family of concepts and practices that ultimately become significant in Europe and North America. That is, these things are "Western" not so much because of where they started out, but because of where they ended up. When we talk about "East" meeting "West," we are evoking something pseudo-geographical (both of these terms, like "Orient" and "Occident," are more objects of imagination than they are physical realities) that we hope will serve as useful "verbal handles" for the reader. We are not speaking of absolute origins, and we are certainly not making claims to cultural purity or authenticity. This is true of the South Asian side of the exchange as well. No tradition—no culture—operates in a hermetically sealed container.

And so, we arrive at the main argument of this book. Or at least we arrive at what the argument is *not*. We are not seeking to uncover the pure, authentic Kuṇḍalinī—not the model and not the experience. Indeed, if we are here to argue anything, it's that such a model and such an experience don't exist. This is true today, just as it was true in the eighth century, when we first begin to see the term appearing in Sanskrit sources. Kuṇḍalinī, modern and premodern, exists at the intersection of several symbolic systems, of which the serpent is only one strand—or rather set of strands, since the serpent too, as we'll quickly see, is very much plural.

The basic trouble is this: even if we limit ourselves to the premodern South Asian sources, we find that Kuṇḍalinī is a term that has been applied to a variety of concepts and phenomena (some incompatible if not outright contradictory with one another), and there are a number of concepts and phenomena that have not been called "Kuṇḍalinī," but which nevertheless seem to share with it some undeniable likeness. And then, of course, we have to account for the Western side of the conversation. If we simply look for the first time that Kuṇḍalinī appears in an English-language source, then we are liable to find it attached to a complex set of assumptions that seem to come out of nowhere. In order to make sense of how nineteenth-century Western authors would have understood Kuṇḍalinī, we need to look at Kuṇḍalinī through their eyes. That is, we need to ask: What in the Western tradition is Kuṇḍalinī most *like*? Because of course this is how human cognition works. We make the strange familiar by comparing.

In this sense, images may actually serve us better than words. As we try to follow the various strands of our contemporary idea of Kuṇḍalinī, we find that the image of a feminine serpentine energy is indeed the thing that allows all of these concepts to cluster together across time and space.[5] Still, we should not take this too far, for an image too is never the thing itself. As Jeffrey J. Kripal writes, in a book appropriately titled *The Serpent's Gift*, "poetically speaking, gnostic thought recognizes that religious expressions function as symbols and, as such, are simultaneously true and false, that they both reveal and conceal."[6]

This is the function of the fiery, feminine serpent. As a symbol, the serpent reveals to us the paths history has taken to produce today's "standard model" of Kuṇḍalinī. It may even reveal something *about* Kuṇḍalinī, both as a concept and as an experience. The serpent leads us to a labyrinth of stories, spanning out in both directions ("East" and "West") that seem to tell us about the intimate link between the human and the divine, body and cosmos. Indeed, they promise us a map for how the divine becomes human and how the human might become divine.

Interestingly, both sets of stories have alchemy as their medieval cornerstone. Here, the inorganic chemistry of minerals reflects both the organic processes of life and the spiritual truths of the cosmos. Mercury and sulfur, which produce the Latin *lapis philosophorum*, the "Philosopher's Stone," or the Sanskrit *rasa-rasayana*, the "Elixir of Elixirs," work like semen and menstrual blood—which produce life. Except here's the catch: the meaning assigned to this combination is wholly reversed from East to West. In India, sulfur is *rajas*, the fiery material that embodies the creative energy (*śakti*) of the Goddess. These things are all feminine. Mercury, on the other hand, is the passive essence of pure unmanifest consciousness associated with the god Śiva. Its organic correspondent is semen, which collects in the moon's crescent as in a bowl, and so it's indelibly masculine. But look over to Europe and it's the cold and wet moon that's correlated to feminine passivity, whereas the hot sun represents the dynamic masculine principle. This causes poor Carl Jung no shortage of trouble as he's forced to insist, in his lectures on Kuṇḍalinī, that the Indians must be wrong about their own cultural symbolism. The moon *must* be associated with the lower *cakras*, which must in turn symbolize the watery depths of primordial chaos (despite the fact that Indian sources clearly associate this anatomical area with the digestive fire that correlates to the consuming natural force of the sun as time, and it absolutely must be feminine).

So much for symbols, then. This is not to say that symbols are meaningless, but only that they speak to us in ways that are shaped by our own cultural stories. Symbols are like gender—they are cultural constructs that spin meaning out of lived experience. But the thing is, mercury can be either masculine or feminine, yet it'll still react with sulfur.

Actually, alchemy gives us a fairly compelling logic for approaching religious thought, and indeed religious experience.[7] Rather than searching for the one "authentic" top-down model, we might look at the primordial chaos of what *is* and what people do with it. This, in a sense, is the logic of the book in front of you now. Instead of grounding Kuṇḍalinī in some lineage of authoritative tradition, we invite the reader to treat the multiplicity of sources we present in this book (ancient and modern alike) as so many ingredients in an alchemical laboratory. As we follow the story of Kuṇḍalinī, we witness elements of culture and experience get combined and recombined to produce something that is not quite reducible to the sum of its parts. And sometimes things explode.

Another way to approach Kuṇḍalinī is to think of it as the story itself. Experience is an event.[8] It is something that happens, and some of that, at least, must be objective—a reconfiguration of atoms and molecules. But experience is also a story we tell ourselves and maybe try to tell others. Kuṇḍalinī, after all, is not simply a word or even an image that we can only track through static sources. Kuṇḍalinī would seem to be rooted in a very specific psycho-physical experience. You feel it, or you don't. And if you're not sure whether you feel it, then you probably don't. After all, it seems difficult to miss a fiery serpent shooting up one's spinal column, or the throbbing of the cosmos inside one's heart. And yet, experience is never actually this simple. Quite a few teachers, including Indian ones, who speak of Kuṇḍalinī say that it isn't necessary to *feel* Kuṇḍalinī at all. And even when Kuṇḍalinī is felt, She emerges as a constellation of bodily sensations. Sometimes these are directed by willful practice. Sometimes they seem to occur spontaneously. All we can really get at, then, is the story that the experiencer ends up sharing with us about how—and along what lines—these sensations come to make sense to them. How the spiritual comes to matter.

For this reason, a substantial portion of the sources we'll examine in this book will be textual. There is a "canon" to the modern Kuṇḍalinī experience. This is, perhaps, appropriate since the etymology of "tantra" (the body of traditions where we first encounter Kuṇḍalinī as a term), like our English word "text," ultimately means "to weave."[9] As we'll see, with modern Kuṇḍalinī lore, text becomes its own kind of transmission—perhaps not quite an initiatory mechanism, but certainly a map to lend order to the rough terrain of human embodied experience.

And, more and more, we will find that the question that haunts this network of textual strands—this web of stories—is the very same one that will trouble our own book. Is there one Kuṇḍalinī, or many? On the one hand, Kuṇḍalinī is a culturally specific model grounded in religion (particularly the followings of certain goddesses), philosophy, and ways of understanding the body. On the other hand, Kuṇḍalinī is an experience—a phenomenon that spontaneously arises within the human organism—and, as such, it must be as universal as human anatomy or the basic mechanics of human cognition.

So, what do we do when our story doesn't seem to follow the standard narrative?

SRAVANA'S STORY

Walter H. Capps writes, "What the scholar does within the subject-field depends upon where he is standing. Where he stands influences what he discovers. Furthermore, where he stands and what he discovers are implicit in what he is trying to do."[10]

This book is a product of a "stir-churn-rise." I am a scholar-practitioner of Śākta tantra. I am from Assam. I was initiated into the Kāmākhyā lineage at the age of eight, and at the time of writing, I am fifty years old, which means I have been a practitioner for forty-two years and counting. It was after twenty-seven years, in 2010, that I started my PhD studies in the United States. From the first day of joining the PhD program, I became intensely aware of a large constituent of people who seemed to be obsessed with Kuṇḍalinī. To be perfectly honest, this was rather perplexing as the tradition of which I am a practitioner seldom uses the term Kuṇḍalinī, and there are zero "Kuṇḍalinī yoga" practices. I identify myself as a woman, and so I chose to focus on Kuṇḍalinī rising in women's bodies, including mine, in the ritual world of Śākta tantra as a way of resolving this confusion.

Such a double project requires a double lens. Kripal, whom we cited earlier on the nature of symbols, repeatedly makes the radical claim that one's personal religious experiences and professional scholarship are not mutually exclusive, that they deeply inform one another, and so to understand one requires an understanding of the other. In my own terms, I would say that when a student embarks on a journey to study religion, she either loses her religion or she must find a way to transform it. If she manages to do the latter, she finds a rich new meaning in her religious practices. Such a field of study can lead to a deep-seated, honest union of the personal and the professional.

This was the beginning of the "stir" within, a journey that would unravel multiple facets of my existence and turn my investigation inward. I speak Assamese, Bengali, and Hindi fluently. I am a Brahmin woman. I am an initiated member of Śākta tantra. These simple existential facts have opened all sorts of doors for my research. Still, it is important to note that my access is geographically curtailed. For example, I do not believe I would have achieved the same amount of access in other parts of India as I enjoyed in Assam and West Bengal. It would have taken many years and formidable language skills to gain that access, if at all.

Other complications quickly arose. Soon after I had access to these communities, for example, I was faced with the classic dilemma that many scholars of religion are faced with: Am I an insider or an outsider? I soon discovered that it was one of the most challenging questions I would have to answer. My quest did not fit into a simple split of either/or. The more I gained access to these communities, the more I felt conflicted. The question of belonging and boundaries ran deep. Every fieldwork trip (and I have made many) intensified this tension. The scholar and the practitioner within me fought and argued.

The scholar recognized that the groundbreaking information I was gathering was available to me only because I was a practitioner. Having said all of that, the dilemma inherent to being a scholar-practitioner had three additional layers of complexity. First, I was born into the tradition. Second, I was initiated at the age of thirteen. I did not know back then that I would pursue an academic career researching the living tradition of Kuṇḍalinī. How could I have? Third, the guru who initiated me was dead. Thus proceeded the "churning."

After much contemplation and soul-searching, I have come to define myself as an insider with an outsider's lens. The "insider" has helped me enormously in gaining access and getting accepted in communities that are governed by secrecy and in which knowledge of certain rituals and practices are kept *gupt*, that is, "secret." I believe this orientation has given me some modest success in transmitting the voices of Hindu Śākta tantric adepts and practitioners in a way that is more faithful to what they do and believe. Many of them have been relegated to the margins of modern Indian society, often misrepresented and maligned by modernist, rationalist, and mainline voices. My objective in this research work is to allow these silenced voices to be heard. My academic training provides me with a strong double lens. From one side, I see through an "outsider lens" that is attuned to the historical and constructed nature of the tradition. From another side, I am deeply sympathetic to the symbols and mythologies of the tradition as possible translations or mediations of some other reality or aspect of being. This double theoretical framework enables me to look at the traditions in question critically and to challenge some of their accepted norms and narratives, even as it also empowers me to look at academic methods critically and to challenge some of their accepted norms and narratives. It is an ongoing two-way journey.

I began by saying that Kuṇḍalinī was not something I understood to be part of my tradition when I embarked upon my studies. Needless to say, this view has been qualified in important and complex ways. One of the most challenging tasks I was given along the way was defining "tantra." As a practitioner, it had never occurred to me to do this; as a scholar, I was told that I must. And so, after a good long while, and drawing upon a number of other scholarly definitions,[11] I arrived at the following. I consider a ritual space, philosophical thought, and/or a text to be tantric, if that space/thought/text engages the following features:

1. The human body is not rejected, including its fluids (those things so often considered most impure); in fact, these are essential.

2. There is an activation of subtle esoteric anatomies—*cakras*, *nāḍīs*, Kuṇḍalinī energy, and so on—which become the catalyst to engage with the divine, with the intention of dissolving all binaries, such as sacred and profane, birth and death, beautiful and ugly, male and female, and so forth.
3. The practitioner engages with ritual tools—such as *mantra*, *maṇḍala*, and *yantra*—to transcend the divide between microcosm and macrocosm. The divine macrocosm resides within the microcosm of all beings. So, we are the divine as much as the divine is us.
4. All the above features can be put into the service of liberation, which is to be achieved while living—that is, *jīvanmukti*.[12]

Arriving at these four bullet points was part of the "rise"—the consummation of what it has meant for me to be a scholar of my own tradition. Kuṇḍalinī is, in central ways, a tantric concept, and so I present this definition as a way to frame the key assumptions that inform how my coauthor and I approach not only the sources from which Kuṇḍalinī emerges, but the places we ultimately understand it to be going.

ANYA'S STORY

In a sense, it feels like I've written the same book four times now. Perhaps I invited this upon myself when, in the preface of my first book, I referred to the text as "a personal ouroboros." They are not all the same book, of course. Still, each of them has retread the same (hi)stories, perhaps not in a circle but in a spiral, each time getting just a bit closer to *something*.

I come to this project as a historian (as well as a practitioner) of yoga but, really, above all as a comparativist. "Transmission is a constant act of translation,"[13] I said, back when I was circling the story for a second time, working on the Western history of modern yoga that would become my second book, *Inhaling Spirit*. It occurred to me, a bit belatedly after the manuscript was already in production, that it actually seemed rather odd to talk about the development of modern yoga practice as an act of translation because, on a very literal level, translation was precisely what the term had resisted. Perhaps it would be more accurate to say that the simple adoption of the term *yoga* (which, I think, is one reason why practitioners are still uncritically quoting Patañjali's *Yoga Sūtras* in classes that consist mostly of creative sequences of lunges) belies a multitude of smaller translations.[14] The translations are conceptual as much as they are linguistic. They happen across cultures: between South Asian idioms and Western ones; between Sanskrit and English. But they also happen across time: between the premodern and the modern. Something changes when we render *prāṇa* as breath. But then, something also changes when we render *spiritus* (or "spirit," for that matter) as breath.

Perhaps this was why translation became for me, in that book, about something more fundamental. It became about comparison. Back in 1982, historian Jonathan Z. Smith infamously declared: "In Comparison a Magic Dwells."[15] For Smith, this was not a good thing. He described comparative scholarship, like magic, as founded on a relationship of similarity (initially a product of the scholar's own subjectivity) developed into a relationship of historical contiguity. Comparison is therefore not the discovery of a connection but the invention of one. When I quoted Smith on this point in *Inhaling Spirit*, I said that I did not entirely disagree with him (though people who believed in magic surely would). Now, I am not so sure. At least not when it comes to my own scholarship. Since finishing that second book, I have come to grapple much more seriously with the implications of my own embodied experiences, including my own postural yoga practice. Perhaps I should just admit that I've come to believe in magic—at least in a specific kind. At the very least, I will say this: I believe interpreting experience (including our own) requires comparison. And I do not think that we can write good histories of experientially based phenomena without at least trying to understand the experiences themselves.

Untangling the history of modern postural yoga meant looking at how bodies could look like they're doing the same thing on the outside—even something so apparently simple as straightening the torso—while actually trying to accomplish vastly different things on the inside. In attempting to untangle Kuṇḍalinī, I've had to grapple with the possibility that bodies could be doing vastly different things on the outside and somehow have the same internal experience. . . . Maybe? But how could we ever know?

I should say, I have never considered myself to be a practitioner (or experiencer) of Kuṇḍalinī. Perhaps my closest personal connection to this content is the "East–West" nature of it. Being Russian, if I can find any mirror in this book, it's probably Helena Blavatsky. But that's another story. And yet, as I began reading the material on Kuṇḍalinī—especially the narratives of experience—I felt it in my body. I am unsure of how to explain or qualify that statement, except to say that it helped me grasp theoretical points that would have otherwise surely eluded me.

Thus, thinking about Kuṇḍalinī forces us to engage in the most radical act of comparison. It is radical in part because it requires us to rely on what Wouter Hanegraaff has called "rejected knowledge."[16] Kuṇḍalinī dwells in the domain of the mystical, the occult, the irrational, the gnostic (or the hermetic, depending on one's preferences for both worldviews and degree of precision in language). When I say "dwells," I mean that these are the sorts of subject matter with which Kuṇḍalinī might be grouped, but I also mean to say that these are the capacities—the *methods*—that we must rely on, or at least take seriously, if we are to give the topic its due. If we want to understand Kuṇḍalinī in any way that goes beyond historical trends and a surface comparison of concepts and images, we need to tap into our own experiential sensibilities. The only way to understand Kuṇḍalinī experience, in the final analysis, is by comparing it with our own. We have to get subjective, and intuitive, and perhaps even a bit irrational. "Hic sunt dracones,"[17] says Hanegraaff of this kind of study. *Here be dragons*. Well, he's right. Literally.

I don't claim to have figured out how to do that last part, much less how to do it well. But I like to think that writing this book has brought me closer to it. Scholarship is also a form of practice.

THE STRUCTURE AND CONTENT OF THIS BOOK

Here we are, then. This is a book written by two authors of very different personal backgrounds—though both immigrants, incidentally, and so both familiar with the dance that occurs in the marriage of cultures. And both of us have chosen to commit ourselves to another sort of boundary-crossing as well: the interplay of the scholar and the practitioner. The book holds these tensions, both cultural and personal. This is not a book that speaks in a single voice.

Actually, we mean that last bit in more ways than one. By the time the reader makes their journey from the first chapter to the last, they may feel that they are reading an entirely different book. This is intentional. The opening chapters are fairly technical. We felt it was important to lay a proper historical foundation for Kuṇḍalinī, and this requires looking closely at the medieval primary sources where the term first appears, as well as taking in the broad sweep of culturally and historically specific concepts, practices, and frameworks that feed into everything that Kuṇḍalinī becomes on the modern global landscape. We do not shy away from Sanskrit terminology where we deem it useful to representing the tradition. We likewise dwell quite extensively on the nineteenth-century English-language literature where "East" and "West" become so indelibly entangled. In order to identify—much less untangle—these strands, attention to such detail is important.

As the chapters progress, however, the subject matter moves closer to us—in time, but also in its very nature. It moves closer to us, the authors, because it becomes more inextricably tangled with things that we have spent our lives not only studying but practicing. And it also moves closer to you, the reader, regardless of whether you have ever studied or practiced such things, but simply because you are human. More and more, we are dealing with first-person (indeed, often rather intimate) experiences and, if such things are to be understood, they must be met on terms that are, at least in part, personal. As a result, the style of our text becomes more fluid, the tone becomes more conversational.

As for content, the arc of our "tale" proceeds as follows.

Chapter 1 lays out the South Asian roots of Kuṇḍalinī, broadly speaking. Here, the "canonical" sources of nondual Kaula Śaiva traditions ultimately culminate in a rich idea of Kuṇḍalinī as a coiled energy associated with the power of the divine feminine (*śakti*), which the practitioner must raise from its resting place within the body up toward the divine masculine principle located in or just beyond the crown of the head. In Buddhist traditions, She is known as *caṇḍalī* (the "Fiery One"). This suggestive name might point to the concept's complex origins. Kuṇḍalinī is said to reside at the opening of the body's central channel, the *suṣumnā nāḍī*, which later texts (including most modern understandings) tend to locate at the base of the spine. However, some earlier texts importantly talk about the central channel as stemming from the heart, likely echoing ancient notions of the heart as the homologue of the sun and the residence of the self. Other texts place the channel's opening in the space just below the heart, in the navel, possibly incorporating the notion of the destructive force of the digestive fire.

In short, there is no standard model, even if we limit ourselves to things that are explicitly called "Kuṇḍalinī." And so, we will instead examine not only the multiplicity of such models, but also the cultural symbols and tropes that have informed them, focusing on two fundamental images that will persist into the modern day: serpents and fire. In addition to providing background for the nonspecialist reader, we present this historical overview as an antidote to the quest for "authenticity," or the idea that there has ever been an agreed-upon and static model of Kuṇḍalinī from which modern practitioners are diverging.

Chapter 2 presents a "Western" strand of themes that help lend context to how and why Kuṇḍalinī as a concept that has its roots in South Asian tantra has become a compelling touchstone to experiencers in Europe and North America. Here, beginning with the diverse religious and philosophical landscape of the ancient Mediterranean basin, we find an analogous tradition of the soul's ascent. The human soul finds its path of return to the divine realm whence it originated, carried through the seven planetary spheres by a luminous subtle body. A number of these traditions also rely on the symbolism of serpents, some biblical, but also other imagery associated with non-Christian figures such as Asclepius and especially Hermes/Mercury. These frameworks persist into early modern Europe by way of the alchemical tradition, but also in the practices of Christian mystics.

Chapter 3 examines the earliest appearances of Kuṇḍalinī within sources by Western authors, from Her first brief appearances in the works of the Theosophists to later and more complex hybrid models. The Theosophical hybrids usually blend Kuṇḍalinī with exactly the sort of Gnostic and Hermetic systems of subtle ascent that we reviewed in chapter 2, a tendency we also see in the psychological framework of Carl Jung. We finish by looking at the single "Western" source that is still most often evoked when talking about Kuṇḍalinī today: Arthur Avalon's *The Serpent Power* (1919). Avalon's account goes to pains to distance itself from Theosophical models and to offer a faithful account of a specific sixteenth-century Kaula tantric text, the *Ṣaṭcakra Nirūpaṇa*, and the Indian tradition from which it arises. However, as it refutes Theosophical hybrids, *The Serpent Power* helps cement an equally important modern phenomenon—the idea of a single authentic model of Kuṇḍalinī tied to the system of the seven *cakras*.

Chapter 4 looks at the centrality of Kuṇḍalinī to another "East-West" phenomenon: yoga. Beginning with none other than Swami Vivekananda—the oft-proclaimed "father" of modern yoga himself—we see that Indian modernizers of yogic practice, both in South Asia and in the West, attempted to square the metaphysical claims of historical traditions with modern understandings of anatomy and physiology. In this project, Kuṇḍalinī often ended up front and center. Though they have rarely been considered from this angle, many of the first popularizing works on yoga written in English, from Vivekananda's *Raja Yoga* (1896) to the Kriya Yoga lineage referenced in Paramahansa Yogananda's famous *Autobiography of a Yogi* (1946), feature systems that involve the raising of Kuṇḍalinī. But the demands of scientific rationalism leave little room for abstract talk of ultimate reality. Of course, some teachers of yoga simply declared that the subtle spiritual dimensions of yoga exist beyond the sphere of the physical. However, those who attempted to nevertheless bridge the two generally proceeded in one of two ways. Some reduced Kuṇḍalinī down to an entirely physical mechanism—a move that, as we'll see, will have important implications later in the twentieth century. Others, meanwhile, suggested that the physical is in fact destined to literally evolve into the spiritual.

Chapter 5 acts as the neck of the hourglass. Here we make a case study of the experience of one of Kuṇḍalinī's most important modern popularizers: Gopi Krishna. Though Gopi Krishna's works are still widely read today as popular guides on Kuṇḍalinī, the personal experience in which they are grounded was neither intentional nor straightforward. Relying on Gopi Krishna's letters and telegrams to Sri Aurobindo in February–March 1938, sent over the weeks where he found himself in agony and desperate for guidance, we follow the gradual process of interpretation that gives shape to raw and unfiltered experience. As we'll see, Gopi Krishna was familiar with the popularly available literature on Kuṇḍalinī, but he nevertheless struggled to bridge the gap between those sources and the reality taking shape inside his body. When his interpretation coalesces into the narrative published decades later as the classic *Kundalini: The Evolutionary Energy in Man* (1967), it forms a complex node of synthesis, representing how diffuse cultural streams of knowledge and experience are received, shaped, and transmitted anew. While Gopi Krishna's work is grounded in the immediate physical reality of his experience, his understanding of Kuṇḍalinī points at something much larger. Indeed, his argument that Kuṇḍalinī is the "evolutionary energy in man"—the bridge between the physical and the spiritual—is the culmination of a century's worth of modern synthesis. It is also the departure point for what Kuṇḍalinī would become in the decades to come.

Chapter 6 digs into case studies of several global gurus who made Kuṇḍalinī central to their teachings. By the mid-twentieth century, the "standard model" of Kuṇḍalinī had generally been established. And so, far more than their predecessors, the gurus of the 1960s and onward became actors in a marketplace where they were competing to differentiate their teachings from that standard, but also from each other. As Kuṇḍalinī became a commonly understood currency of spiritual experience, each teacher strived to present his particular approach to it as superior. On the one hand, we see the "Kundalini Yoga" of Yogi Bhajan become an easily reproducible branded method that presents itself as placing the control in the hands of the practitioner. On the other hand, we have the spontaneous *śaktipāt* of teachers like Swami Muktananda, which asks the practitioner to surrender to the guru, to the energy (*śakti*), and ultimately to the divine. In both cases, however, Kuṇḍalinī begins to act more and more like a commodity.

Chapter 7, then, looks at the "consumer base" of all those gurus in the counterculture of 1960s and 1970s North America. We have arrived now at both a standard model and a canon (on that front, inevitably, all strands seem to lead back to Avalon). And so, a diverse range of interested subgroups—Euro-American students who have become gurus in their own right, human potential visionaries, psychiatric professionals, and above all spiritual seekers—each begin to draw this model into a wide range of interpretive frameworks. And yet, as we've seen, there is no standardizing Kuṇḍalinī. Even the seemingly singular image of the rising serpent still masks something much more plural. Thus we see an inevitable and growing tension between the obvious diversity of the Kuṇḍalinī phenomenon and the desire for a standard framework, prompted especially by the explosion of different experience narratives and the attempts to both document and (scientifically) explain them.

Finally, chapter 8 turns to Kuṇḍalinī in the contemporary world, offering a "state of the field" through the lens of three domains: academic and clinical research, Internet media, and ethnographic accounts of contemporary Indian practitioners of Goddess tantra. This chapter is as close to a conclusion as we are comfortable embracing. Somewhere at the meeting point of the TikTok feed and the charnel grounds of West Bengal, the serpent bites its own tail.

SOME WORDS OF GRATITUDE

Sravana

I can comfortably say that it took a village and almost twelve years to bring this book into reality.

I want to begin by paying homage to my Guru and my Baba. Both have now transitioned from this world. So, wherever you are, know that not a single day goes by when I do not think of you fondly.

I have been very blessed to have not one but several mentors. At Rice University, where I did my PhD, Jeffrey J. Kripal, Anne C. Klein, William B. Parsons, and Elora Shehabuddin (now at the University of California, Berkley) not only shaped my critical thinking, they, along with Hugh B. Urban, saw this book intertwined in my PhD thesis. At that point, I did not. And here we are seven years after that day.

David Gordon White, Frederick M. Smith, and Loriliai Biernacki have helped me find my "voice," so to speak. They have been and continue to be there in my life in beautiful and meaningful ways. June McDaniel and I spoke of this book a few times and explored ways to write it.

Peter Heehs and Richard Hartz, two scholars and generous humans in Pondicherry, helped me get the scans of the letters and telegrams written by Gopi Krishna to Sri Aurobindo. I still remember the day when the scans arrived digitally. #Surreal.

Finally, there are thanks to my family of three. My best friend and husband, Anshul Varma. He listens to my endless stories from the field, supports my penchant for field trips, and complains minimally when I clean and reorganize our home before writing. Our daughter, Faith, received the most amount of stress-induced reactions from me. Thank you for being such a trouper. I marvel at the fact that we have a joyous mother-daughter relationship. And finally, our dear, dear puppy Leo Varma, who has patiently sat through these twelve years staring at the computer screen as I type, be it at 3 a.m. or 3 p.m.

Anya

My journey with this book is perhaps not quite so lengthy as my coauthor's. Technically, from the inception of the project, over a glass of wine at the annual meeting of the American Academy of Religion, to the moment I sit here, writing this in November 2023, a mere half-decade has passed. For a long time, this was just an article. Which seems downright laughable in retrospect.

As I said above, though, in some ways I've been writing this book for far longer. It seems redundant, now, to thank everyone who has helped and encouraged me through the entirety of my academic career, but that feels like the only appropriate thing to do. I will, however, single out two people whose work has been core to shaping my thinking (and writing) basically since the moment I set foot in grad school: David Gordon White and Jeffrey J. Kripal. It's impossible to overstate how much my scholarship owes to their complementary influence.

Though she is due another joint acknowledgement below, I also want to offer my personal thanks to Marleen Thaler, my fellow *śakti*, who has gone on this wild journey with me over the last eighteen months. Kuṇḍalinī works in mysterious ways.

Finally, in addition to the many friends and colleagues who continue to offer me their invaluable support—and who have had to endure so much of my rambling in response to their well-intentioned questions of how the book is going or, worse yet, "So, what *is* Kuṇḍalinī again?"—my deepest gratitude is reserved for my partner and forever-best-friend, Brooks. Thanks, too, to my precious canine muse Baggins, who has taught me more about the dynamics of energy transfer than any book ever could, and to our chaotic puppy, Macaron, who is much younger than this project.

Another round of joint thanks to Marleen Thaler, for being a fine friend and collaborator, for kindly sharing with us advance copies of her work, and especially for the invaluable labor she carried out on the Esalen catalog archives. Joseph Alter, Pallabi Chakravorty, Fredrik Gregorius, Ruth Westoby, and a number of other colleagues offered kind corrections, suggestions, and support. We also offer our deepest thanks to Michael Murphy, for much, but most presently for the hours he dedicated to speaking with us about Esalen, Kuṇḍalinī, and all manner of other things.

1

SOUTH ASIAN ROOTS

Serpents, Fire, and the Ascent of Kuṇḍalinī

O great deep ocean,
the lord entered into you,
mixed and churned you,
deprived you of your nectar.
That lord of illusion
entered into me too,
churned me,
drained me of my essence.
Go to the serpent
who is the lord's couch,
tell him of my endless sorrow
that he may plead for me.

—ĀṆṬĀḶ, *TIRUPPĀVAI*

There are two ways to trace Kuṇḍalinī across the sources of Her native South Asia. One would be to look for occurrences of the actual word—provided that the word means something close to what we're looking for (a consistency that words have a habit of evading). This would place the earliest textual evidence for Kuṇḍalinī sometime in the seventh or eighth century of the Common Era. But this approach ignores the rich tangle of concepts, practices, and symbolic images that stretch back centuries, if not millennia, earlier.

Manipulating Kuṇḍalinī as energy within the body became the signature feature of a system known as *haṭha* yoga, which arose in South Asia around the thirteenth century. Yet it is nearly impossible to make sense of the *haṭha* texts without understanding the multitude of prior traditions, sources, and cultural tropes on which they draw. We first encounter Kuṇḍalinī in the context of tantric traditions. There, She is divine energy—a goddess—that may be visualized as inhabiting special locations within the human body. However, even less so than later *haṭha*-based understandings, tantric ideas of the body cannot be reduced to simple physiological realities. In fact, the physiological (and especially the anatomical) is not their primary referent. Instead, these are visionary or "imaginal" (not to be confused with what we commonly mean by "imaginary") realities,[1] to be used as tools during meditative practice, to help the practitioner chart his ascent through the macrocosm of creation as it mirrors a microcosmic ascent through the body-mind continuum culminating in the true self.

As Mark Singleton and James Mallinson have pointed out in their analysis of the foundational texts of yoga, "although ascent through the central channel is a shared feature across yoga traditions, there is, in practice, considerable diversity in conceptions of what ascends: the soul or self'—designated *jīva* (life essence') or *haṃsa* (the gander')—vital air (*prāṇa*), seed or seminal essence (*bindu*), mantric resonance, Kuṇḍalinī, or, in Buddhist tantric systems of yoga, the fiery energy known as Caṇḍālī."[2] Caṇḍālī, it's worth noting, is not described as a serpent.[3] And as we will see, some texts that address Kuṇḍalinī, like the *Pādma Saṃhitā* or the *Netra Tantra*, treat it not as an engine of transcendence, but rather as an obstruction or a blockage that must be unwound.[4] Thus, not every account of ascending energy historically falls under the label of Kuṇḍalinī, and not every mention of Kuṇḍalinī refers to ascending energy.

In other words, there is no single "authentic" model of Kuṇḍalinī—what it is, where it rests, how and why and to what end it rises—in premodern South Asian sources, so we will not go looking for one. Instead, our goal in this chapter is to provide an overview of some general themes as well as specific texts and images that have contributed to the "standard model" of Kuṇḍalinī that we often see today.

FOUNDATIONAL SERPENTS

First, let us address the image of Kuṇḍalinī as a serpent. Most of the important snakes in South Asian culture, imagery, and lore can be identified with the Nāgas, a class of divine serpentine shape-shifters. Nāgas are found across South Asia within Hindu, Jain, and Buddhist traditions, and share commonalities with other mythic serpents in the traditions of East and South East Asia.[5] An important exception is the Vedic serpent Vṛtra, famously defeated by the storm god Indra, who is not identified as a Nāga. Vṛtra is an *ahi*, a Sanskrit word for "snake" that shares roots with similar terms found in other Indo-European languages and therefore also with their respective mythic serpents.[6] However, some of Vṛtra's key characteristics, like his control of the waters and his enmity with the great eagle of the heavens (also an Indo-European motif) are carried over into the later stories of Nāgas.

The Nāga as a particularly special kind of snake first appeared during the Vedic period in the *Śatapatha Brāhmaṇa*.[7] These figures and their mythologies were then elaborated in the epic *Mahābhārata* as well as the Purāṇas. The cosmic serpent Śeṣa, who drifts upon the ocean of milk, carrying the slumbering Viṣṇu—he is a Nāga. Vāsuki, the serpent who deigns to adorn Śiva's body and serves as the rope in the famous tale of the churning of the cosmic ocean—also a Nāga. Even Patañjali, the semidivine sage to whom the authorship of the *Yoga Sūtras* is conventionally attributed, is often identified as a Nāga.

Kuṇḍalinī, though, is not a Nāga. Nāgas are associated with water, but Kuṇḍalinī is a fiery force. The most famous Nāgas are male, whereas Kuṇḍalinī is a goddess, or *śakti*. Nevertheless, just as our examination of Western serpents will involve following a thematic continuity characterized by reinterpretations and recombinations, so too it is worth briefly considering those most famous Nāgas, namely Śeṣa and Vāsuki, who have undoubtedly contributed to some of Kuṇḍalinī's serpentine characteristics.

In Purāṇic accounts, Śeṣa ("The Remainder," figure 1.1) supports the cosmic egg on his coiled body, composed of calcinated ash, the

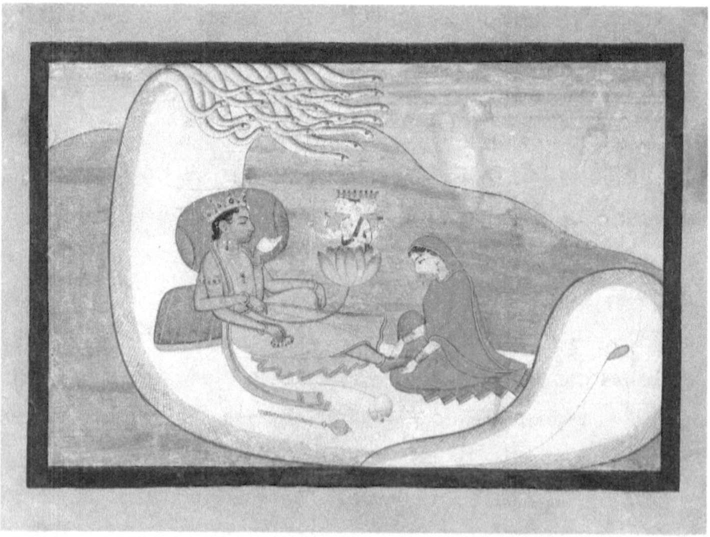

FIGURE 1.1 A depiction of Viṣṇu resting upon the many-headed primordial serpent Ananta-Śeṣa. Himachal Pradesh, Guler, 1775–1800.

Courtesy of The Walters Art Museum

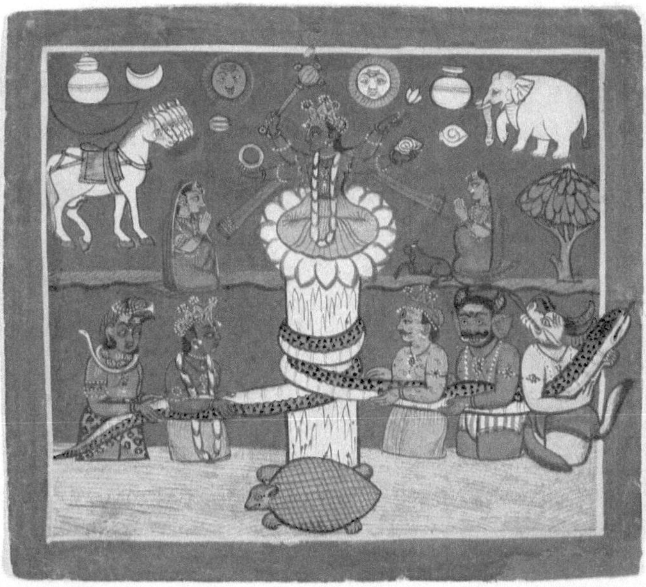

FIGURE 1.2 The great serpent Vāsuki serving as the churning rope. Viṣṇu is depicted in his Kurma (Tortoise) form at the base as well as seated on a lotus at the top of the mountain (Mandara or Meru) that acts as the churning rod. *Haṭha* yogic texts often identify Mount Meru, the mythic axis of the cosmos, with the spine. Punjab Hill, Mandi, 1780–1790.

Courtesy of the Metropolitan Museum of Art

residue of all past cycles of creation. These ashes, produced by the fire of Kālāgnirudra ("The Howler Who Is the Fire of Time," or Śiva in his destructive mode), were washed away by the waters of cosmic dissolution to settle as Śeṣa's body in the deep.[8] Because of this, he is also called Ananta ("The Endless"). Śeṣa thus represents the abiding eternal essence of the cosmos. Vāsuki (figure 1.2), meanwhile, serves as the churning rope in the famous episode that describes the release of the immortal nectar, *amṛta*, from the cosmic waters. As the story goes, at the dawn of time, the gods churned the cosmic ocean to obtain the precious nectar. However, along with the nectar, came Vāsuki's venom, which would have destroyed the universe had Śiva not swallowed it.[9] Thus in both of these narratives, we can see the common themes of creation and destruction, death and immortality, which will become central to conceptions of Kuṇḍalinī.

FIRE, UP ABOVE AND DOWN BELOW

In addition to serpents, there is another key force representing both life and death, creation and destruction that is central to understanding Kuṇḍalinī: fire. In the later Vedic period, as represented by the Upaniṣads beginning around 700 BCE, the year was balanced between the cool and wet seasons, during which the swelling moon would gather and pour out its cooling moisture in the form of rain, and the hot and dry seasons, when the sun would dry it out again.[10] In this same manner, upon death, human souls would go up to the moon as smoke or vapor, condense there, and then come back down as rain. Rain would beget plants, plants would be consumed by male animals, and from their semen souls would be reborn into the wombs of females. In this model of the cosmos, true immortality, and therefore freedom, lay beyond the disk of the sun. Those who managed to free themselves from the cycle of rebirth would pass through the fiery disk of the sun at death, never to return.[11] This cosmic cyclicality had its analog inside the microcosm, or the "little world," of the human body. There, food would be distilled by the digestive fire into increasingly more refined vital constituents (*dhātus*), all the way up to semen, which was the purest concentrate of vital energy. Later yogic traditions put the matter even more explicitly in saying that this vital fluid, which they often refer to as *bindu* (the seminal drop), drips down from its proper reservoir in the head into the abdominal pit housing the digestive fire, where it feeds the lifecycle that inevitably ends in death and rebirth.

And so, within the human body as within the world, twin fires burned above and below. The sun, representing life but also the passage of time to which all life is subject, sent its fire down to heat the earth and to cook the vital materials of the human body. The moon, for its part, served as the reservoir of that elusive immortal nectar—the *amṛta* of which human semen was the bodily counterpart, forever destined to drip downward, like grains of sand in an hourglass, counting down to the moment of death when the glass would be turned again. Ascetic (*śramana*) traditions developing within the northeastern region of Greater Magadha (modern-day Bihar and eastern Uttar Pradesh) around this time attempted to address this situation by mortifying the body. Perceiving the bonds of *karma*, the law of action and reaction, to be the ontological basis of the self's entrapment in the cycle of rebirth, they sought to arrest the accumulation of karmic seeds, as well as to destroy the storehouse already acquired, which meant manipulating both the body's external actions as well as its internal processes.[12]

In these traditions, we find physical and mental techniques referred to as *tapas*, a term which we often translate as "asceticism," but which literally means something like "heat." *Tapas* can refer to the heat generated within the body by various forms of physical and mental discipline but, more broadly, it also signifies natural heat in the form of the sun or fire, as well as the analogous generative heat associated with fertility and gestation.[13] Ascetic techniques, ranging from restricting movement and food intake, to breath-control (*prāṇāyāma*) and meditation (*dhyāna*), sought to repurpose this natural heat, by amplifying its destructive (rather than creative) effects and using it to dry up and bake the body's impure vital constituents, as a way of breaking down karmic bonds. To this same end, such practitioners employed techniques to arrest and even reverse (for instance by literally turning the body upside down) the downward flow of semen, to keep it in its upper reservoir and subvert the natural progression of the lifecycle.[14]

The tradition of the Upaniṣads, though intimately connected with these ascetic movements, took a slightly different approach to the project of liberation. In the Upaniṣads, we see the world-affirming language associated with the creative potential of the Vedic fire sacrifice reshaped into an internal ritual of visionary ascent for self-realization and self-liberation. Such innovations also likely draw on even earlier Vedic narratives about the battlefield apotheosis of warriors, whose glorious deaths would allow them to ride a celestial replica of their earthly chariots up through the disk of the sun. In making an argument for this connection, David Gordon White directs our attention to a famous aphorism found across a variety of sources early in the first millennium of the Common Era: "These are the two people in this world who pierce the solar disk: the wanderer (*parivrāj*) and the *yogayukta* [warrior] who is slain [while] facing [his enemies] on the field of battle."[15] Unlike the warrior's external ascent, hitched upon his celestial chariot (the literal meaning of *yogayukta*), the yogi's ascent was an internal one, effected by way of visionary gnosis (*jñāna*). Piercing the solar disk now involved finding the self (*ātman*), hidden in the cave of the heart, as a path to the greater eternal reality of *brahman* beyond.

From the time of the Upaniṣads, we increasingly find a common image of the heart as an inverted lotus bud, with its stem running upward to the head.[16] It is in that enclosed space that the ultimate essence of existence—the conscious self—is often believed to be housed. And this pocket inside the body, later often referred to as a void (*vyoma*), is also a portal to the self's connection to the cosmos at large. For instance, the *Chāndogya Upaniṣad* (c. 700–500 BCE), tells us:

> Now, these channels [*nāḍīs*] of the heart consist of the finest essence of orange, white, blue, yellow, and red. The sun up there, likewise, is orange, white, blue, yellow, and red. Just as a great road traverses both this village here and that one there, so also these rays of the sun traverse both worlds, the one down here and the one up above. Extending out from the sun up there, they slip into these channels here, and extending out from these channels here, they slip into the sun up there. . . . One hundred and one are the channels of the heart. One of them runs through the crown of the head. Going up by it, he reaches the immortal. The others, in their ascent, spread out in all directions.[17]

Another prime example of this link between the external and internal models of ascent is the second section of the *Śvetāśvatara* (one of the later classical Upaniṣads, possibly composed as late as the first or second century CE), which begins with Savitṛ, a Vedic god sometimes associated with the sun, yoking (from the root √*yuj*, as in "yoga") his mind and extending his thoughts to bring fire and light down to earth. It then proceeds to parallel this to human beings who yoke their minds to the gods to make their offering and identifies the sacrificial ground as the place where the mind is born. Finally, it brings in the physical practice of keeping the body straight and erect, while drawing the senses and the mind into the heart and suppressing the breath along with all bodily movement. A body thus tempered by the "fire of yoga" (*yoga-agni*) is said to be beyond sickness, suffering, and old age and is instead endowed with health, lightness, and purity. But this is only the first step—once the "yoked one" (*yukta*) recognizes the true nature of his self, he is freed from all fetters.

DIVINE ENERGIES AND VISIONARY ASCENTS

Tantric traditions, which began to coalesce around 500 CE, adopted the broad strokes of this model of visionary ascent. However, the tantric cosmos was not only a markedly theistic but also a distinctly gendered one.

Not all Indian philosophical schools gender their metaphysics, but if such distinctions exist (whether implicitly or explicitly), the material world, especially in its manifest form, is generally associated with the feminine principle. Depending on the school of thought, how this principle is understood depends on the answer to some fundamental ontological questions: Is matter the same as consciousness, or are the two eternally distinct? If they are one, is the material world real or only an inferior illusion? Dualistic schools of thought tend to privilege consciousness (often referred to as *puruṣa*, "person," or *ātman*, "self") as the superior reality. Here, the feminine principle might be represented as *prakṛti*, primordial nature that variegates, shifts, and transforms into the many things of our world, entrapping the conscious self's attention like a dancer performing for her audience. Even nondualistic schools of thought like Advaita Vedānta, which insist that matter and consciousness are ultimately one, may nevertheless insist that our material world is not actually real but only a manifestation of *māyā*, an illusory (feminine) power that shrouds the unitary nature of consciousness. In some traditions, however—especially in tantric ones and, within those, especially in ones focused on the worship of goddesses—this power is not illusory, but very real. Indeed, its kaleidoscopic creative dynamism is the necessary opposite pole to the static masculine oneness of the unmanifest self. This is *śakti*, literally "energy" or "power," and it is feminine and fiery, and necessarily both creative and destructive (since the material world, even if it is divine, is never static or permanent).

Tantric cosmologies, though similar in their broad strokes, reflect the complex and ultimately sectarian nature of the medieval Indian cultural and philosophical milieu. The divine energy that pervades the cosmos manifests not only in multilayered metaphysical arrays (called, for instance, *vyūhas* or *tattvas*) but also in expansive arrangements of deities. Tantric ritual diagrams, the *maṇḍala* (circle) or *yantra* (instrument), served as multipurpose maps—they analogized the symbolic geography of the state, complete with its local deities, to a grander understanding of the cosmos, and ultimately to the structure of the human being, placing all three into a single overlapping continuum.[18] Thus, tantric understandings of the body usually don't concern themselves with the physical body as such, but rather they imagine a perfected form that the practitioner meticulously constructs out of the divine energies that pervade the cosmos, charting a course through the features of the universe and the spheres of various deities that control it.

The body thus becomes a ritual medium for interacting with and ultimately controlling these energies. The goal might be liberation, or it might be power, either worldly or transcendental. But in the tantric context, all of these ends tend to imply a kind of ascent to divinity. In any case, as Alexis Sanderson has pointed out, in reading a tantric text, one might find "six seasons,' five knots,' five voids (*vyomas*), nine wheels, eleven wheels, twelve knots, at least three sets of sixteen loci, sixteen knots, twenty-eight vital points (*marmans*), etc."[19] that is to say, tantric traditions have had a vast variety of visionary tools and frameworks at their disposal when it came to charting a course through the body-cum-cosmos.

While the "circles" or *cakras* have become the most widely recognized feature of the tantric body in today's global systems of practice, they are neither the only notable feature of tantric subtle anatomy nor, indeed, a universal one. *Cakras* were originally a way of projecting external arrangements of deities or divine energies onto the human body. Even as they might have been associated with anatomical features, they were generally also identified with specific geographical sites (*pīṭhas*) out in the external world.[20] And just as the geographical locations mirrored culturally and politically significant sites, so too the anatomical locations tended to generally correspond to bodily features deemed significant by contemporary medical theory.[21] But this should not be taken to mean that the *cakras* in question were meant to describe a purely physiological reality. Again, not all tantric systems feature *cakras* and, even when *cakras* are present, they can vary widely from tradition to tradition in number and placement, as well as in their associated characteristics like colors, syllables, and certainly presiding deities.

Allowing, then, for the fact that tantric systems were as a whole incredibly diverse, there is a specific subset of them that tends to yield the concepts that become most central to Kuṇḍalinī. White has argued that the nondual schools of Śaiva (meaning aligned with God as Śiva) and Śākta (holding the Goddess as supreme) tantra, where modern understandings of Kuṇḍalinī primarily originate, have their basis in the ritualized sexual alchemy originally modeled on quasi-mythical encounters between tantric adepts and fierce female goddesses known as Yoginīs. According to White, the Yoginī could play one of two roles. Firstly, descending upon her victim, the *paśu* or sacrificial animal, she could literally tear him limb from limb, extracting his vital fluids, but thereby severing his fetters and allowing him to achieve union (*yoga*) with Śiva. It is for this very reason, the *Netra Tantra* (ninth century) tells us, that they are called Yoginīs: "Those Who Unite."[22] We can see an echo of this imagery in the *Jñāneśvarī* (thirteenth century) of Jñāndev, where Kuṇḍalinī is described as devouring the body's vital components and drinking up its fluids. But, secondly, the Yoginī may also "insanguinate" the male, adept with her own specifically sexual fluids, thereby transmitting the gnosis of her *kula* or "clan," which ultimately connected each member to the divine godhead, whether conceived as the Goddess or the God (usually Śiva) of whom she was a consort. Through contact with the Yoginī, the adept was thus exposed to this fundamentally transformative substance that, acting as a sort of spiritual mutagen, spontaneously granted him divine knowledge and power—a kind of sexually transmitted divinity.[23]

White has also argued the tantric understanding of Kuṇḍalinī as a transformative feminine energy that must be awakened in the practitioner's body and driven upward to unite with the masculine principle is essentially a way of interiorizing—rendering visionary and abstract—this act of sexualized ritual transformation.[24] The external acts of the female Yoginī are replaced by the internal dynamics of the feminine *śakti*. Notably, external rituals (especially rituals of initiation) have remained a feature of many tantric traditions, though the transmission and subsequent transformation within the practitioner are physically affected not by a female divinity but by the (usually though not always male) guru. Tantric initiation has been, and in some traditions remains, an embodied ritual in which the guru spiritually penetrates and enters the body of the disciple, clearing it of impurities and imbuing it with the *śakti* that his status as an accomplished practitioner allows him to wield.[25] This is also the logic behind the modern practice of *śaktipāt* (a descent or a casting down of energy), which has been popularized by several twentieth-century global gurus. We will return to this in chapter 6.

In its interiorized form, this tantric logic reaches its most elaborate physical form in the practices of *haṭha* yoga. According to Mallinson, the distinguishing feature of *haṭha* yoga is the use of physical techniques like *mudrās* and *bandhas* ("seals" and "locks," respectively), thus distinguishing it from tantric *laya* yoga, which is characterized by the visionary *saṃketas* ("methods"). Mallinson traces these physical techniques to earlier forms of ascetic practice, grounded in the idea of *tapas*, arguing that medieval *haṭha* texts represent a newly written record of old techniques that were gradually being reinterpreted and repurposed toward new goals.[26]

The term *haṭha* is usually translated as "forceful," though it is not always clear to what this adjective refers. One hypothesis is that the practice requires forceful effort, though historical sources suggest that this is often not understood to be the case. Another, more likely possibility is that the qualifier refers to the force the practice applies to the body's vital energies—for instance, forcefully moving the *bindu* upward through the body's central channel. The texts themselves offer an esoteric definition, which designates the syllables *ha* and *ṭha* as corresponding to the sun and moon.[27] *Haṭha* yoga is their union. This correspondence is linked up with a number of other pairs, such as the in- and out-breaths, the *iḍā* and *piṅgalā* channels of the body (see more below), and so on, with the goal of effecting a union of opposites.

Here we find much of the symbolism that has characterized South Asian understandings of the body since at least Upaniṣadic times. First and foremost, of course, is the lunar/solar duality which here exists on both axes—left/right as well as top/bottom. The moon is associated with the cranium, but also with the *iḍā* channel (*nāḍī*) that runs along the left side of the body. The sun, meanwhile, is located in the lower torso and occasionally in the stomach, suggesting a direct analogy to the digestive fire, but is also associated with the right-side, *piṅgalā nāḍī*. When depicted, the *iḍā* and *piṅgalā* are typically drawn as straight lines on either side of the central channel or else the column of *cakras*, not the winding caduceus-like helix found in many modern illustrations (figure 1.3). And, interestingly, the gendering of these features is somewhat ambiguous. For instance, insofar as they are analogized to rivers (associated with goddesses), the forces represented by the *iḍā* and *piṅgalā* are both feminine.[28] Insofar as they, as the sun and moon, are celestial deities, they are both masculine, as the gods Sūrya and Candra invariably are.

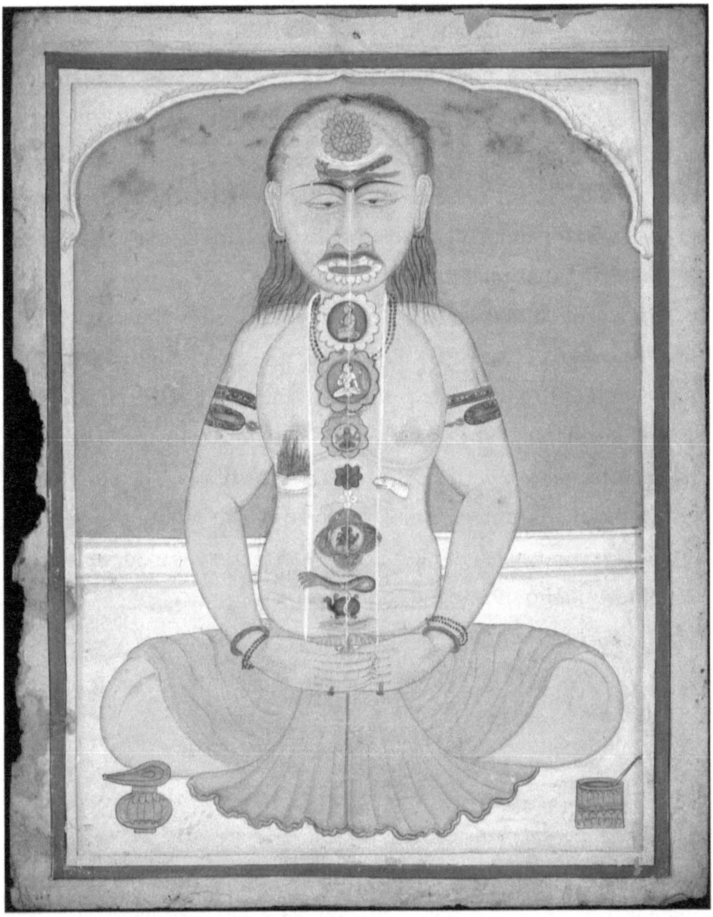

FIGURE 1.3 A tantric depiction of the subtle body, featuring *cakras*. The three primary *nāḍīs* are depicted. The winding detail at the bottom of the central channel may be a gesture toward depicting Kuṇḍalinī, although its positioning upon the tortoise makes it just as likely a reference to the myth of the churning of the Ocean of Milk. Unknown artist, likely nineteenth century.

Courtesy of the Wellcome Collection

Alchemically speaking, though, the solar principle, associated with fiery sulfur and the bodily essence of the Goddess, is feminine. On the other hand, the moon has its analog in mercury and semen, representing the masculine pole of Śiva.[29] (Note that this gendering of both the metals and their astrological analogs is the reverse of Western alchemical symbolism.) In light of the traditional *haṭha* emphasis on the union of opposites, it is perhaps this latter alchemical gendering that must take priority.

The central *suṣumnā* channel, meanwhile, is sometimes associated with the union of these various opposing principles, but sometimes with a kind of fire that stands distinct from the fire of the sun. (For instance, the fourteenth-century *Śiva Saṃhitā* tells us, "The three channels face downward and resemble lotus fibres. They are joined to the spinal column and take the form of the moon, the sun and fire.")[30] It seems especially significant, then, that it is along this channel that Kuṇḍalinī is understood to rise.

SHE WHO COILS

The earliest known textual references to Kuṇḍalinī date to approximately the eighth century, in Śaiva tantric compositions such as the *Sārdhatriśatikālottara Tantra*, which mentions a "primordial coil' (*ādyā kuṇḍalinī*) in the heart,[31] and the *Tantra Sadbhāva*, which likewise refers to a "coiled energy" (*kuṇḍalī śakti*) within the heart:

> Enclosing within herself the *bindu* of the heart, her aspect is that of a snake lying in deep sleep . . . she is awakened by the supreme sound whose nature is knowledge, being churned by the *bindu* resting in her womb. . . . Awakened by this [luminous throbbing], the subtle force (*kalā*), Kuṇḍalī, is aroused. The sovereign *bindu* (Śiva), who is in the womb of Śakti, is possessed of a fourfold force

> (*kalā*). By the union of the Churner and of She that is being churned this [Kuṇḍalinī] becomes straight. This [Śakti], when she abides between the two *bindus*, is called Jyeṣṭhā. . . . In the heart, she is said to be of one atom. In the throat she is of two atoms. She is known as being of three atoms when permanently abiding on the tip of the tongue.[32]

The references to sound here are very characteristic of the nondual Śaiva traditions with which the *Tantra Sadbhāva* is associated. There, creation is emitted as a vibrating progression of sounds—the syllables that make up the Sanskrit alphabet. In all instances, it's important to remember that the meaning of the heart here is metaphysical and symbolic more so than it is anatomical (though the language of the text suggests that we are also meant to consider the literal anatomy of the body as we follow Kuṇḍalinī's progression). Echoing earlier conceptions of the self as residing in the cave or the lotus-bud of the heart, the heart becomes home to the power that drives cosmic expansion (creation) as well as contraction (dissolution). This latter passage may also be the first reference to Kuṇḍalinī as a serpent.[33]

Other roughly contemporaneous sources may place Kuṇḍalinī in the slightly lower region corresponding to the location of the gastric fire. This is true of the *Pādma Saṃhitā*, a Vaiṣṇava (meaning aligned with God as Viṣṇu) tantric text dating from *circa* the sixth to tenth century, which tells us:

> Above and to the side of [the navel *cakra* in the middle of the bulb] is the place of Kuṇḍalī. Taking the form of the eight constituents of matter she is eightfold and coiled. Located all around the edge of the bulb, she constantly blocks the correct movement of the breath and the regular [functioning of] fire and so forth, and thus covers the opening of the aperture of Brahmā with her mouth.

> And when, during yoga, she has risen because of the breath together with fire, she bursts forth into the void of the heart in the form of a snake, blazing brightly.[34]

A very similar passage appears in the later *Vasiṣṭha Saṃhitā*, a thirteenth-century *haṭha* text that notably likewise leans Vaiṣṇava, except there Kuṇḍalinī is located "below and to the side of the navel."[35] Notably, here, the default state of Kuṇḍalinī is obstructive, and something that must be corrected through practice. This is similar to contemporaneous conceptions of *granthis* ("knots") within the body that must be broken or pierced so that the self can ascend to its unconstrained divine state. This can be done by using the breath to push through the blockages in the body's subtle channels (*nāḍīs*), such that the subsequent process of dissolving the body's fundamental elements can flow unimpeded.[36]

Still, other texts reflect the lower position that will eventually become a more or less standard in the global literature. For instance, the *Saṃgīta Ratnākara* (thirteenth century) says: "Between the anus and penis is the *cakra* called the Base (*ādhāra*), which has four petals. . . . In the Base lotus is Kuṇḍalinī, the *śakti* of Brahman. When she straightens as far as the aperture of Brahman she bestows the nectar of immortality."[37] Similarly, the *Śiva Saṃhitā* (fourteenth century) declares: "Two fingers above the anus and one finger below the penis is a single flat bulb four fingers across. Facing backward in the space between the anus and the penis is the Yoni. In it is said to be the bulb (*kanda*). Kuṇḍalinī resides there at all times. She is found at the opening of Suṣumnā. She encircles all the channels, is coiled three and a half times and has inserted her tail into her mouth. She is like a sleeping serpent and sparkles with her own light."[38]

Importantly, positioning Kuṇḍalinī in the lowest part of the torso is characteristic of the system we find in the influential texts of the Kaula Śaiva tradition, whose branches have spread and endured due to their association with India's most prominent and still-active orders of ascetic yogis. This includes the *Kubjikāmata Tantra* (most likely dated to the tenth century) of the school's Western Transmission, which is associated with goddess Kubjikā ("the Crooked One"), and perhaps even more importantly the sixteenth-century *Ṣaṭcakra Nirūpaṇa* ("The Description of the Six *Cakras*"). This text from the Kaula school's Southern Transmission, associated with the goddess Tripurasundarī ("the Beautiful One of the Three Citadels") and known today most popularly as Śrīvidyā, became a crucial touchpoint for modern accounts of Kuṇḍalinī when an English translation of it appeared in 1919 as part of *The Serpent Power* by Arthur Avalon.[39]

However, it is also within these Kaula Śaiva traditions that the role of Kuṇḍalinī is most central, and therefore Her nature and relative positioning becomes most complex. For example, Abhinavagupta, a tenth-century philosopher and a core theoretician of the nondual Śaiva tradition, speaks of three Kuṇḍalinīs: *prāṇakuṇḍalinī*, associated with life force; *śaktikuṇḍalinī*, who acts as the power of creation; and *parākuṇḍalinī*, who is the supreme Goddess.[40] The significantly later *Siddhasiddhānta Paddhati*, an eighteenth-century text belonging to the Nāth tradition and therefore descended from the same Kaula roots, adopts this triadic Kuṇḍalinī, identifying Her as the supreme Goddess, who is one but manifests as central, upper, and lower and therefore has three names. The lower goddess resides at the base (*mūlādhāra*) and is made to ascend through contraction of the root lock (a physical technique of the pelvic floor), while the descent of the upper goddess who resides in the "nameless supreme place" destroys the delusion of duality. In Her gross form, the text tells us, She "wanders through different objects in the form of consciousness" and is identified as the individual soul. But in Her subtle form, She is everywhere, and "she does not pervade nor is she pervaded."[41] The text's most precise physiological template is represented by its sixteen "supports" (*ādhāras*), which refer to specific parts of the anatomy (the big toe, the base, the rectum, the penis, and so on), and the practices one should apply to them. However, it does also offer up a system of nine *cakras*, which remain more visionary even as they are imagined within the body. Of these, "the third is the navel (*nābhi*) *cakra*, which is coiled round like a snake five times. In the middle of it visualize the goddess Kuṇḍalinī as being like ten million rising suns. She is the central goddess (*madhyā śakti*), who bestows all the supernatural powers."[42]

On the whole, this diversity of depictions represents the entangling of two important (and inherently paradoxical) pre-existing concepts. The first is the simultaneously creative and destructive nature of fire. The second is the similarly dual character of mythic serpents. They form the foundation of the world, down in the deep primordial waters, but they are also known to cause trouble—blocking up those life-giving waters at their will. Their essence is both deadly venom and divine nectar. This is to say, serpents and fire alike must be handled with care.

RAISING KUṆḌALINĪ

Raising Kuṇḍalinī (or Caṇḍalī) though the *cakras* in a visionary ascent through the layers of reality first emerged in the context of certain Śaiva and Buddhist tantric schools as a method of *laya* yoga, the yoga of dissolution, which involved dissolving—or, more literally, "reabsorbing"—the mind (*cittalaya*) into the unitary reality of Śiva.[43] Such schools prescribed a variety of specific techniques (called *saṃketas* or "methods") for how to achieve this goal, many of which had to do with the cultivation of internal sounds (*nāda*) that would act like a meditative tuning device to guide the practitioner's ascent.[44]

Depending on the specific text, Kuṇḍalinī might be used to serve what are effectively ascetic goals. The practitioner might drive Her upward through the body, drying up the body's moist vital substances (*dhātus*) as a kind of *tapas*-oriented practice. For example, texts like the *Gorakṣa Śataka* (thirteenth century) describe how Kuṇḍalinī scorches Her way up through the *cakras*, eventually drying up even the moon, and then, having embraced Śiva at the top, disappears.[45] This is also the account given by the *Jñāneśvarī*, which we'll examine more closely below. Kuṇḍalinī's ascent collapses the practitioner's very essences (the elements of earth, water, and so on) in a reversal of cosmic creation. On the other hand, other texts, like the Buddhist *Hevajra Tantra* (dated between the eighth and tenth century) describe the fiery energy's return as She floods the body with the cooling immortal nectar now released from the storehouse of the cranial vault, rendering the body essentially superhuman. As the *Hevajra Tantra* tells us, "Caṇḍalī, blazing in the navel, burns up the five Tathāgatas and burns up Locanā and the other [goddesses]. When [the syllable] ham is burnt the moon flows."[46]

This latter version of events becomes more typical in texts characteristic of what Mallinson has designated as "classical" *haṭha* yoga, beginning chiefly in the fifteenth century. The synthesis represented by these texts also signals an increasingly physiological understanding of Kuṇḍalinī as well as the *cakras* through which She travels. There we find ascetic physical techniques that were originally geared at keeping *bindu* (a specifically physical substance signifying semen) trapped in its reservoir in the cranial vault being repurposed as techniques for awakening and raising Kuṇḍalinī.[47] As a result of this fusion, Kuṇḍalinī, which would have previously been, like the *cakras*, a visionary entity to be used for mentally bridging the internal ascent with a cosmic journey through reality, becomes understood as a physical force actually inside the body.

In some sources, Kuṇḍalinī may be associated with the digestive fire (chiefly by virtue of its location) but generally remains distinct from it. Often, texts may say that by manipulating the body's internal forces, specifically the fire and the breath, one stimulates Kuṇḍalinī to action. Even as She becomes understood in increasingly physical terms, She nevertheless remains a manifestation of *śakti* and therefore of the Goddess. Likewise, even as Kuṇḍalinī may take on a more central role in some tantric texts, as late as the eighteenth century, we have other texts such as the *Siddhasiddhānta Paddhati* that name Her as only one element among many within an intricate yogic body that is both biological and visionary.

Let us close by taking a closer look at an account of Kuṇḍalinī rising as it is presented in the *Jñāneśvarī*. The *Jñāneśvarī*, which probably hails from the late thirteenth century, is remarkable for a number of reasons. Unlike most of the contemporaneous tantric literature on Kuṇḍalinī, which is written in Sanskrit, it is composed in old Marathi. It is a commentary on the *Bhagavad Gītā*, which is, of course, a Vaiṣṇava text, but Jñāndev traces his roots to the Śaiva Nāth tradition.[48] Most importantly, scholar and translator Catharina Kiehnle has described the text as "most probably the first one in history that sounds personal' rather than systematic or stereotyped. It is so vivid that there can be no doubt that the author himself was a practicing *yogī*."[49]

The text is not only vivid in its imagery but also rather detailed in its description of the physical practice, and so it gives us a good idea of what historical methods of raising Kuṇḍalinī might have looked like. The verses, which are framed as instructions from the divine Kṛṣṇa to his now-disciple Arjuna, direct the practitioner to settle himself in a suitable location and then proceed thus:

> Join the thighs with the calves of the legs, put the slanted, well-joined, firm soles of the feet at the foot of the tree of the *ādhāra*

> [*chakra*]. The right [leg] is put at the base, thereby the perineum is pressed then the left foot sits easily on it. Between anus and penis there are exactly four fingers breadth, here, leaving one and a half [on one side] and one and a half [on the other] within [that] area, one finger['s breadth] is left in between. There, by the upper part of the heel [the perineum] is pushed, with the body balanced on top.[50]

As is typical of such premodern sources, the male body is assumed by default, though none of the details here would preclude the technique from being applied to female anatomy. This first *mudrā* is identified with the *mūla-bandha*, the "root lock," and also *vajrāsana*. The *mūla-bandha* restricts the path of the breath in the lower body and so internalizes the *apāna*, the downward and outward breath force. Then, with the eyes resting half-open, the practitioner bends his neck and presses his chin down into his chest, commonly known as the *jālaṅdhara-bandha* or "throat lock." As a result, "the navel is pushed up, the belly disappears inside, [and] the casket of the heart expands."[51]

The physical practices—that is, the *bandhas*—serve as instigators to disrupt the typical homeostasis of the body by restricting both the body's internal circulatory processes and also its channels of exchange with the outside world, acting like a kind of shell of armor. This "breaks the strength of the facult[ies] of the mind" such that "imagination subsides, the outgoing activit[ies of the mind] calm down, [and] the mind naturally takes rest."[52] In this state, the body requires neither food nor sleep.

The *apāna*, meanwhile, enters a state of derangement and begins to wage battle with the body's internal processes and vital components. Restricted by the *mūla-bandha*, instead of moving downward toward the penis and anus as it typically would when serving its excretory functions, it now enters the stomach and scours the bodily humors. This effectively results in a sort of *dhātu*-cleanse, clearing away fat, drawing out marrow, releasing the veins, and loosening the limbs. At this point, the text reassures the reader that, although this bodily experience "frightens the practitioner," there is "nothing to be feared."[53] The purifying process only reveals diseases so that it may immediately clear them away.

As the *mūla-bandha* is stimulating this *apāna*-driven cleanse, the *jālaṅdhara-bandha* is ratcheting up the body's internal heat. It is this effect that catalyzes the phenomenon we are most interested in: the awakening of Kuṇḍalinī. The text describes Her just so:

> As the young one of a snake, bathed with saffron, curled up, come to its bed, like that is this *kuṇḍalinī* asleep, exactly in three and a half coils, the she-serpent with her head downward, like a ring of a creeper of lightning, a rope of flaming fire, [or] an ingot of pure best-quality gold.[54] There, like a star traveling along, or [like] the seat of the sun undone/changed (by the movement of the sun), [like] a seed of light grown into sprouts—like that loosening her coils, out of curiosity relaxing [her] body, the *śakti* is seen mounted on the *kanda*.[55]

The newly awakened Kuṇḍalinī then goes on to purify the body a second time. After Her long slumber, She is famished. With Her flaming mouth, the serpent begins to devour the practitioner's flesh, taking a morsel out of every part of the body. She proceeds to draw the essence out from the nails, the feet . . . and She finally becomes one with the skeleton of the practitioner. She then takes a big gulp of the body's seven constituents, which produces an intense dry heat in the practitioner's body. He, meanwhile, must endure this heat and not allow it to break his concentration. If he is successful, then his body slowly begins to cool down, fundamentally transforming itself in the process: "The paths of the subtle veins break, the distinction of the nine breaths disappears, therefore the qualities of the body exist no more."[56]

Jñāndev devotes a significant number of lines to metaphors that attempt to capture this transformation, which must ultimately be beyond ordinary embodied experience. The result, as is typical within such traditions, is a perfected body capable of an array of *siddhis* ("accomplishments," which amount to nothing less than superpowers). Finally, he describes the entry of Kuṇḍalinī into the practitioner's heart:

> Be it as it may—[when] this *kuṇḍalinī* [has come] into the heart, then she prattles with the words of the unstruck sound. This was faintly heard [by] the intellect [that] had become pure consciousness, stuck to the body of the *śakti*.[57] . . . This has to be imagined, then it is known—but from where is it now brought [to the mind] by someone who imagines [it]? Therefore we do not know what sounds in that place.[58] . . . Listen, [where] the light of the *śakti* disappears, there the form of the body vanishes. Then it hides in the eyes of the world. This would mean that the body becomes invisible. Otherwise it (the body) is still as in the beginning, with members, but as if woven of wind, or [like] the inner [hollow] of a banana tree, standing after having discarded its cover, or a part of the sky, separated [from it]. When the body becomes like that, then it is called sky-walking.' When this state is reached, the body brings about miracles.[59]

When Kuṇḍalinī enters the heart, the body that was woven of *tattvas* or the "elements" begins to dissolve, and finally, the air, the most subtle of the elements, merges with the heavens. This is the final trajectory of Kuṇḍalinī, who now leaves the heart and bursts upward through the head. When that happens, She is no longer called Kuṇḍalinī, but Mārutī, "She of the Wind." Mārutī remains *śakti* until

She merges into Śiva, the final destination. The account concludes with Kṛṣṇa informing Arjuna that yogis who are successful in this practice become equal to Kṛṣṇa himself—in other words, divine.

Though we began this chapter by stating that we were not on a search for a "standard model," we end with the *Jñāneśvarī* because it gets us the closest we can come to such a thing. We say this (with care) for a couple of reasons. One is that the *Jñāneśvarī* reflects the Kaula traditions where Kuṇḍalinī takes on her most elaborate form. If we are looking for a model that is, if not standard, then at least a good representative, then it makes sense to adopt one that is on the richer end. The second, and perhaps more important reason, is that the *Jñāneśvarī* becomes a popular source referenced by modern authors (both Indian and Euro-American) speaking about Kuṇḍalinī from the nineteenth century onward. Thus, even if it was not a "standard" model in its own historical and cultural context, it would be treated as such by later readers. And so, it becomes a crucial thread in the narrative web of Kuṇḍalinī.

2

WESTERN ROOTS

Subtle Bodies, Mystical Ascents, and Assorted Serpents

Perhaps thou shalt not die, perhaps the fact
Is not so heinous now, foretasted fruit,
Profaned first by the serpent, by him first
Made common, and unhallowed ere our taste;
Nor yet on him found deadly; yet he lives;
Lives, as thou saidst, and gains to live, as Man,
Higher degree of life; inducement strong
To us, as likely tasting to attain
Proportional ascent; which cannot be
But to be Gods, or Angels, Demi-Gods.

—JOHN MILTON, *PARADISE LOST*

Modern understandings of Kuṇḍalinī, especially when they occur in a Western context, represent an intimate fusion of already diverse Indian models with an equally complex body of Western images and concepts. As we mentioned in our prologue, we are using "Western" here as a kind of shorthand—a catchall term that, throughout this chapter, signifies a body of entangled traditions that span across the ancient Mediterranean world (including Europe, but also northern Africa and the Near East), touch the vastness of the medieval Islamic empire, and ground themselves in Western Europe from the Renaissance onward, thence diffusing along colonial channels of transmission.

Though origins are nearly impossible to pin down when it comes to history so ancient, it's also worth noting that these Western traditions share certain elements with their South Asian counterparts due to a common Indo-European lineage, but also that they likely owe much to a range of African traditions. The serpent emerges as a convenient emblem here, for one need only think of the West African traditions that contribute to modern-day Voodoo images of the doubled cosmic serpents—the feminine "Rainbow Serpent" Ayida Wedo and the masculine Damballah Wedo—to see that this story is infinitely more complicated than what we are able to present here.[1] And, in a sense, the synthesis that occurs when Kuṇḍalinī enters the imaginations of European and North American occultists in the later nineteenth century is hardly the first instance of such a fusion. We can find striking instances of tantric ideas of the subtle body as a medium for spiritual ascent blending with Sufi Muslim ideas of the same when the two come into contact in thirteenth-century Bengal, for instance.[2]

In any case, in this loosely "Western" body of thought, we find ideas that are both similar in form and analogous in function to those that had contributed to the shaping of Kuṇḍalinī traditions in South Asia. First and foremost, two common features stand out: the symbolism of the serpent intersecting with dueling ideas of obstruction as well as divinity and immortality; and ideas of a subtle body conceived both as luminous energy (again, fire or light) and a map of the cosmos that carries the soul on a journey of divine ascent.

Again, it is not impossible—indeed, it's perhaps quite likely—that these ideas share some common ancient roots or that, at the very least, they were formed not in isolation from one another but rather under the constant influence of cultural diffusion and exchange.

Though the modes in and speed at which we are now able to transmit information certainly differ, the cultures of the ancient world were no more akin to hermetically sealed bubbles than our modern cultures are today. Through a series of migrations and invasions and, perhaps even more importantly, centuries upon centuries of trade along the many land and maritime routes that comprised the famous Silk Road, we can imagine a constant and multidirectional dispersion not only of goods but of ideas all across Eurasia.[3] In this chapter, we are not concerned with recovering these points of contact. Rather, we'll provide an overview of the relevant themes as they developed in the West from antiquity and the Middle Ages through to the eighteenth century, setting the stage for a discussion of the more focused modern exchanges that would take Kuṇḍalinī experiences and practices global.

THE GNOSTIC SAVIOR SERPENT

A superficial look at Western, especially Christian, religion would suggest that the serpent is a generally negative image associated with transgression and indeed with the Fall of humanity. The serpent is the original villain who tempts the first woman with forbidden knowledge, thus leading to humankind's banishment from divine paradise and the "necessary evil" of sex as a feeble counter to the curse of human mortality. (To gesture ahead, for just a moment, it is no coincidence that Western practitioners have been so keen to associate a serpentine Kuṇḍalinī with the redemptive potential of sex—both of these are attempts to subvert the idea of original sin.) In the end, though, a broader and more careful look at Christian understandings of this narrative shows that they tend to reflect the biblical narrative of disobedience, drawing on Jewish tradition, but also the Hellenic and especially Platonic understandings of the soul's fall from divinity and its eventual return. In other words, there is more than one fall to consider. But also, as we will see, this fall has not always been thought of as a curse.

Granted, in the case of the ancient Greek philosopher Plato (c. 428–348 BCE), the fall was likewise not a great thing. In his *Phaedrus* (245c–249d), Plato likened the soul to a chariot, governed by a charioteer who wields the reins of two winged horses. One horse is white, well-bred, honorable, and obedient. The other horse is a malformed lumbering animal, not only insolent and prideful but deaf. Zeus, in his winged chariot, leads the other gods in a circuit around the heavens. The gods' chariots glide around the heavenly spheres evenly and with ease. The human soul, however, is unable to control the unruly horse and so is pulled downward until it loses sight of the supercelestial world of "Forms." On its downward fall, it sheds the wings that are a marker of its divinity. Having dropped to the earth, it forgets the world of Forms altogether. Followers of Plato's thought thus considered the human soul to have fallen from the divine abode of the Good, which was its true home, and so maintained that it must seek to return there once more—to regrow its wings and reascend.

Under this template, the world of matter was often regarded as inferior, if not altogether evil. The latter view appeared most frequently among a variety of individual sects that scholars have collected under the label of "Gnosticism." Gnosis, cognate with our verb "to know" (and, incidentally, also with the Sanskrit *jñāna*), referred to salvific knowledge received through revelation rather than philosophical reasoning. The general tendency toward Gnostic thinking can be found among Jewish, Christian, as well as pagan groups, all of whom generated complex mythological narratives to explain the prevailing philosophical idea of matter as evil. Though the particular actors of these myths varied with each sect, they usually shared the following basic form: there is a transcendent god who created a perfect divine world, which was the original home of the human soul. But then something went wrong, and this led to the rise of an evil demiurge (often associated with the creator god of Genesis and usually birthed by a feminine intermediary) who created the material world, into which the human soul fell, forgetting its divine origins.

However, the Gnostics were a diverse bunch, and they elaborated on this basic narrative structure in a vast variety of ways. When it comes to the role of the serpent, it is the sects commonly referred to as the Ophites (derived from the Greek *ophis*, or serpent) that warrant particular attention. Scattered across a variety of often-conflicting sources, the most complete version of the Ophite teaching ran as follows. In the beginning was the First Man. The First Man produced thought, which was the Second Man, or else the Son of Man. From this came the First Woman or the Holy Spirit, who united with the First and Second Man to produce the Third Man, Christ. Then, overflowing with light, the First Woman produced Sophia ("Wisdom") who fell down below and birthed the demiurge, Ialdabaoth. Ialdabaoth, endowed with Sophia's power, produced six offspring who, together with him, became the rulers of the seven planetary spheres. Finding himself at war with his children, Ialdabaoth also produced the serpent, who became the source of the soul and of all otherworldly things, good and evil alike. Ialdabaoth, notably, claimed himself to be the one and only God, ignoring his predecessors and implicitly identifying himself with the creator god of Genesis. Then came a drawn-out struggle between Sophia, Ialdabaoth, and his six children, which resulted, among other things, in the creation of Adam and Eve. In a modified version of the more familiar Genesis narrative, it was Sophia who caused Ialdabaoth to breathe divine power into Adam (a sort of "pneumatic seed," the key to human salvation), and likewise, Sophia who recruited the serpent to advise Eve to disobey Ialdabaoth and eat from the infamous tree.[4]

In this account, the serpent, being a child of the malevolent Ialdabaoth, is still technically a negative figure. However, in becoming an unwitting agent of Sophia, the serpent's advice and the subsequent act of disobedience by Adam and Eve are both seen as positive and salvific. Other Ophite sources went even further in identifying the serpent with Jesus, or else saying that Sophia herself became the serpent. Even when the serpent remained tied to a negative and antagonistic power (the Devil), it was often simultaneously seen as a medium of revelation and a symbol of wisdom.[5] Similarly, building on contemporary Greek and especially Middle Platonic and Neoplatonic motifs, the serpent was identified with the World Soul, its imprint clearly present in the human body as the serpentine shape of the intestines.[6] Because the Gnostics were pessimists when it came to the nature of the material world, these were not necessarily positive associations. And yet, they still positioned the serpent as central to both the soul's entrapment in matter as well as its escape.

THE MANY PATHS OF PNEUMATIC ASCENT

Alongside the Gnostics, however, there were also two other important groups that deserve mention if we are to understand how ideas surrounding the soul's divine destiny ultimately evolved over the succeeding centuries. First, there were the Neoplatonists: philosophers and mystics who elaborated on Plato's thought, while blending it with other contemporary schools, especially Stoicism, Aristotelianism, and Pythagoreanism. The Neoplatonists varied in their opinions regarding the material world, though most also viewed it, at best, as an inferior manifestation of the divine One that undergirds the whole of reality. In contrast to the Gnostics, Neoplatonic thinkers tended to rely on less elaborate mythologies when it came to the origins of the cosmos and also to place more emphasis on rational philosophy over revelatory *gnosis*. And then, there were the Hermetists (followers of the way of Hermes), who, likewise quite opposite to the Gnostics, tended to view the material world not as an evil prison but as a beautiful creation of the transcendent God (the One), the first reflection of his image, and infused everywhere with his presence.[7]

It's worth noting that the practical distinctions between these three groups would almost certainly look blurry even if we were not separated from them by nearly two millennia. All three (and others besides) were products of the same basic cultural soil—the same rough time and place, where they shared many of the same basic assumptions about the world and were responding to the same basic questions and concerns, often in conversation with and reaction to one another. For instance, while they may have disagreed about the value of the material world, they all agreed that the human soul's ultimate destiny was to ascend beyond its immediate limitations. And, while they may have differed on the best method (philosophical, revelatory, or ritual) to attain this goal, they nevertheless tracked its progress using a common map.

Gnostic, Neoplatonic, and Hermetic understandings of salvation—the soul's reascension—were deeply grounded in ancient Hellenic cosmology. In other words, the soul's journey back to the divine realm of the Good was also mapped as a journey through the cosmos and its seven planetary spheres. Plato and Aristotle both subscribed to a geocentric cosmos where the Earth, or the terrestrial sphere, lay at the center, followed by the two "luminaries" of the Moon and the Sun, then the proper "wanderers" or *planetes*, and finally the fixed stars. The eventual accepted order would be the one put forth by the Alexandrian astronomer Ptolemy (c. 100–170 CE). Ptolemy placed the Sun in the middle of the sequence of celestial bodies, rendering the order as it progressed outward from the Earth: Moon, Mercury, Venus, Sun, Mars, Jupiter, Saturn.[8] The Sun's "central" place was not simply due to empirical reasons owing to contemporary astrological understandings, but also because it matched and reinforced the reigning philosophical and religious frameworks of the time. Gods associated with the sun (Apollo, Mithras, and the supreme gods of the Chaldeans and the Neo-Zoroastrians) were often elevated above all others. Likewise, references to the sun as the "heart of the universe" and the "king of the visible universe" were a standard feature of philosophical tracts.[9] Thus, though the divine realm of God was understood to lie beyond the planetary spheres, the actual doorway to it tended to be through the sun.

As early as Plato, Western thought has tended to imagine the human being as consisting of three parts. Plato identified these as reason (the charioteer of his chariot parable for the soul's fall from the divine), spirit (the white horse), and appetite (the dark horse). He considered reason to be rational and immortal, while the latter two were ultimately irrational and mortal products of the lower world. Aristotle (384–322 BCE), partially following Plato, elaborated on this basic division. In his *De anima* ("On the Soul"), he described the nutritive (later also called "vegetative") soul, responsible for generation and growth and found in all living organisms including plants; the sensitive soul, responsible for movement and perception and found only in animals; and the rational soul, responsible for intellect, which was exclusive to humans. A third version of this division can be found in the work of the Greek physician Galen of Pergamon (129–210 CE). Galen's system, in particular, would be elaborated on extensively by later thinkers in the Hellenic, Islamic, and Medieval European worlds, becoming the core canon of premodern medicine. Drawing on the models of both Plato and Aristotle, among others, Galen rearticulated the three capacities of the soul as three types of *pneuma*—a way of thinking about the human organism that would persist well into the early modern era in the form of physiological spirits. These *pneuma* (or *spiritus*) were called psychic (after the Greek *psyche*, or later animal, after the Latin *anima*, but in any case, both words for "soul"), associated with sensation and voluntary motion in the brain; vital, associated with the heat of the heart; and natural, associated with the nutritive function of the liver.

Though this tripartite division was fairly widely accepted, scholars of the ancient Greek world disagreed about which of them took precedence as the ultimate "control center" of the human being and the seat of the soul. Galen's system placed this function in the brain, just as Plato had associated the brain with the immortal, rational capacity of the soul. But Aristotle and some other philosophical schools such as the Stoics actually located these things in the heart.[10] This latter view, of course, would have correlated with the larger spiritual and philosophical importance of the heart as we reviewed it above. Just as the sun was viewed as the heart of the cosmos, so too the heart was viewed as the life-giving center of the human body. And so, if the way to the soul's divine abode ran through the sun, it also ran through the heart.

Over the first three centuries of the Common Era, a blend of Platonic, Aristotelian, and Stoic thought yielded the idea of a subtle body, variously referred to as the "ethereal" (*aitherodes*), "pneumatic" (*pneumatikos*), or "astral" (*astroeides*) body.[11] As the aforementioned terms may indicate, this body was composed of *pneuma*, a term that initially refers to something like breath (and specifically the living breath of animals). However, beginning with the writings of Aristotle, *pneuma* was also theorized as the soul's "instrumental body"—indeed, it was the thing that ultimately allowed the soul to literally "form" the body.[12] It shared qualities with the elements of air and fire, being somewhat akin to hot air, but was ultimately not identical to either element, nor precisely the combination of the two, or indeed any of the other four terrestrial elements. Instead, as Aristotle stated, it was the "counterpart" of the special element that comprised the stars and heavenly bodies—*aither* (or "ether")—hence the adjectives of "ethereal" and "astral."[13] On the most basic level, this subtle body provided an intermediary mechanism through which the immaterial soul could act on the material organism and external world. For the Neoplatonists, Hermetists, Gnostics, and their ilk, however, it became an instrument that could also be used to accomplish the opposite. The *ochema pneuma*, literally the "spirit vehicle," was the thing that carried the soul through the planetary spheres, beyond the astral realm, and back to its divine source.[14]

This practice of ascent was sometimes referred to as "theurgy" (*theourgia*), literally something like "god-work," referring to the notion of both interacting with divine beings and ascending to the status of one.[15] Like tantric yoga and Kuṇḍalinī-based practices, theurgic ascent had both a contemplative visionary and a distinct ritual (that is, physical) component. For instance, Iamblichus of Chalsis (c. 245–325 CE), a Syrian Neoplatonist, explained that theurgic invocation of the appropriate deity would heat the soul with its divine presence. Analyzing Iamblichus's writings, Gregory Shaw has suggested that the soul's subtle body owed its heating and luminous incandescence to the physical breath, or *pneuma*. Shaw goes so far as to liken this "heating" of the soul through breath with the yogic understandings of *tapas* (ascetic heat).[16] Likewise, translating the remaining fragments of the *Chaldean Oracles*, Ruth Majercik has postulated that (possibly in conjunction with other symbolic rites such as figurative death by burial), "the initiate himself would aid in releasing the soul by engaging in certain breathing exercises." Collating a number of these fragments, Majercik describes the soul as being "thrust forth" by "inhaling," and subsequently that the soul (at a higher level of ascent) "draws in" the "flowering flames" which descend "from the Father." The soul enters or "hastens" toward the streams of light, is drawn upward, "mingles" with the solar "channels" or "rays" and is ultimately established in the sun itself—"the seven-rayed god."[17] The slightly later Mithras Liturgy (tentatively dated to Egypt around the fourth century) similarly instructed the practitioner to "draw in breath from the [sun's] rays, drawing in three times as much as you can, and you will see yourself lifted up and ascending to the height so that you seem to be in midair."[18] Once there, the practitioner would ascend upward via a pipe (*aulos*) extending out from the sun, or else via a fiery conduit (*ochetos*).[19] Here, of course, we might remember the image, given to us in South Asia by the much earlier *Chāndogya Upaniṣad*, of a channel that runs from the heart, up through the crown of the head, and toward immortality through the disk of the sun.

Mirroring the divide between positive and negative understandings of matter, in some early-Common Era sources, the planetary spheres and their ruling deities (the planetary bodies understood as *daimones*) were deceitful forces to be conquered, while in other sources they were helpful guides along the soul's path. In the latter case, the theurgic ritual would have relied on the use of tools—material objects like stones, herbs, aromatics, and also animals, and less material things such as spells, chants, and melodies—that were seen as bearing the symbols or tokens (*sunthemata*) of the gods. Lists upon lists of such correspondences can be found in the Hermetica, the magical papyri, assorted texts on the properties of stones, and astrological guides of the era. The idea was that the benevolent *daimones* had seeded signs of themselves, like breadcrumbs, throughout the world, and thus harmonizing the soul with such objects via ritual would show it the way to its own divine nature.[20] Conversely, in sects where the material world was regarded as evil, the practitioner would seek to use chants, seals, and the like as "passwords" (again, *sunthemata*) to assert authority over and secure safe passage from hostile divinities.[21] Beyond this, the exact path through the planets also varied from sect to sect. Indeed, April DeConick has suggested that we should think of the different ascent patterns as the "trade secret" of each individual sect or "initiatory guild."[22] In other words, because ascending through the spheres was not simply a matter of passing through them in sequence, but rather something closer to navigating a maze to find the right door, religious communities who were otherwise drawing on very similar ideas could set themselves apart by claiming to know the best route.

In chapter 1, we noted that there is no single standard formulation of the *cakras* in premodern South Asia. The *cakras*, even when they do appear as the primary way of organizing the visionary body, vary wildly in terms of number, placement, and their various associations with colors, syllables, deities, and so on. What the systems have in common is direction. The practitioner's visionary journey through these centers takes him upward to the very top. In the ancient Western context, we see something similar, if also rather the reverse. The path out of the cosmos consists of a standard map of celestial bodies, namely the seven planets and twelve constellations of the zodiac. However, the sequence of these bodies that the soul must traverse on its outward route is the thing that varies.

Another helpful way to think about the logics of theurgy is that they are "harmonial." Neoplatonic thought, in particular, borrowed a lot from the Pythagoreans, for whom cosmogony was arithmogony and reality was on a fundamental level numerical. The One (*to hen*, equated to the intellect or *nous*) generates all other numbers just as the creative fire that burns at the center of the cosmos generates all other celestial bodies—even the One itself is a *harmonia*, or a "fitting together" of the odd and the even, the limited and the unlimited. Thus, as far back as Plato himself, we find the physical structure of the universe being imagined as identical to the diatonic octave of musical theory, the latter's mathematical proportions determining the distances between the celestial bodies such that their *harmonia* results in a sort of cosmic symphony.[23] This is what is known as "the music of the spheres." From the standpoint of theurgy, then, the celestial spheres may have had a set order, but the key to navigating them was to play their notes in a specific sequence—that is, to find the right melody.

What we find, then, among the traditions of the ancient Mediterranean world is a common conception of a hot and luminous subtle body, possibly connected to the drawing in of breath, that was supposed to raise the soul through the planetary spheres into the divine realms. This model did not need to involve the serpent, but in Gnostic variants it often did.

OTHER FAMOUS SERPENTS AND THE GODS THEY OUTLASTED

As for the serpent, biblical scholar James H. Charlesworth has shown that not only were serpents (those that were good, bad, and everything in between) ubiquitous in ancient Near Eastern and Mediterranean iconography, but that even in (non-Gnostic) biblical sources the serpent is a far more multivalent figure than a simple reading of the Genesis narrative would suggest. Often, though certainly not always, serpents were understood as chthonic creatures, living beneath the earth and associated with both death and rebirth.[24] For our intents and purposes, however, the most important ancient serpents might be the ones that wind their way around the staffs of Asclepius and Hermes, as well as the one that winds around itself: the self-consuming coil of the ouroboros.

Hermes is perhaps one of the oldest gods of the Greek pantheon and scholars continue to debate his origins,[25] including the likely but tangled narrative (common with popular and long-surviving gods) of how multiple regionally specific deities may have coalesced to produce the figure with whom we are familiar today. Hermes was a god of travelers, which made him a god of the crossroads and the herald of the gods. Over time, Hermes came to acquire several other associations, becoming the crafty god of merchants and thieves but also the inventor of various arts and sciences.[26] He was the only Olympian who was able to enter and depart the underworld—the realm of Hades and of the dead—at will, and thus he was also understood as a psychopomp, a "guide of souls."[27]

In addition to his winged sandals and his traveler's cap, Hermes's signature possession was his caduceus, the winged staff of twin entwining serpents. The caduceus is literally (that is, etymologically) the staff of the herald but, in keeping with its possessor's complex image, it also became representative of Hermes's more mystical functions. For example, Homer's *Odyssey* describes Hermes's caduceus as "the wand he uses to enchant men's eyes to sleep or wake as he desires."[28]

However, Hermes acquired an added level of complexity when he became identified with the Egyptian moon god Thoth, another herald, psychopomp, and inventor of sciences. As Hermes-Thoth, he became a god of magic, a development that came to the fore when he was reinvented yet again over the first couple of centuries of the Common Era as Hermes Trismegistus, the "Thrice-Great Hermes": not a god now but a sage come to teach humanity the mysteries of the cosmos.[29]

Asclepius, meanwhile, was probably a god of healing early on, and perhaps originally an earth deity or spirit (*daimon*) who specialized in healing the sick. At times, Asclepius would literally appear as a giant snake. In his humanoid form, he was nearly always depicted bearing a staff encircled by a single serpent.[30] Traditionally, devotees would visit and sleep inside the god's temple, where they would receive their cure by way of a dream.[31] Though, like Hermes, he was worshipped for centuries in the ancient Greek and Roman world, Asclepius persisted into the later centuries of the Common Era primarily through a text, the eponymous *Asclepius*, a fairly liberal Latin translation of the lost Greek *Logos Teleios* ("Perfect Revelation"), likely authored in Alexandria sometime during the second or third century.[32] This text belonged particularly to the Hermetic tradition. Structured as a discussion between Hermes and Asclepius, along with Tat (another re-rendering of the Egyptian Thoth) and Ammon (Egyptian Amun), the *Asclepius* treats in loosely associative fashion topics like the structure of the universe, matter and the soul, gods, demons, the practices of theurgy, and the special nature and destiny of the human being.[33]

Indeed, in his guise as Hermes Trismegistus, Hermes became associated with a whole body of wisdom texts (the Hermetica) treating subjects like alchemy, astrology, theurgy, and various other types of occult arts and sciences. Asclepius was often depicted as Hermes's disciple but also as a teacher in his own right. Most importantly, however, such depictions meant that when the *Asclepius* and other Hermetic texts experienced a revival in twelfth-century Europe, Christian thinkers were able to position Hermes not as a pagan god (which would have made any wisdom he imparted deeply suspect) but as an ancient sage and a contemporary of Moses. Alchemy and astrology, grounded in the classical wisdom of the Hermetica, thus become the twin sciences of the Renaissance. And, as such, they bridged practical earthly wisdom (proto-biology, chemistry, and physics, culminating especially in medical applications) that governed the workings of our world with spiritual wisdom that ultimately reflected the divine order of the cosmos and the journey of the human soul.

Thus, Hermetic ideas not only survived but thrived, even against a backdrop of Catholic orthodoxy. And, along with them, so did the images. Hermes Trismegistus, unlike his more divine alter ego, was only rarely pictured with the caduceus. More commonly he appeared with an armillary sphere, an instrument representing a model of the solar system (not coincidentally, the very same map through which

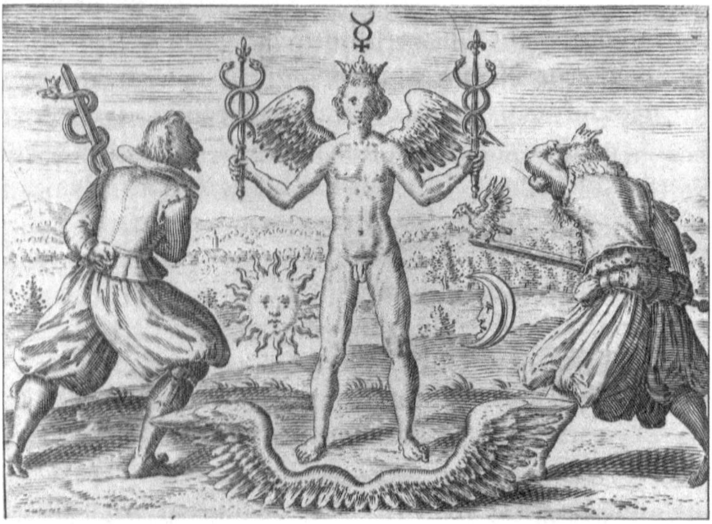

FIGURE 2.1 Mercury (designated with the astrological symbol overhead) stands holding a caduceus in each hand. He is flanked by the Sun and Moon, and likewise by two warring figures—one whose sword supports a bird and another whose sword is encircled by a serpent—indicating the conjunction of opposites. The Second Key from *The Twelve Keys of Basilius Valentinus*, 1599.

Reproduced in Musaeum Hermeticum reformatum et amplificatum (Frankfurt, 1678)

the soul made its ascent). The divine aspect of Hermes persisted instead under his Latin name, Mercurius, which made him more or less identical to the *prima materia* (the primal matter) of the cosmos, and one of the three basic substances employed in alchemy—the element mercury. The astrological symbol for mercury (☿) is in fact derived from the shape of the caduceus, and the symbol thus persisted in this abstract form, as well as in more traditional, literal renderings (see figure 2.1).

The symbolism of the caduceus's twin snakes overlaps significantly with that of another famous serpent—the self-devouring ouroboros. The ouroboros (the "tail-eating" one) can be traced to an

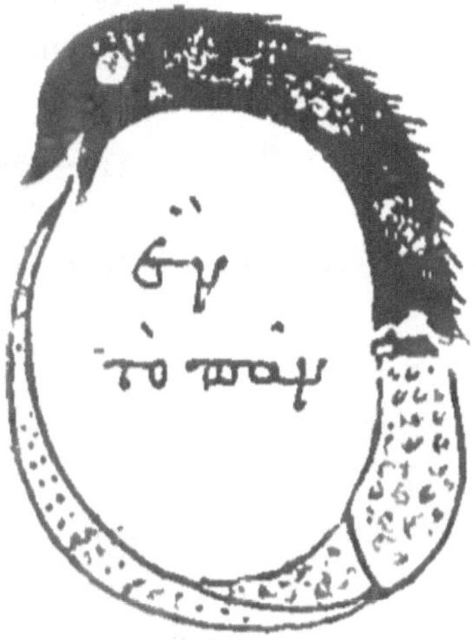

FIGURE 2.2 The ouroboros from the "Chrysopoeia of Cleopatra."
Reproduced in Marcellin Berthelot, *Collection des anciens alchimistes grecs* (Paris, 1888)

ancient Egyptian motif signifying eternity, or else the boundary between cosmic order and the chaos beyond, and the image continued to be used for both symbolic and practical purposes (such as the binding of demons) into the Common Era.[34] However, the cornerstone of the ouroboros's alchemical meanings is perhaps in the "Chrysopoeia of Cleopatra," a single page of symbols attributed to the *circa* third-century Alexandrian alchemist Cleopatra and preserved in the tenth- to eleventh-century Marcianus graecus 299 manuscript, alongside the writings of several other important alchemists. The specific image in question is a rough drawing of a serpent, half-dark and half-light, biting its own tail (see figure 2.2). Inside the serpent coil is written "One the All" (*hen to pan*), gesturing to the philosophical notion of the single self-recycling substance that underlies the entire world.[35]

The world-negative Gnostic texts, despite attributing salvific revelation to the serpent in paradise, nevertheless tended to imagine the material realm as encircled by a malevolent ouroboros, which they named, after the biblical fashion, Leviathan. If, on its path through the planetary spheres, the soul's knowledge was found lacking, it would be swallowed by the world's dragon-like captor and returned into an animal body through its phallus.[36] This, of course, matched the Gnostic view of the material world as an evil prison that the soul must fully escape. On the other hand, the alchemical understanding of the ouroboros was more closely in line with the Hermetic world-positive reasoning that matter is ultimately a manifestation of divinity (meaning, the One is the All), and though the soul must still ascend, this is less an escape and more a realization.

In the Hermetica, the ouroboros is sometimes also associated with Agathodaimon (literally, the "Good Spirit"), another ancient Greek serpentine deity who was originally worshipped as a protector and a god of good fortune.[37] Like Asclepius and Hermes, Agathodaimon underwent significant transformations as a result of his time spent in the Alexandrian melting pot. In Hermetic texts, he emerged as a revealer of occult secrets on a level with Hermes himself.[38] The ouroboros thus became ubiquitous in Renaissance alchemical literature. There it usually took the form of a dragon, sometimes winged. Or else two dragons who similarly formed a circle by biting one another's tails. Like the caduceus, the self-devouring dragon was a symbol of the *prima materia*. Signifying the ultimate oneness and continuity of natural creation, it gestured at the divine order underlying the material world.

SUBTLE ENERGIES AND VISIONARY JOURNEYS IN EARLY MODERN EUROPE

As we've seen, spiritual ascent has a long history in Western traditions. Some of the most famous cases appear more as mystical travel narratives, rather than accounts of embodied experience and practice. For instance, Arthur Versluis points us to the dream-like visionary journeys of Ibn Sina (980–1037) and Dante Alighieri (1265–1321), whose otherworldly experiences are depicted as more or less literal treks to other worlds.[39] However, we also find accounts by mystics whose private writings offer us insight into how such journeys of the soul were understood as elements of intentional and inwardly experienced practice. One especially rich example can be found in the life and work of Johann Georg Gichtel (1638–1710), a German mystic, whose diagrams of the visionary subtle body would be somewhat misleadingly incorporated into the Theosophist Charles Leadbeater's *The Chakras* (1927) some three and a half centuries later.

Gichtel was heavily influenced by the work of fellow German philosopher, mystic, and Lutheran theologian Jakob Böhme (1575–1624), but his own thought displays undertones of Gnosticism even beyond those found in that of his predecessor. Gichtel understood his practice as a form of spiritual self-mastery that ultimately resulted in a transcendent transformation. And his journey along this path began with a striking experience—one that overtook him while he was imprisoned for thirteen weeks on charges of heresy—which he described thus:

> In 1664 I lay in prison and was wrestling with Satan . . . I suddenly fell to earth, and [was] exalted into the spirit, saw a large serpent lying in a three-fold coil around my heart; but in the midst of the circle, it became quite light, and in the light appeared the Lord in the form described by John under the seven candlesticks, who spoke with a deep sigh: If thy mercy, O Lord, were not my comfort, I should perish in my misery.
>
> After these words, the serpent was cut up into innumerable pieces, and cast like a flash so sensibly into the darkness of the entrails, that I thought all my insides were broken to bits.

> Whereupon I recovered, feeling great strength of faith indeed, but learning that this was merely laying the ground to a bloody struggle, which has indeed continued until this hour, and it would take a book rather than a letter, were I to tell of it.[40]

In the midst of the striking imagery, laden as it is with deep symbolism, it is easy to miss the immediate physicality of Gichtel's description—the "flash" that travels through his body, its force so great that he feels his insides have shattered. This initial experience appears to have been both disarmingly spontaneous and overwhelmingly corporeal, much like the one we will see Gopi Krishna describe in chapter 5. And, as in the case of Gopi Krishna, it was not an end but rather the beginning of what would become a lifelong journey.

This breakthrough, which Gichtel conceptualized as the destruction of the serpent binding the heart and its relegation to the "darkness of the entrails," manifested explicitly in his later diagramming of his spiritual progress. The entrails stand for the lowest part of the torso which in Gichtel's time was associated with the lowest physical sphere of the cosmos (as opposed to the middle astral/ethereal and higher empyrean worlds associated with the mid-torso and the head).[41] In his natural state, man is wholly absorbed in his physical life, ruled by the influence of the planetary spheres and constellations and the bodily and emotional states they inspire within him. In a manner strongly evocative of ancient Gnostic planetary maps, Gichtel draws a visionary path that travels like a spiral through the body, beginning with Saturn at the head, to the Moon in the lower abdomen, Jupiter at the forehead, Mercury at the navel, Mars at the upper sternum, Venus at the lower sternum, and culminating with the Sun, encircled by a serpent, in the heart (figure 2.3).[42]

The process of spiritual awakening is effected as one follows this path through the use of the imagination, which here should not be

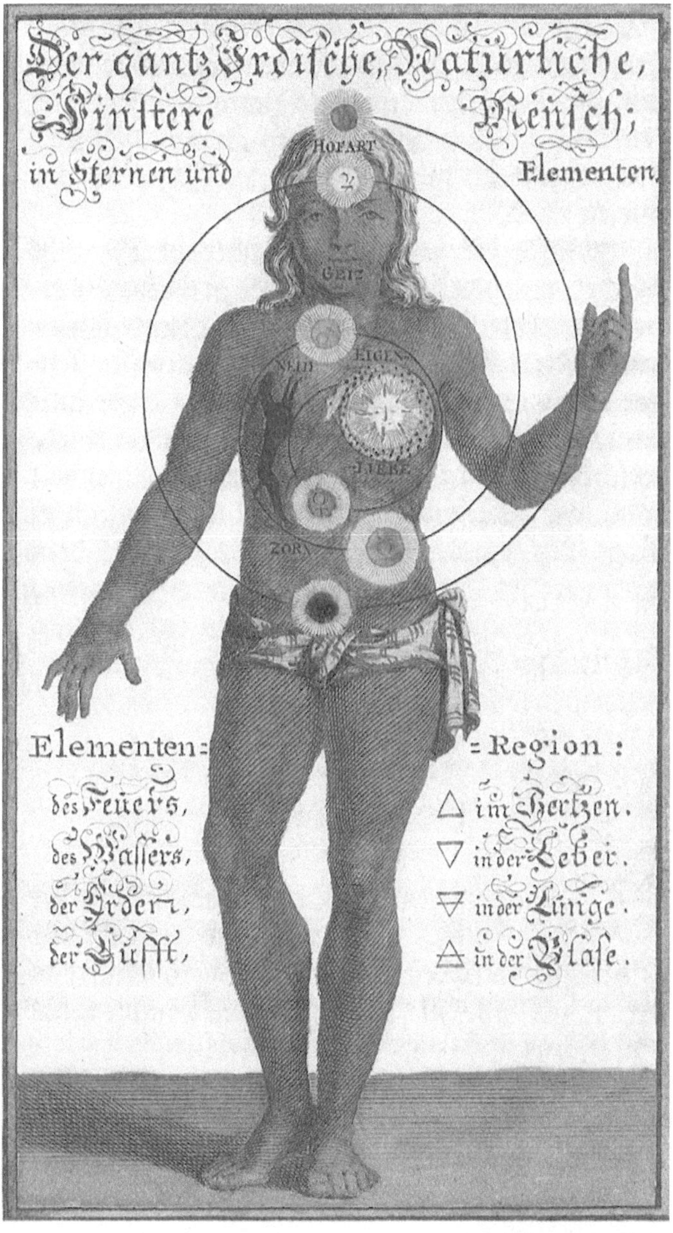

FIGURE 2.3 Gichtel's diagram of the "Earthly Dark Man" charting a visionary course for the soul's ascent by linking bodily and planetary symbolism.

Reprinted in *Theosophia practica* (Leiden, 1723)

understood in the weak sense we normally use today, but rather as an intentional and sustained focusing of the mind, not unlike meditation.[43] If the practitioner is successful, he is able to ascend into the higher and deeper reality that lies beyond the physical and astral spheres—in other words, into the divine realm. This ascent is understood in visionary and cosmic terms, but Gichtel's imagery also makes it very clear that this is a process that happens within and is mapped onto the body. As spiritual awakening occurs, the serpent's hold is broken and a winged bird rises from the Sun in the heart, where blood rains down, to be received by a black sun (*sol niger*) which has taken the place of Mercury in the abdomen. Indeed, the imagery of Gichtel's illustration is deeply evocative of an embodied alchemy. At last, in the body of the spiritually awakened man, the physical world is relegated to the lowest torso along with Gichtel's visionary serpent, Jehova sits at the navel, the Holy Spirit fills the head, Sophia abides in the throat and upper chest, and Jesus shines forth in the heart.

We might also consider the writings of the Swedish theologian and mystic Emanuel Swedenborg (1688–1772). Swedenborg began his career as a scientist who, at one point, had hoped to uncover an anatomical explanation of the soul, a project that was interrupted by a series of dreams and visions that fundamentally altered the trajectory of his life. Some portions of Swedenborg's vast body of published work recount his visionary journeys to what he understood to be other planets, cataloging the physical features and levels of spiritual advancement common to their inhabitants. Other portions, however, give insight into a more embodied kind of mysticism. Swedenborg understood God as manifesting as the divine cosmic body of a Grand Man. This body was composed of the intricate communities of angels—divine beings whose subtle heavenly existence was also the ultimate destiny of human man.[44]

Like Gichtel, Swedenborg conceived of the soul's ascent as happening inside the body, declaring: "Be it known that although I was in heaven, I was nevertheless not out of myself, but in the body, for heaven is within man."[45] Swedenborg, however, understood this journey not as an application of willful imagination but rather as a result of controlling and "internalizing" his breathing. He focused especially on the activity of the heart and the lungs, which he correlated to the celestial and spiritual kingdoms of heaven as the Grand Man. His experiences taught him that the celestial kingdom, associated with will and with the heart, pulses with a "tacit and gentle" movement. The spiritual kingdom meanwhile is associated with understanding and with the lungs, and its pulsations are "strong and vibratory." The pulse of the first flows down into the second and from thence passes into nature and the physical world.[46] Physical external respiration is thus only the physical manifestation of a much more profound subtle internal process. When the practitioner experiences this internal dimension, he is able to dwell in his divine heavenly nature.

BETWEEN THE HEAD AND THE HEART

The dueling primacy of the head and the heart percolated through the European Renaissance and onward in two correlating and sometimes overlapping tracks. On the one hand, in the evolving sphere of the sciences—from the practical medical to the theoretical physical—subtle energies and vital fluids continued to serve as an explanatory mechanism for the mechanics of the world and of the human body alike, and especially for the interaction between the two. On the other hand, mystics and occultists persisted in centering these two loci within the human body, sometimes privileging one and sometimes the other, as the nexus points of the physical, the spiritual, and the divine.

Though medical understandings of agency and cognition had swung in the direction of the head, the upper torso persisted as the secondary center. By the dawning of the modern age the chief anatomical feature there was no longer the muscle of the heart, but its closest nerve cluster: the celiac, or "solar," plexus. Writing in 1780, the famous German anatomist Heinrich August Wrisberg (1739–1808) stated this understanding of the celiac plexus as a simple matter of fact: "*Cerebrum abdominale appellatus est*" (It is called the abdominal brain).[47]

As we've seen, however, in the sphere of mysticism it was not uncommon to find this lower anatomical location continually elevated as the primary locus of spiritual realization. An interesting midpoint between the medical and the mystical can be found in the work of the magnetic physician Franz Anton Mesmer (1734–1815). Unlike Gichtel's willful application of the visionary imagination and Swedenborg's quiet absorption in the dynamics of internal breath, Mesmer's original practice was based on inducing a crisis state of manic enthusiasm. There is reason to believe that, at a critical moment in his life, Mesmer had likewise experienced something of the sort himself, and this experience must have surely influenced his later work.[48]

Mesmer's system was based on his theories of a subtle and pervasive energetic fluid (following historical understandings of ether), which built on contemporary understandings of gravitation and electromagnetism to propose an "animal magnetism" ("animal" once again from the Latin *anima*, so literally something like "soul magnetism") that was capable of acting on the body's nervous system. Mesmer was far from original or unique in his adherence to this model;[49] however, he was the most prominent theoretician to put his ideas into striking practice. Robert Darnton describes Mesmer's treatments as follows:

> Everything in Mesmer's indoor clinic was designed to produce a crisis in the patient. Heavy carpets, weird, astrological

> wall-decorations, and drawn curtains shut him off from the outside world and muffled the occasional words, screams, and bursts of hysterical laughter that broke the habitual heavy silence. Shafts of fluid struck him constantly in the sombre light reflected by strategically placed mirrors. Soft music, played on wind instruments, a pianoforte, or the glass "harmonica" that Mesmer helped to introduce in France, sent reinforced waves of fluid deep into his soul. Every so often fellow patients collapsed, writhing on the floor, and were carried by Antoine, the mesmerist-valet, into the crisis room; and if his spine still failed to tingle, his hands to tremble, his hypochondria to quiver, Mesmer himself would approach, dressed in a lilac taffeta robe, and drill fluid into the patient from his hands, his imperial eye, and his mesmerized wand.[50]

This, however, was not the format in which magnetism—or mesmerism, as it widely came to be called—endured after Mesmer's death. Under the guiding hand of one of Mesmer's principal disciples, the Marquis de Puységur, Amand Marie Jacques de Chastenet (1751–1825), the practice became abstracted, psychologized, and dissociated from any notion of a physical fluid, which was proving increasingly untenable from a scientific perspective. It also moved away from Mesmer's dramatic focus on enthusiastic crisis and began to emphasize instead the passive somnambulistic state.[51]

In some ways, however, this new understanding of magnetism was even more mystically inclined than Mesmer's original model. The Puységur school tapped into existing understandings of physiology to emphasize the division of labor between the body's two "brains." On the one hand, there were the rational and conscious capacities of perception, discernment, and will, which were associated with the actual brain. But on the other hand, there were the unconscious capacities of the "abdominal brain" or the celiac plexus.

And, while this latter anatomical feature's general status was a commonly acknowledged fact among the ascending medical profession, the magnetists went further in associating it with the subconscious soul and its visionary, intuitive, and therapeutic capacities. Mesmeric practitioners thus believed that activating this upper abdominal center could not only induce healing within the body but also bring on clairvoyance.[52]

It is for this reason that the solar plexus emerged as a principal feature of nineteenth- and early twentieth-century theories of embodied mystical experiences, including those that increasingly claimed connections to South Asian models. As Karl Baier has pointed out in examining early Western appropriations of *cakras*, it was only natural that Western mesmerists and other occultists drew parallels between their magnetic practices and what they learned of yogic and tantric systems, and that they interpreted the latter based on their own cultural understandings of the subtle body ranging from contemporary talk of magnetism and nerve force to ancient Greek speculations on the seat of the soul.[53] By the nineteenth century, sectarian distinctions between Gnostics, Hermetists, and Ophites had all but vanished from the minds of esoteric thinkers interested in the universality of mystical knowledge. In such contexts, the single winding serpent of Asclepius's staff was easily conflated with the winged twin helix of Hermes's caduceus. And both become symbols of the Gnostic wisdom-granting serpent, the emissary of Sophia, who, of course, likewise readily merged with the similarly feminine Kuṇḍalinī. Moreover, practical instruction on how to awaken and raise Kuṇḍalinī, such as was incorporated into the teachings of early global yogis, would have been easy to translate into familiar notions of clairvoyant awakening associated with domestic notions of magnetism and its larger implications as tapping into the divine ascent of the soul.

3

WEST MEETS EAST

Kuṇḍalinī and the Serpent Power

'Then said I: It is good, pass on. I, Quetzalcoatl, will go down. Sleep thou the sleep without dreams. Farewell at the cross-roads, Brother Jesus.

'He said: Oh, Quetzalcoatl! They have forgotten thee. The feathered snake! The serpent—silent bird! They are asking for none of thee.

'I said: Go thy way, for the dust of earth is in thy eyes and on thy lips. For me the serpent of middle-earth sleeps in my loins and my belly, the bird of the outer air perches on my brow and sweeps her bill across my breast. But I, I am lord of two ways. I am master of up and down. I am as a man who is a new man, with new limbs and life, and the light of the Morning Star in his eyes. Lo! I am I! The lord of both ways. Thou wert lord of the one way. Now it leads thee to the sleep. Farewell!

'So Jesus went on towards the sleep. And Mary the Mother of Sorrows lay down on the bed of the white moon, weary beyond any more tears.

'And I, I am on the threshold. I am stepping across the border. I am Quetzalcoatl, lord of both ways, star between day and the dark.

—D. H. LAWRENCE, *THE PLUMED SERPENT*

We now make our way to the earliest Western encounters with Kuṇḍalinī. In these sources She is often used to refer to—and occasionally to give a slightly new shape to—the web of overlapping but not entirely identical concepts we reviewed in chapter 2. In some cases, the references perhaps amount to no more than a superficial dalliance. For instance, the Austrian occultist Rudolf Steiner first adopted the term in 1903 and continued to use it until roughly 1909, a historical period that roughly overlaps with his involvement in the Theosophical Society. After this time, Steiner began replacing references to Kuṇḍalinī (which he had often framed as "kundalini light" or "kundalini fire") with alternate terms like "power of perception," "higher life element," "organ of perception," or "element of higher substance."[1] In 1912, Steiner formally broke with the Theosophical Society to found his own Anthroposophical Society, which significantly leaned away from Theosophy's Orientalism to foreground Western frameworks. Other thinkers showed more commitment.

Though Western engagements with Kuṇḍalinī are certainly not limited to members of the Theosophical Society, an esoteric organization founded in New York in 1875, Theosophical authors provide a foundational context for such thought. Theosophical sources establish some of the earliest and most enduring imagery that continues to characterize Kuṇḍalinī globally, but especially in the West. A particularly striking example of this is Kuṇḍalinī's serpentine form, reinforced by a visual link with the winged caduceus of Mercury (Roman Hermes), a comparison referenced by nearly every Western Theosophist writing on the subject.

One might look askance at such cultural borrowing and blending, and with good reason. One of the most influential early modern writers on Kuṇḍalinī, Arthur Avalon—a tricky figure whom we'll meet at the tail end of this chapter—criticized the Theosophists on precisely these grounds when he wrote that "though 'Theosophical' teaching is largely inspired by Indian ideas, the meaning which it attributes to the Indian terms which it employs is not always that given to these terms by Indians themselves. This is sometimes confusing and misleading, a result which would have been avoided had the writers of this school adopted in all cases their own nomenclature and definitions."[2] If we are being more generous, however, we might regard these adoptions not as scholarly attempts to faithfully represent the Indian Kuṇḍalinī traditions and practices, but rather as novel spiritual explorations—ones that occur in and rely on a primarily Western conceptual framework but nevertheless seek to build comparative bridges to Indian traditions. Sometimes, such usages are ornamental, and therefore perhaps appropriative (especially when considering their historical context, which is indelibly marked by the realities of colonialism). However, at other times, they represent true instances of conceptual as well as experiential synthesis and fusion.

It is also worth noting that the Theosophical authors in question were not uniformly Westerners. As Julian Strube has convincingly argued in his historical study of global tantra, when disagreements arose, they did not do so simply along East–West lines. Nor was influence a one-way street. As we'll see in chapter 4, Indian yogis grounded in (and ultimately committed to) fundamentally Indian frameworks nevertheless engaged in active synthesis and likewise reimagined Kuṇḍalinī with Western ideas in mind.

Most importantly, what we see in these new English-language sources is the beginning of a textual web that ensnares every future discussion of Kuṇḍalinī. These are the sources that future accounts of Kuṇḍalinī (even Indian ones) will unavoidably reference.

THEOSOPHICAL KUṆḌALINĪ: "SERPENT POWER" OR "MYSTIC FIRE"?

As we've already indicated, Kuṇḍalinī first began appearing in Western sources in the work of authors associated with the Theosophical Society. The Theosophists, led by Russian occultist Helena Petrovna Blavatsky (1831–1891) and American Spiritualist Henry Steel Olcott (1832–1907), were primarily grounded in Western esoteric thought, and especially Gnostic, Hermetic, and Neoplatonic ideas. However, their universalist impulses—the search for a *prisca theologia*, the one true ancient theology at the base of all the world's religions, manifesting as a *philosophia perennis* or perennial philosophy that crops up in slightly different forms across time and space—led them to look for reflections of their own ideas in the traditions of others.

Upon the founding of their society, Blavatsky and Olcott located the fount of ancient wisdom in Egypt and Chaldea (an ancient state approximately overlapping with modern-day Iraq). This would have been true to their Western occultist, especially Hermetic, intellectual roots. Over the course of the Theosophical Society's nascent years, however, their gaze shifted to India.[3] In 1882, the Society's headquarters were relocated from New York to Adyar, in modern-day Chennai. It is thus undeniable that the Theosophical Society represented a colonial movement, fundamentally Orientalist in its interests and goals. Nevertheless, the organization attracted a number of Indian thinkers who approached its comparative project from the standpoint of their own traditions and so provided a crucial stream of translations of and expositions upon Indian religious and philosophical texts.

Indeed, it is within this body of sources that Kuṇḍalinī makes its earliest meaningful appearances. Translations of Sanskrit texts produced by Indian scholars and disseminated by the Theosophical

Society, such as Manilal N. Dvivedi's translation of the "Yajnavalkyas-amhita" (1891),[4] were no doubt a crucial resource for Western Theosophists. Moreover, it's likely that the model of Kuṇḍalinī as a natural force akin to electromagnetism first emerged in the writings of Indian Theosophists who formulated arguments to reclaim and rehabilitate tantra from the poor reputation it had acquired at the hands of colonial scholars and Indian reformers alike.[5]

One such early example is an 1881 essay by Tallapragada Subba Row (1856–1890), which actually had precious little to say on the topic of Kuṇḍalinī as such, focusing instead on a syncretic analysis of the occult meanings of the Zodiac. In the course of this analysis, however, Row cites Kuṇḍalinī as one of the "six primary forces in Nature" (or *śaktis*) represented by the astrological sign of Kanyā or Virgo. In a lengthy footnote, he describes Kuṇḍalinī as the "universal life-principle," which governs all forces of repulsions and attraction, and of which electricity and electromagnetism are mere manifestations. Even further, Row identifies Kuṇḍalinī as the natural force that the yogi must subjugate if he is to achieve liberation, ultimately equating it with "the great serpent of the Bible."[6]

This very passage was later quoted by Blavatsky herself in *The Secret Doctrine*, her magnum opus of Theosophical thought.[7] And yet, despite seemingly singling out Kuṇḍalinī as a force central to spiritual pursuits, neither Row nor Blavatsky saw fit to expound on the matter beyond a single footnote. This is perhaps not so odd in the case of Row—after all, an exploration of Kuṇḍalinī hardly falls within the purview of a short article on astrology. The omission is more striking in Blavatsky's *The Secret Doctrine*, which, despite running on for over 1,500 pages, likewise limits its treatment of Kuṇḍalinī to barely a gloss. This isn't to say that there are no snakes to be found in those pages. Indeed, the text is replete with serpents, remaining faithful to both their ubiquity and their multivalence. Especially frequent are references to the Gnostic serpent, as well as to the infinite ouroboros, which comprised a part of the Theosophical Society's seal, and which Blavatsky continuously links to Ananta-Śeṣa, the great Nāga that supports Viṣṇu as he slumbers adrift on the Cosmic Ocean. In light of this, it seems that, in the years when she was working on *The Secret Doctrine*, Blavatsky had neither any great familiarity with Kuṇḍalinī nor any pressing interest in Her functions.

This changed somewhat in *The Voice of the Silence*, authored after Blavatsky's return to Europe and published in 1889. Unlike Blavatsky's earlier writings, which are meant to be expository and even encyclopedic in nature, this is a text that is explicitly intended for practitioners. The title page indicates that it is meant "for the daily use of lanoos (disciples)." The book is not a manual, per se, but—in the words of Charles Leadbeater—it is one of "three treatises which occupy a unique position in our Theosophical literature—directions from those who have trodden the Path to those who desire to tread it."[8] In her preface to the text, Blavatsky indicates that it is derived from an ancient work known as "The Book of the Golden Precepts," delivered to the Buddhist Nāgārjuna by the Nāgas or "Serpents"—not literal serpents, Blavatsky clarifies, but rather ancient "Initiates." However, Blavatsky also carefully notes that the "maxims and ideas [of 'The Book of the Golden Precepts'], however noble and original, are often found under different forms in Sanskrit works, such as the *Dnyaneshwari* [i.e. *Jñāneśvarī*]."[9]

The Voice of the Silence engages with Kuṇḍalinī more meaningfully than Blavatsky's previous work, though the references remain brief. Kuṇḍalinī is named as the "Serpent Power" or "mystic fire."[10] Describing a sort of mystical ascent, the text extolls: "Let not thy 'Heaven-born,' merged in the sea of Maya, break from the Universal Parent (SOUL), but let the fiery power retire into the inmost chamber, the chamber of the Heart and the abode of the World's Mother. Then from the heart that Power shall rise into the sixth, the middle region, the place between thine eyes, when it becomes the breath of the ONE-SOUL, the voice which filleth all, thy Master's voice."[11] In a note accompanying this passage, Blavatsky further explains: "The 'Power' and the 'World-mother' are names given to Kundalini—one of the mystic 'Yogi powers.' It is *Buddhi* considered as an active instead of a passive principle (which it is generally, when regarded only as the vehicle, or casket of the Supreme Spirit ATMA). It is an electro-spiritual force, a creative power which when aroused into action can as easily kill as it can create."[12] Here, Blavatsky was most likely drawing on a source that first appeared outside of the Theosophical fold, and which Karl Baier has identified as perhaps the first mention of Kuṇḍalinī in an English-language text.[13] Indeed, it is a source that her own preface to *The Voice of the Silence* appears to reference, though in a roundabout sort of way.

Between 1853 and 1854, the Dublin University Magazine published a serialized work of anonymous authorship called *The Dream of Ravan: A Mystery*. Though the text was clearly grounded in the Indian *Rāmāyāṇa* epic—indicated by its title's reference to the epic's chief antagonist—it was littered with references to Western traditions such as Gnosticism and Rosicrucianism. Among a number of interpolated passages, it also quoted from Jnānadeva's *Jñāneśvarī*, the thirteenth-century tantric commentary on the *Bhagavad Gītā* we discussed in chapter 1. This quoted passage spoke of a "Power" in the body's "middle chamber," with regards to which the modern author clarified (again in a footnote) that "this extraordinary Power, who is termed elsewhere the 'World Mother'—the 'Casket of Supreme Spirit,'—is technically called Kundalini, which may be rendered serpentine, or annular. Some things related of it would make one imagine it to be electricity personified."[14]

This tangle of references suggests the existence of conversations—ones that precede the founding of the Theosophical Society by at least two decades—that had already forged substantial links between South Asian and Western occult frameworks, including understandings of Kuṇḍalinī. Especially influential would be the notion of Kuṇḍalinī as a power either identical with or akin to electricity. The anonymous author of *The Dream of Ravan* was ahead of their time, on this count. Magnetism had by then long been a point of convergence of the natural and occult sciences. However, in the mid-nineteenth century, electricity was only beginning to make headway into the popular imagination. First elaborated by German Pietist theologians a century prior, it was interpreted as a kind of primordial creative fire.[15] In some ways, this was a novel formulation. Yet, in others, it followed directly from classical understandings of ether. And, just as ether found its human analog in *pneuma*—the luminous substance, derived from breath, that formed the subtle body of theurgic assent—so too electricity became instantiated in the vital functions of human bodies, gross and subtle.

Thus, Blavatsky's work, insofar as it addresses Kuṇḍalinī at all, does not offer any original elaborations or synthesis. Again, her handful of references to Kuṇḍalinī—barely more than footnotes—are themselves drawn from footnotes, one in Row's article on the Zodiac and another in *The Dream of Ravan*. Certainly, Blavatsky had much to say regarding serpents, as well as the sacred fire, of which she understood electricity to be an aspect. However, if she ever accorded a central role to Kuṇḍalinī as such, it would have been only toward the very end of her life. Moreover, any practical instructions would have been made known only to members of her Inner Group within the Theosophical Society's Esoteric Section, which Blavatsky formed in 1890 with the ostensible goal of not only investigating esotericism but putting it into practice.[16]

The Inner Group, which consisted of Blavatsky herself along with twelve disciples—six men and six women—met for less than a year between its founding and Blavatsky's death in May 1891. While one of its most prominent members, Annie Besant, subsequently went on to publish a number of the instructions released to the larger

Esoteric Section, no complete and systematic record of the Inner Group's actual practices remains. Kurt Leland has nevertheless attempted to reconstruct, based on transcripts and other available sources, what Blavatsky's version of Kuṇḍalinī practice must have looked like.[17] The model is theurgic and harmonial; in short, it is Western. Its practices rely on a visionary ascent through seven principles correlated with the seven planetary spheres, the seven musical notes, and the seven colors of the visible electromagnetic spectrum—which was itself a fundamentally harmonial system formalized by Isaac Newton based on its divisions corresponding to the seven intervals of the diatonic octave.[18] Assuming that Leland's account presents an accurate picture of the Inner Group's understanding of Kuṇḍalinī, there is every reason to say that, if Theosophists like James Pryse, Charles Leadbeater, and George Arundale had ever been exposed to these teachings, they elaborated on them extensively when drawing up their own models. Notably, none of these men were an official member of the Inner Group.

What we have, then, beginning in the second half of the nineteenth century, is an emerging textual narrative of the Kuṇḍalinī concept in English-language sources—what it is, how it works, why it matters. Many, though not all, of these sources were produced by authors affiliated with the Theosophical Society and thus invested in its project of comparative esotericism. The Kuṇḍalinī narrative, on the whole, remained piecemeal and blurry. The emerging consensus depicted Kuṇḍalinī as a "power," articulated in quasi-scientific language as a natural force akin, but not exactly identical, to electromagnetism. Insofar as it was related to electricity, this force was fiery. Insofar as it moved in a circular or curved path, it was snake-like. All of these features are captured by Blavatsky's own references.

At the same time, we also have the on-the-ground reality of Kuṇḍalinī practice. As we will see in subsequent chapters, the traditional South Asian forms of Kuṇḍalinī practice (diverse though they were) likely persisted into the twentieth century with little disruption. There is little divergence between the medieval literature and the systems presented by early popularizers of modern yoga. And yet, we also have a growing number of Westerners who are clearly practicing—and, even more importantly, experiencing—*something.* They call this something "Kuṇḍalinī," but often as one name among others, and the resulting systems prove just as complex and diverse as the historical variety of South Asian Kuṇḍalinī models.

HYBRID SERPENTS AND SOLAR POWER

We turn now to three essentially hybrid models of Kuṇḍalinī that represent the innovations of the early twentieth-century Theosophical authors James Pryse, Charles Leadbeater, and George Arundale. They are worthy of being singled out for the way that they are in fact accounts of Kuṇḍalinī—that is, they focus on the awakening and raising of Kuṇḍalinī as the central feature of spiritual progress. Indeed, Kuṇḍalinī is at the core of their cosmologies, amounting to a fundamental feature of their understanding of the world. And yet, they are undeniably hybrids, and ones that privilege the Western side of their parentage.

The sun features prominently in all three models. Identifying Kuṇḍalinī with the sun is certainly not unprecedented in South Asian sources, but the identification here is different and has a distinctly Western feel (flavored either Gnostic or Hermetic, depending on where one looks). Another prominent feature is the Logos, literally the "Word," which mainstream Christian sources typically identify with Jesus Christ, but which Theosophical thought tends to understand along more Hermetic lines as the creative power of the material cosmos. Finally, we see an emerging focus on individual experience, nearly to the exclusion of traditional (especially textual) authority. Theosophical authors like Leadbeater and his student Arundale are not particularly concerned that their portrayals of Kuṇḍalinī are inconsistent with traditional sources, or even among and within themselves. Thus it is important to note that the experiences—or what we can glean of them from the spare details provided by these authors—are not strictly identical. And yet all describe a violent force—fiery, flashing, electric—that fundamentally transforms the body as it is normally felt and inhabited.

James Pryse: The Apocalyptic Serpent

James Morgan Pryse (1859–1942) was an American Theosophist who, along with his brother John Morgan Pryse (1863–1952), ran Theosophical printing presses first in the United States and then, at Blavatsky's own behest, in London during the late 1880s and early 1890s. The elder Pryse was close to Blavatsky, who, even over the short period of their acquaintance, became "like a mother" to him. In fact, Pryse, who was raised in a Welsh community in Minnesota where belief in and open discussion of faeries, ghosts, and all manner of occult experiences were no uncommon thing, reports encountering Blavatsky on the astral plane several years before meeting her in the flesh.[19]

Pryse left the Theosophical Society after Blavatsky's death, frustrated by the schisms and infighting that followed. The two Pryse brothers would go on to found the Gnostic Society in Los Angeles in 1928. This, apparently, was John's idea, and one from which James vehemently tried to dissuade him. James, who claimed to "have a poor opinion of the Gnostics," wrote that he found the name, in particular, to be "inappropriate and misleading."[20] It is therefore perhaps ironic that James Pryse's 1910 work, *Apocalypse Unsealed*, bears all the hallmarks of a latter-day Gnostic treatise.

The book is framed as an esoteric commentary on the Book of Revelation, which Pryse calls instead "The Initiation of Iôannês," after the Greek name of the text's purported author, John. Pryse's book interprets the Apocalypse (from the Greek *apokalypsis*, literally "revelation" or "unveiling") not as a work of history or prophesy but as a "manual of spiritual development."[21] The "Gnôsis" (which Pryse translates as "sacred science") contained in its pages is common to "all the old religions and philosophies, constituting, in fact, their common esoteric basis."[22] In this particular iteration, it presents itself as a numerologically coded roadmap that charts a journey through the microcosm of the practitioner's mind–body complex, mirrored in a macrocosmic journey through the signs of the Zodiac (see figure 3.1).

To this end, Pryse evokes a "spiritual" or "*pneuma*tic" body, which he describes as a sort of causal ovum that contains within itself the "paraklete" (*paraklêtos*, the "helper," usually linked in biblical discourse with the Holy Spirit). Pryse also identifies this paraklete as "the light of the Logos" and "living, conscious electricity," noting that it is "the 'good serpent' of ancient symbology . . . It is called in the Sanskrit writings *kundalinî*, the annular or ring-form force, and in the Greek *speirêma*, the serpent-coil."[23] In Pryse's view, this is the most perfect body—divine and immortal in its nature, circular in its form, self-luminous like the sun. This perfect solar body is the archetype from which the lower bodies (the subtle psychic and the gross physical) emerge, and so, terming it the "causal body," Pryse links it to the *kārana śarīra* of Upaniṣadic exegesis (that is, Vedānta).

The seven churches addressed in the Book of Revelation become the seven planetary spheres of the Western system, as well as the seven *cakras* of the Indian system. Pryse correlates both of these frameworks to various psychophysical capacities, from the

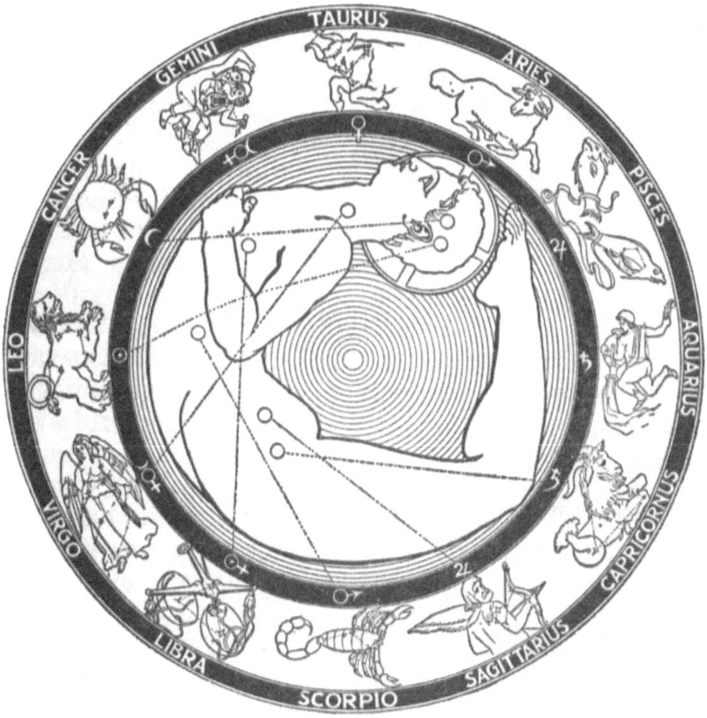

FIGURE 3.1 "The Apocalyptic Zodiac" from James Pryse's *Apocalypse Unsealed* (1910).

intellectual to the generative, which correspond to certain nerve centers or ganglia throughout the physical body. It is along this bodily map that Kuṇḍalinī travels. Pryse explains:

> The latent *kundalinî* (*speirêma*), which in the *Upanishads* is poetically said to lie coiled up like a slumbering serpent, is aroused to activity, it displaces the slow-moving nervous force or neuricity and becomes the agent of telestic or perfecting work. As it passes from one ganglion to another its voltage is raised, the ganglia

> being like so many electric cells coupled for intensity; and moreover in each ganglion, or *chakra*, it liberates and partakes of the quality peculiar to that centre, and it is then said to "conquer" the *chakra*.[24]

The language of "conquering" the *cakras* (or, really, the deities enthroned within them) is a fairly common feature of South Asian tantric systems. This was the language used by Sabhapati Swami, a Tamil yogi whose teachings Pryse may have encountered through Blavatsky or else through the Theosophical Society more broadly.[25] However, it also evokes the Gnostic *archons*, or rulers, who guard the gates of the Zodiac and whom the practitioner must conquer to successfully complete his cosmic ascent.[26]

There are other ways that Pryse's account of Kuṇḍalinī rising markedly departs from South Asian trends. For instance, he emphasizes focusing attention not on the central channel of the *suṣumṇā*, but rather on the two side channels of the *iḍā* and *piṅgalā* (which Pryse associates with the left and right sides of the sympathetic nervous system, respectively). Indeed, he insists that the *suṣumṇā* must be initially ignored, because it cannot be energized alone and instead is only activated when the positive and negative currents have begun to flow along the side channels—a statement for which Arthur Avalon will later rebuke him. In Pryse's system, however, this is all entirely logical, for it allows him to give Kuṇḍalinī the particular cruciform shape that corresponds to his ultimately Christian framework (figure 3.2). He tells us:

> These two currents, on reaching the sixth *chakra*, situated back of the nasal passages, radiate to the right and left, along the line of the eyebrows; then the *sushumnâ*, starting at the base of the spinal cord, proceeds along the spinal marrow, its passage through each section thereof corresponding to a sympathetic

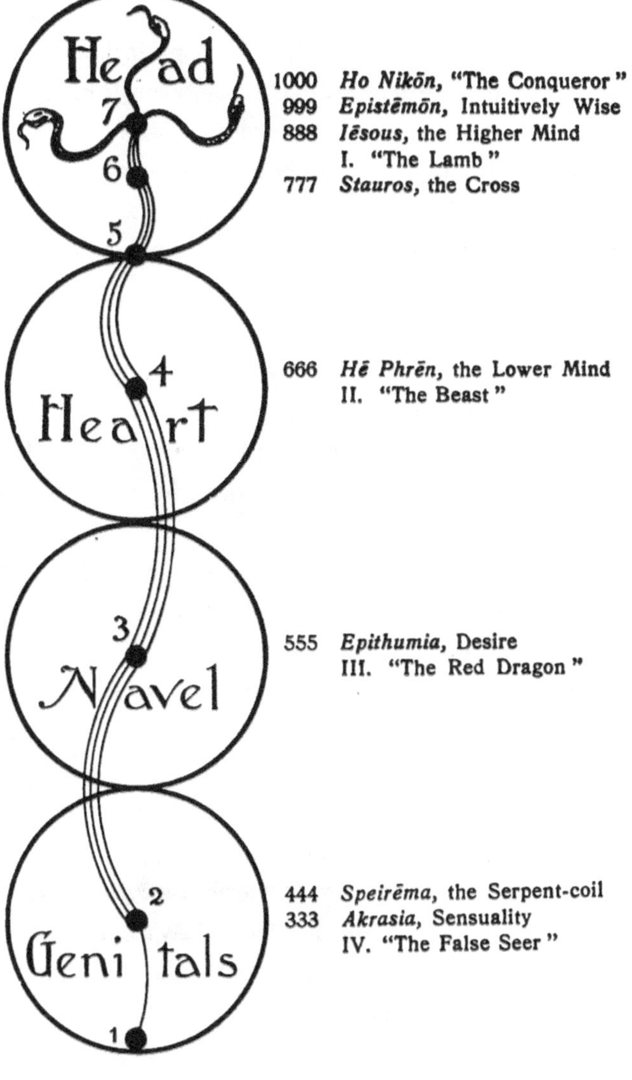

FIGURE 3.2 "The Gnostic Chart Concealed in the Apocalypse" from James Pryse's *Apocalypse Unsealed* (1910).

> ganglion being accompanied by a violent shock, or rushing sensation, due to the accession of force—increased "voltage"—until it reaches the conarium, and thence passes outward through the *brahmarandra*, the three currents thus forming a *cross* in the brain. In the initial stage the seven psychic colors are seen, and when the *sushumnâ* impinges upon the brain there follows the lofty consciousness of the seer, whose mystic "third eye" now becomes, as it has been poetically expressed, "a window into space."[27]

The experience is an undeniably powerful one—both earth-shattering and mind-blowing. Having endured the ascent of this fiery power, and having felt his brain crucified, as it were, the practitioner finds himself in a world fundamentally changed. The window into space casts his mind out of contact with ordinary matter, "as if the earth crumbled instantly to nothingness, and sun, moon and stars were swept from the sky, so that he suddenly found himself to be but an unbodied soul alone in the black abyss of empty space, struggling against dread and terror unutterable."[28] This is why, Pryse clarifies, the Book of Revelation has come to be understood as narrating the end of the world. And yet, it is instead the beginning stage of a process of self-perfection that culminates in rebirth into an immortal "solar body" (*soma heliakon*). This, Pryse argues, is the true "Apocalypse" or occult revelation.[29]

As for Pryse's usage of the peculiar term *speirēma*, this appears to be his own original invention. It is most likely a straightforward translation of Kuṇḍalinī ("the coiled one"), possibly relying on a biblical dictionary, which would have been conventional in the practice of contemporary biblical exegesis.[30] Though coiling serpents are not uncommon in Western esotericism, especially of the Gnostic variety, they are never referred to by this term. Nor does the term really catch on, with one very notable exception that begins to reveal the phantom textual web we spoke of earlier.

Nearly half a century later, in her iconic *Yoga for Americans*, Indra Devi (1899–2002, born in Riga as Eugenia Vasilyeva Peterson) would go on to compare Kuṇḍalinī to the coiled serpent in the Genesis "Tree of Knowledge" narrative, calling the latter "speirema."[31] Indra Devi, though, did not pick up the term from Pryse himself. Rather, she came to it indirectly by grasping the end of the same thread of transmission that, some twenty years later, would also capture the attention of Gopi Krishna. Indra Devi's reference was drawn from Hereward Carrington's *Higher Physical Development* (1920), which couched an intensive treatment of Kuṇḍalinī (drawing primarily on Avalon's *The Serpent Power*) in a larger framework of Western occultism. Carrington's reference, in turn, came from a rather curious text.

In 1914, the same year that Pryse published an expansion of his esoteric biblical exegesis in the form of *The Restored New Testament*, a printing house in northern New Jersey released an edition of *The Comte de Gabalis* ("The Count of Kabbalah"), a seventeenth-century French esoteric novel detailing its author's initiation into the mysteries of (potentially romantic) congress with alchemical elemental beings. This particular translation was presented alongside a commentary produced by anonymous authors known only as "the Brothers," who reinterpreted the text according to a new occult rubric. In the Brothers' hands, the novel's somewhat fanciful discussion of spiritual alliances with nymphs, sylphs, gnomes, and salamanders became a veiled discourse about awakening the "Solar Force" or "Serpent Fire," which these commentators identified in passing with the *speirēma.*

As in Pryse's work, from which the Brothers quoted explicitly and without attribution, the goal of awakening this force was to produce a deathless "Solar Body." The Solar Force would rise along the ganglia of the cerebrospinal and sympathetic nervous systems, until it reached the centers in the brain, opening up new vistas of divine consciousness. Curiously, despite referencing a variety of religious frameworks, including Indian sources, the Brothers never once used the language of Kuṇḍalinī. And yet, the image is clearly that of a fiery serpent rising up the spine. No surprise, then, that upon perusing the book in 1978, Gopi Krishna was led to remark on "the striking similarity between what I am expounding about Kundalini and the ideas expressed in *Le Comte de Gabalis*."[32]

The relationship between Pryse and the Brothers remains unclear. Their respective works share compelling similarities and equally compelling differences, both in terms of content and style. And, of course, James Pryse did have a brother who shared his occult interests . . .

Charles Leadbeater: The Fire in the Earth

Charles Webster Leadbeater (1954–1934) joined the Theosophical Society in 1883, after a brief stint as an Anglican priest. Of the many books he subsequently published, his 1927 work, titled *The Chakras*, would arguably emerge as by far the most famous. On the surface, its Indian subject matter seems to be a departure from the rest of Leadbeater's work, which is deeply rooted in Western occultism and esoteric Christianity. However, upon closer examination, it quickly becomes apparent that *The Chakras*, which also contains the most developed version of Leadbeater's theory of Kuṇḍalinī, draws its worldview from these same Western and Christian sources far more than from the Indian systems it purports to discuss.

Leadbeater's interest in Kuṇḍalinī first emerged in *The Inner Life* (1911), where he referenced Blavatsky's *The Voice of the Silence*, describing Kuṇḍalinī as "the Fiery Power" and "the World's Mother," before explaining that "there is much reason for these strange names, for it is in truth like liquid fire as it rushes through the body, and the course through which it ought to move is a spiral one like the coils of a serpent. It is called the World's Mother because through it our various vehicles may be vivified, so that the higher worlds may open before us in succession."[33] In *The Chakras*, he elaborated on this framework by systematizing and fleshing out his understanding of Kuṇḍalinī as a force within a larger occult cosmology. Only the final chapter of the book, however, is in any way devoted to Indian sources or models of the *cakras* or Kuṇḍalinī. According to Simon Cox's work on historical models of the subtle body, Leadbeater was arguably the first among the Theosophists to approach such topics not from the standpoint of textual authority, but rather he "opens the door to first-hand experience and phenomenological testimony."[34]

As Kurt Leland has pointed out, Leadbeater's understanding of how energy interacts with and moves through the *cakras* is fundamentally different from premodern Indian models. Leadbeater's *cakras* are like funnels that draw energy into each biophysical plexus to channel it through the corresponding etheric, astral, and mental centers.[35] Rather than signifying visionary circles of deities, or even energetic markers within the body where such divine powers might together form a vertical roadmap to ascension, *cakras* for Leadbeater are individual gateways: not things in and of themselves, but rather openings. He describes them as "simply vortices in the matter of the body—vortices through which all the particles pass in turn—points, perhaps, at which the higher force from planes above impinges upon the astral body."[36] Vivifying these centers of force by means of the "sacred serpent-fire" results in suprasensory phenomena, such as clairvoyance, and lays out the path for human evolution. This, therefore, is the function of the Kuṇḍalinī force. As it moves through the plexuses of the physical body, it activates the organism's lines of connection to higher aspects of reality.

Indeed, Leadbeater also identifies a total of three principal forces that flow through the physical *cakras*, which he correlates to three aspects of the divine Logos: the vital force, the life force, and the

Kuṇḍalinī. The vital and life forces are downward streams that originate from the Second and First aspects of the Logos, respectively. Kuṇḍalinī, meanwhile, becomes for him the returning upward force of the First Outpouring (effected by the Third Logos), which had originally manufactured the chemical elements, creating raw material for the creation of the cosmos.[37] It is important to note, however, that—like the other two forces—Leadbeater's Kuṇḍalinī is a physical phenomenon. The *cakras* can also serve as gateways for more subtle, psychic forces, but the vital, life, and Kuṇḍalinī forces operate on the physical level in particular.

While the vital force flows downward from the sun, Leadbeater's Kuṇḍalinī force "comes from that laboratory of the Holy Ghost deep down in the earth. It belongs to that terrific glowing fire of the underworld."[38] It is not the airy light of the sun, but "much more material, like the fire of red-hot iron, of glowing metal" and an outgrowth of the same force that constitutes elements like radium.[39] Though Leadbeater devotes much attention to the dangers of arousing this force improperly or before one is ready, it is not in itself sinister. He highlights that the ascending Kuṇḍalinī

> works in the bodies of evolving creatures in intimate contact with the primary [life] force already mentioned, the two acting together to bring the creature to the point where it can receive the Outpouring of the First Logos and become an ego, a human being, and still carry on the vehicles even after that. We thus draw God's mighty power from the earth beneath as well as from heaven above; we are children of the earth as well as of the sun. These two meet in us and work together for our evolution. We cannot have one without the other, but if one is greatly in excess there are serious dangers. Hence the risk of any development of the deeper layers of the serpent fire before the life in the man is pure and refined.[40]

Thus, as a strain of Western esoteric thought, Leadbeater's model leans more toward world-affirming Hermeticism than pessimistic variants of Gnosticism. His connection of Kuṇḍalinī with a fire situated deep within the earth has ancient and complex roots. The notion of a fire in the underworld—one intimately connected with and indeed perhaps giving rise to the visible sun—can be found in a variety of ancient mythologies, being central to Babylonian, Egyptian, Greek, and Roman models of the world. The image of a "black sun" (*sol niger*) within the earth, also referred to by a number of other terms including the "central fire" and the "invisible sun," persisted through the alchemical tradition and thence into modern occultism.[41] In Leadbeater's work, this principle similarly emerges as the terrestrial force that ultimately works to elevate the human being to a perfected state.

Following his implicitly Hermetic model of Kuṇḍalinī, Leadbeater understands the force's ascent as happening along a caduceus-like path (figure 3.3). Like Pryse, he places greater-than-traditional importance upon the activity of the two side-channels of the *iḍā* and *piṅgalā*. But, unlike Pryse, this results for him in the image not of the

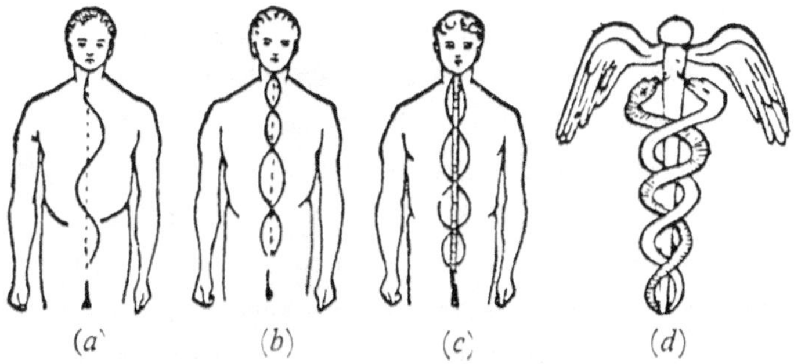

FIGURE 3.3 Leadbeater's illustration of the *iḍā* (a), *piṅgalā* (b), and *suṣumnā* (c) channels, which he directly correlates to "the caduceus of Mercury" (d), from *The Hidden Life in Freemasonry* (1926).

Reprinted in *The Chakras* (1927)

cross but of the winged rod of Hermes. "The spine is called in India the Brahmadanda, the stick of Brahma," writes Leadbeater. "It is also the original of the caduceus of Mercury, the two snakes of which symbolize the kundalini or serpent-fire which is presently to be set in motion along those channels, while the wings typify the power of conscious flight through higher planes which the development of that fire confers."[42]

George Arundale: The Sun in the Body

George Sydney Arundale (1878–1945) was raised by his aunt, a prominent member of the Theosophical Society, and thus Theosophical thought was for him formative in a way that went beyond any other figure discussed in this chapter. Arundale met Blavatsky when he was still a boy and would later report, "I loved her from the moment I saw her."[43] However, it would be Charles Leadbeater, with whom Arundale studied in his childhood and then again in his early adult years, as well as Annie Besant, who would prove to be his chief influences.

In his book *Kundalini: An Occult Experience* (1938), Arundale lays out a vision of Kuṇḍalinī that is deeply indebted to that of his mentor, doubling down and building on the unique aspects of Leadbeater's framework. Even more so than Leadbeater before him, Arundale adopts a kind of world-affirming Hermetic outlook that regards the sun as the living heart of a world suffused with divinity. Like Leadbeater, he imagines a universal "Cosmic Kundalini," embodied in the sun, but also in "whirling wheels of fiery energy"—something like Leadbeater's *cakras*—within the earth.[44] In essence, Kuṇḍalinī is the "Fire of Life" and, as such, it is always already awake everywhere life exists. Thus, in Arundale's view, it is rather a matter of intensifying this force and of directing it toward specific ends.

Elsewhere, Arundale positions the sun and the earth as the two opposing poles of Kuṇḍalinī, one positive and the other negative, and thus the awakening of the force is akin to becoming a human embodiment of the occultist's "Rod of Power" between them.[45] In this sense, the individual instantiation of Kuṇḍalinī does not arise from the body per se, but rather is drawn into it from both the sun and the center of the earth, such that it coalesces and comes to rest at the bottom of the spine. "Each individual Kundalini," Arundale tells us, "in whatever kingdom of nature, in whatever substance—great or small—in whatever world, is part of the Sun-Kundalini."[46]

Like Leadbeater, Arundale posits that there may be multiple forces at work within the body. But, unlike Leadbeater, he resists definitively systematizing these forces. Particularly curious are his cautious attempts to differentiate between Kuṇḍalinī, which he understands as traveling upward as a single spiraling stream, and the "Caduceus Fire," which we can assume is implicitly threefold. Arundale explains:

> The Caduceus Fire and that of Kundalini lie close and together, forming a splendid rainbow of colour. They subserve the same ends—differently. . . . The Caduceus seems independently awakenable, that is to say, stirred into conscious usage on the part of the individual. But its relationship with Kundalini is intimate. . . . The student concerned had the distinct impression that while the Fire of the Caduceus offered a Way of Release, the Fire of Kundalini offered a Way of Fulfilment. Phrases in these regions must never be taken very literally, for here there are no impenetrable compartments, each aloof from all the rest. But it seemed as if Sushumna with its Ida and Pingala aspects, the Caduceus, were a route of release from confinement within the lower bodies, while the Fire of Kundalini is rather in the nature of a witness-guide to identity of the larger with the smaller

> consciousness. The difference *may* be subtle, and from a functional point of view somewhat unreal. Yet it seems definite and probably has foundation in a fact not as yet clearly perceptible. Of some very close relationship between the two Fires there seems no doubt.[47]

This reluctance to issue definitive statements on the nature of Kuṇḍalinī experience is characteristic of the work as a whole; indeed, much of Arundale's writing is striking in its humble and open-ended tone. However, in this case, Arundale's reserve is not simply a matter of affect but crucial to his specific approach to the topic at hand. In following Leadbeater's emphasis on direct experience, Arundale is forced to account for the inevitable diversity that arises from subjective reports. He acknowledges this diversity repeatedly throughout the text, specifying, moreover, that his book is neither a guide to awakening Kuṇḍalinī, nor indeed concerned with knowledge of Kuṇḍalinī as such. Instead, he emphasizes that Kuṇḍalinī is, by nature, a "mystery" and that "all knowledge, for true understanding, must at first be a mystery as well as an experience."[48]

Even so, Arundale does provide a fairly concise, but metaphysically loaded, description of how Kuṇḍalinī operates within the body. Recall that, for Arundale, the essence of Kuṇḍalinī ultimately emanates from the divine effulgence of the sun, and indeed it is omnipresent within the living cosmos. But, Kuṇḍalinī also has a resting seat within the body, where "the globe or sphere at the base of the spine contains within it the Kundalini Fire coiled spherically."[49] And so, Arundale elaborates:

> The prescribed concentration upon the globe, and thus upon the Fire within, begins to stir it into activity, provided the right kind of life has been lived beforehand for a considerable period, which

> is to say provided it is fed with the right kind of fuel.... Assuming the stirring takes place along right lines, there is a gradual dissolution of the globe caused by the frictional energizing of the Fire itself. The Fire is fanned into bright heat and becomes active, forcing its way through the matter in which it lies embedded, burning it up, and causing the globe to become a Radiant Sun, instead of the dull though glowing mass it normally is. This Sun radiates in all directions heat which is physically felt, specially in the surrounding areas of the physical body. This Kundalini Sun would seem to rush upward when it moves fast, as often it does not, along the spine as a bullet passes through a grooved gun-barrel. There is something spiral about the movement. In any case, there seems to be a direct rush upwards, without passing beyond the top of the head, but specially stimulating centres according to the individual's Ray. The sensation is that of pressure, while as regards the centre at the top of the head unusual heat will be felt.[50]

As this happens, the practitioner will experience an expansion of consciousness—and, more mundanely, perhaps some dizziness as the adjustment takes place—as well as a sense of detachment, as if the world were suddenly a thing to be observed from very far away. The body, however, becomes intensely sensitive, especially along the region of the spine. Yet, deferring once more to the subjective nature of such bodily sensations, Arundale clarifies:

> The burning sensation, so usually associated with Kundalini, and by no means confined within the channels of its passage through the body, is not necessarily inevitable. There may be a sensation of cold, of pressure, of a bursting, the latter generally within the head. Some students have experienced an uncomfortable warmth

> throughout the trunk of the body, with extension into the head, so that the whole of the upper part of the body seems intensely hot, streaming forth heat in all directions.[51]

Eventually, "Kundalini pierces its way through and ascends through the top of the head beyond the physical body like a fountain of coloured water."[52]

CARL JUNG AND THE SERPENT IN THE DEEP

Today, Carl Jung (1875–1961) is most famous for his historical role in the development of psychoanalysis, and perhaps especially depth psychology, which emphasizes the role of the unconscious. Of course it is precisely that latter aspect of Jung's theories that most clearly elucidates his concern not only with the psychiatric but also the spiritual. For Jung, the unconscious was not simply an individual repository of suppressed memories and drives, but rather the shared psychic foundation of humanity, primordial and universal: the collective unconscious.

Jung associates serpent symbolism with the lower torso and its organs, but also, and especially, with the body's sympathetic nervous system which he ultimately ties to his idea of the collective unconscious. He explains:

> In the sympathetic nervous system you would experience not as a person but as mankind, or even as belonging to the animal kingdom; you would experience nothing in particular, but the whole phenomena of life as if it were one. . . . But you see, this collective unconscious, in spite of its being everywhere, or in spite of its universal awareness, is located in the body; the sympathetic nervous system of the body is the organ by which you

> have the possibility of such awareness; therefore you can say the collective unconscious is in the lower centers of the brain and the spinal cord and the sympathetic system. Speaking accurately, this is the organ by which you experience the collective unconscious, which means as if there were nothing but you and the world—whether you are the world, or extend over the whole world, or the whole world is in you, is all the same.[53]

Jung's thought is not always systematic and even more rarely static. His use of associative symbolism, especially, tends to shift as he recombines and rearranges which thing stands in for which other. Rather than the collective unconscious as a whole, the serpent also comes to signify his idea of the anima. This, itself, is a slippery subject, which Jung sometimes uses specifically to point to the feminine elements of the male psyche, and at other times positions as a more generic—albeit still feminine—aspect of the unconscious, which serves a role somewhat akin to a mediating subtle body.[54] Mirroring Gnostic imagery, Jung states that "the anima is represented as woman above and serpent below."[55]

Indeed, if there is a single lens that helps to make sense of Jung's thought and especially his use of imagery and symbolism, Gnosticism might well be it. His entry point into the latter was the work of another Theosophist: G. R. S. Mead (1863–1933).[56] Through Mead's work, Jung also dove into the Hermetic and alchemical traditions. Drawing on the deep spiritual symbolism of Renaissance European alchemy, he came to consider the whole enterprise a "Western form of yoga."[57] In truth, for all his engagement with Asian ideas (both Chinese and Indian), Jung was deeply ambivalent about their cross-cultural applications. For instance, because he understood the psychological formation of the "Western mind" to be different from that of its Asian counterparts, he advised that, for the Western practitioner, the methods of Indian yoga were not only inappropriate but dangerous.[58] At this point, it is important to note that Jung was himself a practitioner, of sorts. Ultimately, Jung's psychological framework, not to mention his writings on more esoteric topics, cannot be separated from his personal spiritual explorations.

Serpents troubled Jung. His own mystical experiences as catalogued in *The Red Book*, first made public only in 2009, are swarming with serpents. Thousands of black serpents writhing in a great abyss, blotting out, devouring the sun.[59] A black serpent battling a white.[60] A great black serpent squeezing his body taught as he finds himself crucified, Christ-like, his red blood seeping from his body upon the rocky earth.[61] The black serpent transforming into a white bird that flies up to the heavens and returns with a golden crown.[62] And, perhaps most important of all, the serpent to whom he speaks as his own soul.[63]

Though Jung's body of work is vast, it is arguably in these personal writings that we are able to see into the heart of his thought most clearly. His spiritual journey coalesces as a tale of two primordial principles—pleasure (personified as Salome) and forethought (personified as Elijah)—which are entwined, reciprocal, and ultimately one. And as he narrates his encounters with these spirit guides, he tells us:

> Apart from Elijah and Salome I found the serpent as a third principle. It is a stranger to both principles although it is associated with both. The serpent taught me the unconditional difference in essence between the two principles in me. . . . The serpent is the earthly essence of man of which he is not conscious. Its character changes according to peoples and lands, since it is the mystery that flows to him from the nourishing earth-mother. The earthly (numen loci) separates forethinking and pleasure in man, but not in itself. The serpent has the weight of the earth in itself but also its changeability and germination from which

> everything that becomes emerges. It is always the serpent that causes man to become enslaved now to one, now to the other principle, so that it becomes error. One cannot live with forethinking alone, or with pleasure alone. You need both. But you cannot be in forethinking and in pleasure at the same time, you must take turns being in forethinking and pleasure, obeying the prevailing law, unfaithful to the other so to speak. . . . The way of life writhes like the serpent from right to left and from left to right, from thinking to pleasure and from pleasure to thinking. Thus the serpent is an adversary and a symbol of enmity, but also a wise bridge that connects right and left through longing, much needed by our life.[64]

This basic tripartite schema, a variant of which appears in the thought of Jung's erstwhile mentor and contemporary Sigmund Freud as the id, superego, and ego, is a staple of Western models of the human self at least as far back as Plato, who wrote of the appetitive, rational, and spirited capacities of the soul. What is unusual—if not, strictly speaking, unique—about Jung's model is his resistance to establishing a strict hierarchy among these principles. Jung's Neoplatonist predecessors might have elevated the rational aspect of the soul as the most purely divine, but then, most of them were looking for an escape hatch out of the physical world. Jung, meanwhile, makes it clear that he is interested in *life*. His aim is not absolute transcendence, or even the dazzling astral vistas of the Theosophists, but rather the embodied actualization of the human self, a process he names "individuation."

And so, Jung's own mystical experiences, as represented by his dreams, were profoundly Gnostic (in the broader sense of that term, or perhaps even more meaningfully Hermetic) in their imagery. However, when he interpreted them, he did so through the lens of his psychological framework. Mythic apotheosis, drawn out in fire, and serpents, and men with lions' heads, was for him ultimately a symbolic language for the inner workings of the human self. It was not the historical meanings of these concepts and images with which Jung was concerned, but how they could be used to illustrate his own understandings and theories. If this is true of the Gnostic material, in which Jung was quite profoundly steeped, it is all the truer for the historical meanings of Kuṇḍalinī, with which Jung was only superficially familiar.

In light of his musings on the serpent, it is perhaps not surprising that Kuṇḍalinī became a concept of special interest for Jung. In addition to a full set of Mead's works, Jung's library also contained a heavily annotated copy of *The Serpent Power*.[65] In 1932, Jung held a seminar where he delivered a series of lectures on the topic. In these lectures, he appears to directly borrow Avalon's words, using them rather out of context to describe Kuṇḍalinī as the "Inner Woman."[66] At another point, he goes so far as to unequivocally state: "the anima is the Kundalini."[67] In Jung's understanding,

> to activate the unconscious means to awaken the divine, the devī, Kundalini—to begin the development of the suprapersonal within the individual in order to kindle the light of the gods. Kundalini, which is to be awakened in the sleeping mūlādhāra world, is the suprapersonal, the non-ego, the totality of the psyche through which alone we can attain the higher cakras in a cosmic or metaphysical sense. For this reason Kundalini is the same principle as the Soter, the Saviour Serpent of the Gnostics. This way of looking at the world is the sūkṣma aspect. The sūkṣma aspect is the inner cosmic meaning of events—the "subtle body," the suprapersonal.[68]

And here we come to the crux of Jung's particular brand of mysticism and to the very reason that his treatment of Kuṇḍalinī, though a relatively minor aspect of his larger body of work, forms an integral part of our history.

Gopi Krishna, despite his own rather modern and syncretic understanding of Kuṇḍalinī, criticized Jung's tendency to become so "entirely preoccupied with his own theories about the unconscious" that he is able to find in his Asian sources "only material for the corroboration of his own ideas, and nothing beyond that."[69] The same criticism has subsequently been made by Western scholars.[70] Historian Sonu Shamdasani, on the other hand, proposes that matters may be somewhat more complicated. He writes, "For Jung, the Western 'discovery' of the East constituted a critical chapter in the 'discovery' of the collective unconscious."[71]

In other words, in Jung's understanding, South Asian models of Kuṇḍalinī became another culturally specific data point in a broader theory concerning the psychological process of individuation, which he understood as a universal phenomenon that nevertheless could only be observed when refracted through the lens of the specific cultural and historical context in which it occurred. More angles of approach meant a more accurate picture. However, Shamdasani argues that Jung engaged with his data in an earnest and constructive way. "It would also be a mistake," says Shamdasani, "to view Jung's commentary as consisting in the translation of the terms of Kundalini yoga into psychological concepts whose meaning had already been delimited in advance: for in the course of translating the terms of Kundalini yoga into those of analytical psychology, the latter became altered and extended. At base, the symbolism of the cakras enabled Jung to develop an archetypal regional topography of the psyche and to provide a narration of the process of individuation in terms of the imaginal transit between these regions."[72]

Arguably Jung's framework departs from its Indian point of reference far more drastically than any of the other Western models we have reviewed. And yet, in some ways, this is what makes it crucial to our history. Jung's understanding of Kuṇḍalinī is as revolutionary as his understanding of the subtle body as a whole, and for the same reason. He takes realities that occupied an increasingly tenuous hold on physicality and offers them a new domain: psychology.

THE SERPENT IN AVALON

And so we come now, at this chapter's end, to the source that arguably began much of the creative engagement with Kuṇḍalinī that we have summarized above: Arthur Avalon's *The Serpent Power* (1919). We include Avalon in this chapter not so much because the approach he represents is fundamentally Western (it isn't), but because it was meant to be perceived as such. That Arthur Avalon was the pseudonym of one Sir John George Woodroffe (1865–1936) was a secret so poorly kept, that it should come as no surprise to discover another secret concealed behind it. Namely, that Arthur Avalon was in fact not one person, but several.

Woodroffe's exact birthplace is debated, but he was baptized in January 1866 in Calcutta, where his father then served as a barrister of the High Court. Woodroffe, educated at Oxford, also enjoyed a lengthy legal career in India.[73] It was during his own time as a judge at the Calcutta High Court, beginning in 1904, that Woodroffe likely encountered devotees of tantric gurus—Bengali men who would eventually become his collaborators.[74] The details are difficult to substantiate, but biographer Kathleen Taylor suggests that Woodroffe may have received two tantric initiations. Both came from gurus associated with Atalbihari Ghosh (1864–1936),[75] a Bengali scholar whom Taylor has identified as Woodroffe's primary collaborator behind the Avalon name. Julian Strube, while acknowledging Taylor's arguments regarding Ghosh's importance, goes on to add that "it might be more appropriate to see Avalon not as a duo but as a team of several, and most likely altering, individuals."[76] Among these, Strube names Woodroffe and Ghosh's mutual guru, the Bengali tantric Shivachandra Bhattacharyya Vidyarnava (1860–1913), as well as a number of other Bengali men like Pramathanath Mukhopadhyay and Baradakanta Majumdar, who were authors in their own right.[77]

As both Taylor and Strube assert, though Woodroffe did undertake the study of Sanskrit in earnest, the translations attributed to Avalon were not his. When we say that the approach represented by Avalon is not essentially Western—indeed, that it is Indian—we refer not only to Woodroffe's own involvement and devotion to Indian tantra, but also to the fact that, as a Westerner, he was outnumbered by his Indian collaborators in giving voice to Avalon. Why, then, is Woodroffe's name the one so clearly linked to Avalon—to the point that most of Avalon's publications have been continually printed with his name appended? The "open secret" was likely a strategic move. As Strube has suggested, "there can be little doubt that all those involved were very well aware of the fact that a British judge and Christian would be a more efficient spokesperson for the 'rehabilitation' of tantra than an Indian scholar, let alone a Tantric."[78]

Avalon's name itself, of course, is a deliberate and explicit signal. For anyone familiar with European culture—but especially for those born in the Victorian era, obsessed with all things medieval—"Arthur Avalon" would have immediately summoned up images of magic and esoteric lore, mythical islands hidden in the mists, and legendary quests for the Holy Grail. Indeed, the name was apparently derived from a famous painting by British painter Edward Burne-Jones, titled *The Last Sleep of Arthur in Avalon* (begun in 1881 and left uncompleted upon the artist's death), which was itself based on British poet Alfred Tennyson's "The Passing of Arthur" (part of the cycle comprising *Idylls of the King*, published between 1859 and 1885).[79] In other words, Arthur Avalon's pedigree would have been both obvious and deeply significant: an author steeped in English legend, but writing with authority on colonial India. Thus, Avalon's persona was built to capitalize on both sides of the exchange—an authoritative Western mouthpiece for authentic Indian wisdom.

In one sense, Avalon might stand as a contrast to syncretic and hybrid work like that of the Theosophists insofar as he often remains insistently and indeed righteously faithful to the original texts he's translating and to the Indian systems from which they arise. Such a reading would be supported by Avalon's own statements, such as the one we cited at the outset of this chapter. Indeed, in *The Serpent Power*, Avalon spends considerable time refuting the Theosophists and their understandings of Kuṇḍalinī. However, Strube has demonstrated that John Woodroffe and especially his wife Ellen, who likewise underwent initiations and studied Sanskrit alongside him, were closely involved with the Theosophical Society. So were a number of his collaborators.[80] And, for all its insistence upon tradition, *The Serpent Power* does not shy away from modern readings of Kuṇḍalinī, some of which are rather closely in line with Theosophical models. For instance, on one occasion, Avalon quotes at length from the work of his "friend and collaborator Professor Pramathanatha Mukhyopadhyaya," comparing the relationship of Śiva and Śakti as well as the internal dynamic of the subtle body to the positive-negative polarity of electromagnetism.[81] In other words, things are—as always—quite complicated.

Though Avalon's name appears on a number of works, *The Serpent Power* is arguably the most famous, and almost certainly the one with the biggest footprint. The text is lengthy and, as some scholars have rightfully pointed out,[82] not exactly easy to read. Just under half of its five hundred or so pages are devoted to translations of two Sanskrit texts, the *Ṣaṭcakra Nirūpaṇa* and a much shorter hymn of praise to the guru called the *Pādukā Pañcaka*. The first section of the book is devoted to a lengthy introduction by Avalon himself, which consists of multiple subsections and includes, among other things, a crash course in Indian (and specifically nondual Śaiva) metaphysics.

The *Ṣaṭcakra Nirūpaṇa* ("The Description of the Six *Cakras*") is a sixteenth-century text from the Southern Transmission of the nondual Kaula Śaiva tradition. As its title suggests, the text describes in detail the six primary *cakras*, in the course of which it also treats Kuṇḍalinī. Like some other texts in the Southern Transmission, the *Ṣaṭcakra Nirūpaṇa* also appends to its list of six *cakras* a lotus, which it does not technically refer to as a *cakra*—the luminous and thousand-petaled inverted lotus of the *sahasrāra*, located at the cranial fontanelle or just above it. This formulation, of course, is hugely responsible for the modern-day global ubiquity of the seven-*cakra* system.[83]

The same thing can be said for Avalon's representation of Kuṇḍalinī. As we've seen, the "Serpent Power" was already a popular way to refer to Kuṇḍalinī among the Theosophists—Avalon's book no doubt reinforced this language. Beyond that, Avalon's greatest impact lies perhaps in the general features foregrounded by his work—the centrality of Kuṇḍalinī, the sevenfold nature of the *cakras*—rather than the specific details, which would have been difficult for even an educated reader to penetrate without an extensive background in Indian religious imagery and metaphysics. More than anything else, perhaps, Avalon is responsible for codifying the notion that there is a standard and "authentic" model of Kuṇḍalinī.

This notion—which, as we argued in chapter 1, is wholly inaccurate—is not precisely what Avalon intended to convey. Quite the opposite: Avalon explicitly acknowledges the diversity and frequent inconsistency of textual sources. Indeed, he is very careful in repeating that the account offered in *The Serpent Power* is that of a particular system of yoga, as represented by the *Ṣaṭcakra Nirūpaṇa*. This, however, is belied by the amount of space Avalon devotes to refuting and correcting competing accounts, chiefly those of prominent Theosophical authors.

For instance, after informing his readers that the tantric models he intends to describe have recently received some attention in "Western literature of the occult kind," he immediately bemoans the many inaccuracies littering such sources. The first author Avalon quotes is Pryse, though he is never named. Avalon refutes and corrects Pryse's understanding that the *iḍā* and *piṅgalā* must be "energized" prior to the *suṣumnā* (indeed he takes issues with Pryse's understanding of the nature of *nāḍīs* as a whole), as well as identifying a number of other details in Pryse's description of Kuṇḍalinī experience as inaccurate.[84] He then moves on to a longer refutation of an individual he obliquely calls a "well-known 'Theosophical' author," immediately specifying in a footnote that he is referring to Leadbeater's 1911 book, *The Inner Life*. Avalon opens his treatment of Leadbeater by clarifying that

> his [Leadbeater's] account does not profess to be a representation of the teaching of the Indian Yogis (whose competence for their own Yoga the author somewhat disparages), but that it is put forward as the Author's own original explanation (fortified, as he conceives, by certain portions of Indian teaching) of the personal experience which (he writes) he himself has had. This experience appears to consist in the conscious arousing of the "Serpent Fire," with the enhanced "astral" and mental vision which he believes has shown him what he tells us.[85]

Avalon then proceeds to give a faithful account of Leadbeater's understanding of the *cakras* and Kuṇḍalinī, occupying several pages. The account is so detailed that one begins to forget Avalon means to disagree with its content.

At the very least, then, anyone reading Avalon would also receive a fairly detailed introduction to these competing Theosophical models. Indeed, an inattentive reader may well fail to differentiate them from Avalon's own version. Notably, Avalon never claims that Leadbeater's account of metaphysics in general or the *cakras* in particular is false; he only says that it is not in accordance with the Yoga Śāstra, which he does not always take pains to differentiate from the specific system of the *Ṣaṭcakra Nirūpaṇa* on which *The Serpent Power* is based. And yet, the manner in which he corrects the Theosophists' statements and the space he devotes to doing so implies the existence of an authoritative and authentic system, which Avalon's book will presumably elucidate.

Avalon's position on these Theosophical adaptations is perhaps best exemplified by an anecdote he offers at the conclusion of that first section where he treats them. The account refers to "a European friend" who, being familiar with some translated Sanskrit works, believed he had succeeded in arousing Kuṇḍalinī. This friend described an experience of a multicolored, Caduceus-like rush of fiery energy that culminated in a double-winged radiance in the head. If one were looking for textual connections, this experience would sound very much in line with the descriptions offered by Pryse, Leadbeater, and Arundale. The Indian *pandit* to whom Avalon recounted this experience, however, politely informed him that his friend must have been "confused."[86] The *pandit* deemed it possible that the European practitioner had seen the unaroused Kuṇḍalinī in the root *cakra* but was disoriented as to the location of the vision since it was being perceived with the mind. The details of the experience, however, did not describe the raising of Kuṇḍalinī. Avalon goes on to state (presumably based on the authority of the same *pandit*) that Kuṇḍalinī may produce intense heat in the spot where She is aroused, but She leaves the body "cold and apparently lifeless as a corpse" as She rises, until all that remains is a small spot of warmth at the top of the head.[87] The reported experience of Avalon's friend—just like the Theosophical positions represented in the preceding pages, which it so obviously mirrors—may constitute a "confused" brush with Kuṇḍalinī, but it does not reflect the full and genuine phenomenon of Kuṇḍalinī rising. The implication is, of course, once more, that such a phenomenon follows a single and specific model that Avalon will subsequently go on to expound.

We will not delve here into the specifics of this model, chiefly because it does not substantially differ from the Kaula Śaiva models we have already addressed in chapter 1. However, there is one final thing that does deserve special note. This is Avalon's resistance—quite faithful to the traditional nature of his tantric source material—to physicalize the subtle anatomy of the *cakras* and especially of Kuṇḍalinī. Contra the Theosophists, as well as quite a few Indian authors whom we will encounter in chapter 4, Avalon insistently maintains that these are divine powers and subtle visionary realities, *not* features of the gross body. Though Avalon devotes much space and effort to unpacking the nature and location of the *cakras* (again citing a number of competing accounts), he closes by stating, "One conclusion emerges clearly from all this namely, that the Lotuses [*cakras*] are in the vertebral column in Sushumna, and not in the nerve plexuses which surround it. There in the spinal column they exist as extremely subtle vital centres of Prānashakti and centres of consciousness."[88] He goes on to say, more firmly still, "It is a mistake, therefore, in my opinion, to identify the Chakras with the physical plexuses mentioned. . . . In other words, from an objective standpoint the subtle centres, or Chakras, vitalize and control the gross bodily tracts which are indicated by the various regions of the vertebral column and the ganglia, plexuses, nerves, arteries, and organs, situate in these respective regions."[89]

Through this spatial association, by virtue of the necessary connection between gross and subtle reality, it may be said that the forces of the *cakras* may produce effects upon the physical body, but the *cakras* are not themselves *in* the physical body.

In this sense, Avalon's (fairly traditional Indian) position is perhaps closer to that of Jung (which is anything but) than it is to the hybrid models of the Theosophists and their attempts to reify Kuṇḍalinī as an aspect of the physical body through talk of nerve plexuses and quasi-electromagnetic principles like "neuricity." For Jung, Elijah, Salome, and the serpent are quite real—just as the goddess Kuṇḍalinī and the divinities occupying the *cakras* are real—but they are not literal physical features of the body. Of course, the Gnostic archons that presided over the Zodiac of the premodern Western tradition weren't exactly physical either. And plenty of premodern Indian texts treated Kuṇḍalinī as a physical obstruction. Perhaps, then, the distinction is not so much between East and West, or even premodern and modern.

4

EAST MEETS WEST

Kuṇḍalinī and the Evolution of Modern Yoga

Divine Mother asked me to look and see
If I could find Her close by the hills of Elsinore.
But now I shall seek Her no more
In any other sea-fenced mountain core;
For Dame Divinity I found reigning
Within, without, everywhere—bliss-showers
raining—By enrapturing Encinitas' elysian shore.

—PARAMAHANSA YOGANANDA, *SONGS OF THE SOUL*

There is an oft-repeated, though likely apocryphal story that Swami Dayananda Saraswati, founder of the modern Hindu reformist group Ārya Samāj, once pulled a corpse out of the Ganga and dissected it in search of *cakras*. Upon failing to find any, he chucked his Sanskrit texts on yoga into the river like so much dead weight.[1] Modern innovators of yoga generally went one of two ways when responding to this sort of thing. They either doubled down on the idea that, while the features of the yogic body were indeed physical, the premodern texts could not be taken literally with all their talk of variously petalled lotuses and inscribed phonemes; instead, they insisted, such descriptions should be taken as coded attempts to refer to real physiological features now known to the medical and biological sciences. Or the other option was to affirm a formal split between the physical body and the subtle one.

In any case, with some interpretive license, *cakras* could be associated with anatomical features, such as nerve ganglia or plexuses (or, slightly later, endocrine glands),[2] if not reduced to them entirely. Kuṇḍalinī, however, was not so easily naturalized. As we saw in chapter 3, early Theosophical accounts liken Kuṇḍalinī to a kind of electric force but, in literal terms, this proves untenable even by nineteenth-century standards.

The naturalization of the yogic body arguably began much earlier. As we discussed in chapter 1, Kuṇḍalinī eventually became a prominent feature of the medieval literature on *haṭha* yoga. According to yoga scholar and philologist James Mallinson, the distinguishing feature of *haṭha* yoga is the use of physical techniques like *mudrās* and *bandhas* ("seals" and "locks," respectively). These mark *haṭha* practice as different from other forms of tantric yoga, for instance *laya* yoga, which is characterized by visionary *saṃketas* (methods) such as the cultivation of internal sound. Mallinson argues that these physical techniques first emerged in the context of ascetic practice, where they were used toward specifically physical ends, such as cultivating the heat of *tapas* within the body, or else manipulating the internal flow of *bindu* (semen). In the medieval *haṭha* texts, however, we see these practices repurposed toward new goals—specifically, awakening and raising Kuṇḍalinī.[3] It requires no huge logical leap to imagine that the application of physical practices (as opposed to purely contemplative ones) might make us regard the thing those practices are targeting as more physical. And so, in the *haṭha* texts, we begin to see Kuṇḍalinī and the *cakras* through which it is raised become increasingly associated with features of and experiences in the physical body.

Haṭha yoga, which emerged in the thirteenth century, comes at the tail end of what some have called the Śaiva Age.[4] From a philosophical perspective, this meant that the Śaiva framework was giving way to that of Vedānta. The Upaniṣads were making a comeback. Thus *haṭha* texts, despite their tantric character, often drew on both Śaiva and Vedānta versions of nondualism.[5] In turn, Advaita Vedāntins, who previously had not thought very highly of yogic methods, believing them to depend on ultimately inferior cognitive mechanisms, had a gradual change of heart. For instance, the Yoga Upaniṣads, written largely in this medieval period, borrow from *haṭha* materials and integrate them with Advaita Vedānta.[6]

And so, from the moment of its inception, *haṭha* yoga was a thing caught betwixt and between. It exists as a distinct and stable category only if we limit our reference point to a very specific body of medieval texts—these represent what Mallinson has called "classical" *haṭha* yoga and, for the sake of clarity, this is the sense in which we'll be using the term in this chapter. But, in reality, the messy constellation of conceptual frameworks and practices we call *haṭha* has from the outset been scattered across the contested ground shared by ascetics, Tāntrikas, and Vedāntins. Add to this the impact of British colonialism, which labeled as dangerous and degenerate tantra and asceticism alike, while elevating the ancient wisdom of the Veda and the sophisticated "purity" of classical philosophy.

This background is crucial to understanding why Kuṇḍalinī awakening frequently forms the core teaching of late nineteenth- and early twentieth-century yogis who declare themselves to be Vedāntins while denouncing the ascetic excesses of *haṭha* yoga. Of this trend, Swami Vivekananda, with whom we'll begin our story shortly, is the quintessential example. But although both tantra and *haṭha* yoga had, by his time, become rather infamous brands to evoke, both had so thoroughly soaked into Indian philosophy and religious practice in general and yoga in particular that their implicit influence resisted any explicit denunciations.

The common ambiguity that persists through all these shifts, and reformulations, and changes of terminology can perhaps be summed up as follows: Is Kuṇḍalinī awakening a physical phenomenon or a mental (and therefore metaphysical) one? The visionary techniques of the tantric texts swing toward the latter, whereas the physical *haṭha* techniques would seem to emphasize the importance of the former. Objectively, we might say that it is necessarily both. But, as Kuṇḍalinī emerges into the global imagination where the "modern" must also be the "scientific," this question takes on a new dimension.

VIVEKANANDA AND THE IMPORTANCE OF ROUSING SERPENTS

Swami Vivekananda (1863–1902), born Narendranath Datta in colonial Calcutta, is a tricky figure when it comes to the history of modern yoga. He is widely acclaimed as the father of yoga in the West, a title that grossly oversimplifies the situation but is not without merit. At the same time, he bears a reputation of being downright hostile to physical yoga, which means his authority is often evoked to label modern posture-centric practices as inauthentic. In truth, while Vivekananda indeed did not teach the complex postural practices common to global yoga today (more on this later), his prescribed method was hardly divorced from the physical body. And it was unquestionably a method of raising Kuṇḍalinī.

Vivekananda's seminal status is owed chiefly to two factors. Firstly, he was one of the first (though neither the actual first, nor the only) among early popularizers of yogic concepts and practices in North America. In addition to the media frenzy that surrounded his appearance at the 1893 World's Parliament of Religions in Chicago and subsequent lecture tour, he established the first Vedanta Society in New York in 1894, paving the way for other swamis from the newly founded Ramakrishna Mission to do the same. Arguably the more important factor, however, was the 1896 publication of *Raja Yoga*, which collected Vivekananda's American lectures and placed them alongside a commentary on the classical *Yoga Sūtras* of Patañjali (c. fourth century CE). In the decades following, this text would be referenced, emulated, and occasionally downright plagiarized by spiritual teachers, Western and Indian alike, as well as endlessly referenced by scholars in search of an authoritative source on authentic yoga.

In light of all this, it's significant that, for all that *Raja Yoga* has to say about classical philosophy and contemporary science, its ultimate goal assumes Kuṇḍalinī awakening. As Vivekananda unequivocally states, "the rousing of Kundalini is the one and only way to attaining Divine Wisdom, super-conscious perception, realization of the spirit."[7] The practical scaffolding, though simple, is at least nominally aimed at this eventuality. The same can be said of Vivekananda's public presentations. Contemporary accounts from people who attended Vivekananda's talks describe the practice of "Raja Yogi" as involving the awakening and ascension of the "Kundalina" into the brain via the "sussuma" canal.[8] "We sat in a line or in a circle and breathed deeply," one practitioner reported. "We tried to breathe entirely through the left nostril and concentrated on it until we felt the breath going way down to kindalina [*sic*]." This was accompanied by "exercises in the imagination" in which the practitioners would visualize "a locust [*sic*] on the top of our heads growing brighter and brighter or to imagine that there was a locust in our hearts growing brighter and brighter."[9] (In this case, one only hopes that the obvious mistake was made by the *Chicago Tribune* reporter who recorded the account rather than the practitioner himself. Vivekananda almost certainly instructed his students to visualize a *lotus*, which is both more traditional and more pleasant.) Yet, despite the abundant and occasionally comical misspellings, all this seems to make it clear that Vivekananda was instructing his students in a basic type of *prāṇāyāma* and visualization exercise.

There is some historical ambiguity regarding whether Vivekananda ever received formal initiation from his guru, Ramakrishna, or what his personal spiritual practice and commitments may have entailed.[10] Certainly, the simplicity of his instructions stands at odds with the complexity of both the medieval texts and the methods of his general contemporaries (such as Paramahansa Yogananda) who had firmer ties to a lineage of formal practice. And yet, the practice Vivekananda prescribes is not so unlike the simple meditation that would yield Gopi Krishna's famous Kuṇḍalinī awakening some four decades later.

Indeed, one could deduce this practice from *Raja Yoga*, if so inclined, despite the fact that the book is hardly a manual. Vivekananda very clearly describes a version of what is sometimes known as "alternate-nostril breathing," where the practitioner inhales through one nostril, retains the breath for some time, and then exhales through the opposite nostril. The new cycle of breath begins with an inhale on the side through which the exhale has just passed, so alternating the direction of breath between left and right. Vivekananda instructs:

> Slowly fill the lungs with breath through the Ida, the left nostril, and at the same time concentrate the mind on the nerve current. You are, as it were, sending the nerve current down the spinal column, and striking violently on the last plexus, the basic lotus, which is triangular in form, the seat of the Kundalini. Then hold the current there for some time. Imagine that you are slowly drawing that nerve current with the breath through the other

side, the Pingala, then slowly throw it out through the right nostril.[11]

This technique is usually referred to as *nāḍī śodhana*, or the purification of the channels, because the alternation between left and right is meant to mirror the interplay between the *iḍā* and *piṅgalā nāḍīs*.

And this, incidentally, is where Vivekananda sets about constructing his bridge between a biophysical understanding of the body and the spiritual effects of such a bodily practice. The *iḍā* and *piṅgalā* are understood in physiological terms as nerve currents, whereas the central *nāḍī* of the *suṣumnā* becomes for Vivekananda a kind of hollow canal that runs through the center of the spinal cord. Nerve currents represent the typical function of the mind inside the body. They carry impulses from the central nervous system, traveling along the body's network of nerves like electricity coursing through wires. But just like an electric current—which can be sent along a wire but can also travel freely through natural media—the force of mind can be liberated from its physiological medium. This is precisely what the yogi does. By opening the hollow channel of his *suṣumnā*, he is able to project his mental force beyond the confines of his body.[12] In short, the typical animal mind is a landline. The yogi has WiFi.

Vivekananda's grasp of the science is not rigorously technical, but it is generally in line with the broad understandings of his time. He was not the first to adopt such theories. For instance, his manner of understanding the *cakras* as nerve plexuses follows on the heels of similar speculations by Bamandas Basu.[13] Though Vivekananda's scientific assertions are both vague and speculative, they represent a crucial link in the chain of efforts to bridge notions of Kuṇḍalinī as a spiritual force with the kind of biophysics that would come to occupy later innovators of modern yoga. Far more than any of his predecessors (and indeed many of his successors), Vivekananda advances an attempt to rationalize precisely *how* one might move from the physical to the spiritual. Contrary to historical accounts that emphasize the abstract and contemplative dimensions of Vivekananda's teachings, the core mechanic here is physical breath. Vivekananda explains:

> In the first place, from rhythmical breathing comes a tendency of all the molecules in the body to move in the same direction. When mind changes into will, the nerve currents change into a motion similar to electricity, because the nerves have been proved to show polarity under the action of electric currents. This shows that when the will is transformed into the nerve currents, it is changed into something like electricity. When all the motions of the body have become perfectly rhythmical, the body has, as it were, become a gigantic battery of will. This tremendous will is exactly what the Yogi wants. This is, therefore, a physiological explanation of the breathing exercise. It tends to bring a rhythmic action in the body, and helps us, through the respiratory centre, to control the other centres. The aim of Pranayama here is to rouse the coiled-up power in the Mulâdhâra, called the Kundalini.[14]

Casual practice has its own benefits, says Vivekananda. The body and mind will grow calm. The practitioner will acquire a beautiful voice. But only sustained practice will bring true transformation. And this, only through the awakening of Kuṇḍalinī.

Vivekananda understands Kuṇḍalinī in a rather unique way, as a latent power comprised of accrued action and sensation—something perhaps halfway between traditional Indian notions of *saṃskāras*, and the sort of thing early psychologists would soon dub as the subconscious. In small amounts, Vivekananda tells us, this power is responsible for the phenomena of dreams and imagination. However, if it is augmented and awakened through meditation, it can flood the nervous system to induce a reaction far beyond the mental states made possible by normal sense perception. This is what opens the channel of the *suṣumnā* and allows the yogi to project his mind and will throughout the whole of nature in a manner that is not accessible to ordinary humans. In effect, this is why the yogi has superpowers (*siddhis*).

At this point, it's worth remembering that *Raja Yoga* is derived chiefly from Vivekananda's public talks. This is true even of the commentary on the *Yoga Sūtras*, which is why that commentary occasionally appears so at odds with traditional interpretations of the text, and even with itself. Indeed, it doesn't seem difficult to guess which sections Vivekananda wrote for the book alone. Vivekananda's commentary on the more technical aspects of Patañjali's *sūtras* is brief, and generally quite vague. One of the longest commentaries is attached to a verse on *prāṇāyāma*, and it is replete with the subtle physiology of the *nāḍīs*. Lurking behind Vivekananda's dutiful discussion of *vṛittis* and *saṃskāras* is an occupation with the control of subtle reality. This, it seems, is as good an indication as any of Vivekananda's priorities.

In light of all this, one final passage is worthy of note. Having declared that "the rousing of Kundalini is the one and only way to attaining Divine Wisdom, super-conscious perception, realization of the spirit,"[15] Vivekananda proceeds to elaborate:

> The rousing may come in various ways, through love for God, through the mercy of perfected sages, or through the power of the analytic will of the philosopher. Wherever there was any manifestation of what is ordinarily called supernatural power or wisdom, there a little current of *Kundalini* must have found its way into the *Sushumna*. Only, in the vast majority of such cases,

> people had ignorantly stumbled on some practice which set free a minute portion of the coiled-up *Kundalini*. All worship, consciously or unconsciously, leads to this end. The man who thinks that he is receiving response to his prayers does not know that the fulfilment comes from his own nature, that he has succeeded by the mental attitude of prayer in waking up a bit of this infinite power which is coiled up within himself.[16]

In one sense, this elaboration is a restatement of the original claim: Kuṇḍalinī is the only way to our highest goal. But the reframing is also important for the way that it broadens the scope of what counts as Kuṇḍalinī. Which, to be clear, is basically everything—at least as far as Vivekananda is concerned. Thus Vivekananda is not denying the efficacy of other paths (devotion, grace of the guru, the philosophical gnosis of *jñāna*, and so on). Yet all of these paths are effective not as alternatives to Kuṇḍalinī awakening but because they are alternative ways that the awakening is effected. All paths—if they're done correctly, anyway—lead to the same goal. Keep this in mind as we proceed.

RELE'S NOT-SO-MYSTERIOUS KUṆḌALINĪ

Vivekananda's physicalism builds to its most radical iteration in Vasant G. Rele's *The Mysterious Kundalini* (1927). The book got its start as a short paper, presented by Rele in 1926 before the Bombay Medical Union following a demonstration of feats of strength and acuity by a practitioner of "Yogic Science and Prāṇāyāma," identified only as Deshbandhu. The yogi, Rele reports, was nothing special—"a middle-aged man, of average height, of slender body, with chest not broad enough to compare favourably with an athlete of average development, with long thin legs, and calf muscles showing insufficient physical exercise."[17] And yet, this man was able to break a heavy iron chain with a mere tug of his body. What's more, he was able to stop and restart his pulse, seemingly at will. Rele himself recorded a cessation of arterial pulse in Deshbandhu's wrist for an interval of one minute. This was confirmed with a stethoscope applied directly to the chest.

Rele held a Licentiate in Medicine and Surgery, likely from Grant Medical College in Bombay, as well as a more specialized Fellowship of College of Physicians and Surgeons degree. It is from this perspective that he sets about presenting his theory—and he freely admits it is only a theory—for how Deshbandhu's application of yogic techniques led to these unusual phenomena, chief among them the stopping of the heart, which would require control over typically involuntary physical functions. As the book makes clear, Rele's answer to the mystery is Kuṇḍalinī, which Rele identifies specifically with the right vagus nerve.

Rele's chief expertise might have been in medicine, but he situates himself quite clearly among the contemporary popularizers of yoga and Kuṇḍalinī. He prominently cites both Vivekananda and Arthur Avalon. Indeed, a statement from John Woodroffe is presented as a foreword to the volume. This seems like a particularly interesting move since Woodroffe takes it as an opportunity to openly disagree with Rele. Rele's book thus opens with a traditionalist view that seems to undermine his core argument. Kuṇḍalinī is the "Grand Potential" that cannot be reduced to any of her material products. "She is then not as such, in my view," declares Woodroffe, "a nerve or any other physical substance or mental faculty but the Ground Substance of both which, on being roused, ascends and is merged in the higher Tattvas ending in Shiva-Shakti Tattvas when she is said to be merged in Paramashiva. The Yoga is, in short, an evolutionary movement which is the reverse of the involution into matter which constitutes the Universe. Kundalini is the Dynamic

Real as the residual Power, the Power 'left over' (to use a gross expression, for we can find no others) after the production of Prithivi when she coils herself around the Linga or Static Real and rests."[18] Despite this, Woodroffe recognizes the value of Rele's contribution as a starting point for scientific enquiry. As such, regardless of its correctness, it serves the greater project upon which, it seems, both men can agree—namely, that we must "make *living* for us to-day the Scriptural Texts of the past."[19] Of course one can only assume that even a lukewarm endorsement from the author or *The Serpent Power* must have carried quite a bit of capital.

In fact, the juxtaposition of Woodroffe's dissenting foreword and the main thrust of Rele's text nicely captures the chief tension within attempts to "modernize" Kuṇḍalinī. Insofar as the yogic raising of Kuṇḍalinī is a physical practice, and leads to a physical experience, it must have some corollary phenomenon in the sphere of modern biophysics. Even Woodroffe admits that the vagus nerve may have some central importance in the practice of yoga, even if it is not to be identified with Kuṇḍalinī Herself. And conversely, insofar as the traditional outcomes of Kuṇḍalinī awakening lay claim to far more than extraordinary feats of the body, the matter cannot be described as only physical. This even Rele is forced to admit by the time his book winds to a close.

Still, what's significant, for our purposes, is the utter and complete conviction with which Rele insists on the purely *physiological* nature of Kuṇḍalinī as such. There is nothing visionary or imaginal here. Rele reads the medieval texts, with their talk of suns and moons, lotuses and immortal nectar, as coded discussions of bodily anatomy. Like some of his predecessors, he equates the *cakras* to the six important nerve plexuses of the sympathetic nervous system. The *śaktis* ruling over individual *cakras* become the efferent nerve impulses originating from associated regions of the central nervous system and acting upon the body's various organs. The *suṣumnā* is the spinal cord, while the *iḍā* and *piṅgalā* are the gangliated cords of the sympathetic nervous system. The thousand-petaled *sahasrāra* (the seventh pseudo-*cakra*) is "the plexus of nerves of a thousand branches or the cerebrum,"[20] and thus the divine nectar of *amṛta* becomes cerebrospinal fluid. Perhaps the most unique feature of Rele's argument is his identification of Kuṇḍalinī with the vagus nerve (specifically the right one)—not a dynamic power, but a static organ in the body. And yet, this seems like a logical progression of his predecessors' reinterpretations of the *cakra* system. After all, if one directly equates the *cakras* with the nerve plexuses—not subtle functions that emanate from or are associated with them, but the plexuses themselves—then it also makes perfect sense to identify Kuṇḍalinī with the vagus. It makes for a clean physicalism, though an unprecedented one.

Based on this framework, then, Rele proceeds to reinterpret the awakening of Kuṇḍalinī as a physiological process induced by yogic techniques. By applying *haṭha*-yogic *bandhas* and *mudrās*, together with *prāṇāyāma*, the practitioner is able to stimulate some nervous impulses while inhibiting others, eventually deranging the normal functions of the nervous system in a way that renders normally unconscious bodily processes open to the mind. Notably, in this way, Rele is able to explain everything from the "weird and exaggerated language" (his words not ours) of the *Jñāneśvarī* to the sonic manifestations of *nāda* yoga.

Awakening Kuṇḍalinī effectively means establishing voluntary control over the functions of the vagus nerve. Doing so, Rele claims, should afford complete control over the typically involuntary functions of the parasympathetic nervous system, thus also explaining yogic "miracles" such as stopping the heartbeat. Admittedly, the connection between manipulating the incoming and outgoing impulses of the various nervous plexuses and some of the more colorful yogic feats Rele references, such as knowledge of the past and future or the transmutation of metals,[21] is less obvious. And so too, by the end of Rele's exposition, it remains somewhat unclear how all of this physiological manipulation amounts to a state of being "one with that Cosmic Power which creates and sustains the universe."[22]

Thus, Rele's argument may indeed be—as Woodroffe calls it—"an original one,"[23] but whether it offers a compelling explanation of Kuṇḍalinī is perhaps another matter. To start, Rele's explanations of this process freely mix modern anatomical terminology with the premodern terms used in *haṭha* yoga and Āyurveda in ways that are not often easy to track. Nor are Rele's attempts to map subtle physiology onto gross quite as neat as they appear at first glance. Most troublesome: when forced to explain how the singular Kuṇḍalinī corresponds to the dual (right and left) structure of the vagus, Rele has no choice but to insist (without much evidence) that the left vagus nerve is simply not as important. This, coupled with the vagueness of his references and the overall lack of clinical evidence for the fact that any of these things actually *happen* in the way he describes—that pressing the heel into the perineum, for instance, really does block the efferent nervous impulses of the pelvic plexus while encouraging afferent impulses to rise—makes any objective evaluation of Rele's claims impossible. (On this score, at least, one can't help but agree with Woodroffe.) And then, of course, there is the matter of Kuṇḍalinī's metaphysical import. After all, Kuṇḍalinī is not a device for breaking chains or stopping the heart. She divinizes. She liberates. How does the right vagus nerve allow one to become one with the cosmos?

The closest we get to an explanation is when, in the final section of the book, Rele turns his attention to the eight traditional yogic powers of perfection. Unfortunately, however, the answer is a nonanswer. "The explanation of these *Ashta-siddhis* is beyond the scope of the physiology of the physical body," Rele informs the reader. "A Yogi cannot do or achieve these through the nerve current in his body, but when the Yogi has freed himself from nerve currents, he will be able to achieve the *Ashta-siddhis* by other channels."[24] Here Rele appeals to the "astral body," a concept that he draws, quite explicitly, from Theosophy. Once the practitioner liberates his soul from his physical body, he is free to inhabit the astral body composed of fine ethereal matter. Kuṇḍalinī, however, is only a preparatory mechanism for this process, acting exclusively on the level of the physical anatomy. One can see why Woodroffe, as an admirer of Śākta tantra, might have taken issue with the move. Going from the Goddess to one half of a nerve is quite the demotion. And yet, having rendered Kuṇḍalinī not so mysterious after all, Rele is forced to displace the mystery. Given that it was "Western anatomy and medicine" (as indicated by Rele's subtitle) that thus demystified Her, it is perhaps not surprising that a Western spiritual concept should be brought in to take up the slack.

And, in light of the spirit of Rele's project, neither is it surprising that the final words of his book (with the exception of a brief concluding summary) go to Vivekananda, though updated with a few stealthy revisions. Rele "quotes": "Whenever there is any manifestation of what is ordinarily called supernatural power of wisdom there must have been a little (control over the) current of *Kundalini* which found its way into the *Sushumna*. Only, in the vast majority of such cases of *supernaturalism*, they ignorantly stumbled on some practice which set free, (and made them conscious of) a minute portion (of the control) of the coiled up *Kundalini*."[25] The parenthetical portions are Rele's own additions, made necessary by the ultimate divergence between Vivekananda's understanding of Kuṇḍalinī and his own. After all, it would hardly be possible for the vagus nerve to make its way into the spinal cord.

THE ELUSIVE KUṆḌALINĪ OF POSTURAL YOGA

It seems impossible to understate the influence of Vivekananda's synthesis upon the development of Indian postural yoga. One clear continuity is the standardization of Patañjali's eight-limb system as a pathway to Kuṇḍalinī awakening. Vivekananda was certainly not the first to make this connection. Medieval commentaries on the *Yoga Sūtras* frequently read the verses in light of *haṭha* yogic subtle physiology, despite the absence of such meanings from earlier interpretations.[26] However, Vivekananda's explosive popularity ensured that this rather abstruse text whose dualistic metaphysics actually stand at odds with much of the medieval *haṭha* literature would join a handful of sources from that latter group (most notably, the *Śiva Saṃhitā* and the *Haṭha Pradīpikā*, both of which Vivekananda relied upon in composing his own book)[27], as the ad hoc canon of modern yoga.

Indeed, Vivekananda's layering of a tantric *haṭha* framework onto the philosophical authority of Patañjali's classical text, all the while presenting both under the label of "Rāja Yoga," also standardized one of the *Haṭha Pradīpikā*'s more distinctive statements: "Without Haṭha, Rājayoga does not succeed, and without Rāja, nor does Haṭhayoga."[28] Vivekananda's dismissals of the more specialized techniques of *haṭha* (and of the label as a whole) did little to dissuade this.

Thus, a common trend among early English-language—so, not simply modern, but intended as potentially global—manuals of yoga is a kind of formal nod to the framework of Patañjali's eight limbs, followed by a telescoping expansion of the limbs of *āsana* and *prāṇāyāma*. The proliferation of complex and occasionally dynamic poses was a trend already well underway by the seventeenth century, as indigenous forms of physical culture fed into the newly empowered physical techniques of medieval *haṭha* traditions.[29] However, in the cultural climate of the early twentieth century, these practices became a uniquely accessible dimension of yoga that would be systematized, empiricized, and popularized.

Yoga in the Lab: Swami Kuvalayananda

Swami Kuvalayananda (born Jagannatha Ganesa Gune, 1883–1966) provides us with perhaps the best example of the line increasingly drawn between the benefits of *āsana* and *prāṇāyāma*, which could be scientifically evaluated, and yoga's metaphysical claims. Coming from humble beginnings, Kuvalayananda attained a considerable level of education, which included not only a university degree, but also sustained training in Sikh martial arts and other physical culture, as well as yogic *sādhana* at the feet of a guru. In 1924, he founded the Kaivalyadhanam Ashram in Lonavla. One of the more unique features of the center was scientific laboratories where Kuvalayananda set out on a project investigating the empirical dimensions of yogic practices.[30]

Notably, Kuvalayananda's interest in yoga's scientific foundations seems to have been sparked by a set of unspecified but clearly spiritual—"quite abnormal," as Kuvalayananda described them—experiences which took hold of him when he was training with his guru, Paramahamsa Madhavadasaji of Malsar. As a result of these, "phenomena, physical and mental, that an average man is not able to induce, came slowly under his control."[31] Whether Kuvalayananda understood his experiences as related to Kuṇḍalinī is impossible to say, but it is intriguing that he would go on to frame the effects of yoga practice in these terms. We can, at the very least, say that Kuvalayananda's later gestures toward the spiritual dimensions of yoga were not founded on theory alone.

Whether despite this personal investment, or perhaps precisely because of it, Kuvalayananda worked hard to maintain the line between the scientifically supported nature of yoga's physical techniques, as framed by his research center, and their ends, which he regarded as ultimately spiritual. Intimately familiar with the trend of attempts to map scientifically grounded understandings of physiology and even physics onto yogic metaphysics and subtle anatomy, Kuvalayananda remained politely agnostic as to the ultimate accuracy of such positions.

In a lengthy footnote, appended to a discussion of the *nāḍīs* in a volume of his research center's journal, *Yoga Mīmānsa*, Kuvalayananda reviews the history of attempts to accord the subtle channels with modern anatomical features. Perhaps unsurprisingly, the most abstract iterations actually receive the lightest criticism. These are Bamandas Basu's article in *The Theosophist*, "The Anatomy of the Tantras" (1888), and a section of Brajendranath Seal's *The Positive Sciences of the Ancient Hindus* (1915), both of which identify the six *cakras* with nerve plexuses. Neither, notably, makes any claims with regards to the mechanisms of practice. On Rele's book, for which he provided the illustrations, Kuvalayananda is more ambivalent. "We heartily recommend the book to our readers' attention," he says, before immediately remarking that "we have serious doubts regarding the accuracy of many of his interpretations, and the whole book looks to be of doubtful scientific value."[32] Vivekananda receives the same treatment. Kuvalayananda heaps copious praise upon the "great master," while also making it clear that "the whole structure" of his work "is based upon the treacherous sands of speculation."[33] It's worth specifying that, in the course of all this, Kuvalayananda is also careful to distinguish between "the efficacy of these exercises," in which he professes "adamantine faith," and "the scientific interpretations of the Yogic practices and Yogic anatomy and physiology."[34]

This distinction can help us make sense of the way Kuvalayananda proceeds to compartmentalize his treatment of yoga. As we will see, it is implicitly clear that the "efficacy" of yogic exercises lies precisely in their ability to awaken Kuṇḍalinī. In the greater scheme of things, this is what the exercises are *for*. And yet, if we are to describe the practices from a scientific standpoint, such an interpretation remains always a bit out of reach. Kuvalayananda's clearest statement about Kuṇḍalinī is tucked away in yet another footnote: "According to Yogic teachings Kuṇḍalinī which represents spiritual energy is coiled up in the lower abdomen. The concentration being prescribed is calculated to wake up this Kuṇḍalinī. We have purposely avoided any modern anatomical terms here, simply because we cannot venture any speculative theory in connection with Kuṇḍalinī."[35]

It was common practice among Kuvalayananda's contemporaries to differentiate between dynamic, standing, and other complex postures as promoting the physical health of the body and seated poses as providing a foundation for meditation, with the implicit assumption that the latter represented the more complex level of practice. Kuvalayananda adopts this split, grouping *āsanas* as either "meditative poses" or "cultural poses." However, it's worth noting how his understanding of the cultural poses actually preserves some of the medieval logics that first proposed physical ascetic techniques as effective methods for the awakening of Kuṇḍalinī. "To put the whole thing in a nutshell," Kuvalayananda explains, "we can say that the cultural poses are practised for training the nervous and endocrine systems, whereas the meditative poses are undertaken to eliminate physiological disturbances from mental activity."[36]

The importance of the cultural poses is actually twofold. On the one hand, Kuvalayananda specifies that the brain and the spinal cord "are the most important parts of the nervous system, and the spiritual force of Kuṇḍalinī when awakened works through them."[37] Accordingly, the cultural poses prepare both organs to be able to sustain the interaction with Kuṇḍalinī. On the other hand, certain poses (again following the medieval logic) act on the physical body in ways that actually produce spiritual effects. Specifically, Kuvalayananda explains, "yogic processes practised for the awakening of Kuṇḍalinī are mainly characterized by two features. They either involve the stretching of the spine and its adjacent parts, or are capable of attracting a richer blood supply to the regions roundabout the spinal column, especially in the pelvic and lumbar regions."[38] Still, though such *āsanas* serve an important role, in the end they are subordinate to the effects of *prāṇāyāma*. It is "the high abdominal pressure created in Prāṇāyāma by the action and counteraction of the different anatomical parts together with the upward pull of the crura, [that] is responsible for the awakening of Kuṇḍalinī."[39] Meanwhile, "the aim of the meditative poses is to offer a comfortable posture for Prāṇāyāma, Pratyāhāra, Dhāraṇā etc., and in co-ordination with other Yogic exercises to help the student of Yoga in the awakening of Kuṇḍalinī."[40] What can we conclude from all this? Primarily two things. First, Kuvalayananda clearly views Kuṇḍalinī awakening as a crucial aspect if not the ultimate goal of yoga practice. Second, despite the nod to Patañjali's rubric, the meditative aspects of the eight-limb system are secondary in effect to the physical ones in achieving this end.

This is not to say that Kuvalayananda's understanding of yoga is purely physical and lacks a contemplative dimension. However, this is where his language becomes increasingly vague, as he is unable to moor it in the empirical framework of physiology. Early volumes of his *Yoga-Mīmānsa* journal are packed with tables upon tables of experimental data detailing the effects of *āsana* and *prāṇāyāma*. However, such scientifically demonstrable virtues of yogic practice inevitably stop short of empirically illustrating more transcendent forms of self-realization. Though Kuvalayananda is convinced of the spiritual effects of practices like breathwork—he tells us as much—his explanations of the mechanics stop at speculative references to the potential of nerve stimulation and the newly discovered hormonal fluctuations of the endocrine system to induce psychological changes. The bridge from science to experience remains somewhat shrouded. "Again we are hypothetically satisfied," Kuvalayananda declares, "that the practice of Prāṇāyāma introduces high pressure both in the central canal of the spinal cord and the ventricles of the brain. These pressures centrally stimulate the whole nervous system. Owing to these central and peripheral stimuli, the human consciousness begins to be internalized and supersensuous perceptions begin to be possible. Worlds subtler and still subtler begin to be opened out in proportion to the consciousness itself getting more and more refined, till at last the individual consciousness merges into the cosmic and the individual becomes one with the Infinite."[41] And yet, he never quite explains *how*.

Updating the Medieval Synthesis: Swami Sivananda

This split approach is mirrored by Kuvalayananda's contemporary Swami Sivananda Saraswati (1887–1963). Born in Tamil Nadu as Kuppuswami Iyer, Sivananda left a long and successful career as a medical doctor to start his Divine Life Society in 1936. He ultimately authored over two hundred books on yoga and related subjects, most of which the organization still distributes. His *Kundalini Yoga* (1935) long persisted as the standout practical resource on the eponymous practice.

Sivananda's widely distributed publications, like his *Yogic Home Exercises* (1939), subtitled "Easy Course of Physical Culture for Modern Men and Women," contain only passing references to metaphysical concerns. This is despite the fact that the aforementioned manual incorporates the full range of *bandhas* and *mudrās* that might have traditionally been employed toward Kuṇḍalinī-related ends. For instance, in his description of the "Yoga Mudra," Sivananda states obliquely that it "is very useful for rousing the Kundalini Shakti," before immediately moving on to specify that "this pose removes all kinds of disorders of the abdominal viscera."[42]

These sorts of passing references are not uncommon in twentieth-century literature on postural yoga and, as we will see shortly, not a reliable indication of any deep interest in Kuṇḍalinī. More often than not, they amount only to a kind of lip service to received tradition. But this is not the case with Sivananda, as picking up his *Kundalini Yoga* makes immediately clear. Here we find, clearly articulated, the unspoken assumption behind his other popular practice manuals and the public-facing message of the Divine Life Society: Kuṇḍalinī awakening is essential to Sivananda's whole system. "No superconscious state or Samadhi is possible," says Sivananda, "without awakening this primordial energy, whether it is Raja Yoga, Bhakti Yoga, Hatha Yoga or Jnana Yoga."[43] The latter part of that sentence is crucial, though certainly not unprecedented, given positions such as the one already put forth by Vivekananda. The vast terrain of yoga practice is traversed by so many roads, all leading to the same goal. Sivananda elaborates, "Kundalini can be awakened by Pranayama, Asanas and Mudras by Hatha Yogis; by concentration and training of the mind by Raja Yogis; by devotion and perfect self-surrender by Bhaktas; by analytical will by the Jnanis; by Mantras by the Tantrikas; and by the grace of the Guru (Guru Kripa) through touch, sight or mere Sankalpa."[44] Any of these methods may be sufficient in itself but, for most students, a combination of methods will prove necessary if the ultimate goal is to be attained. Such a personal cocktail of methods should be prescribed by the guru, like medicine by a doctor. This is the logic behind the Divine Life Society's "Yoga of Synthesis." It also explains why Sivananda might have felt comfortable casually offering instructions for Kuṇḍalinī-related practices. In his view, it was highly unlikely that performing a couple of *mudrās* would blast the modern man or woman into full-on Kuṇḍalinī awakening.

Sidelining an Obstruction: The Lineage of Tirumalai Krishnamacharya

Of course, there is no denying the multiplicity and diversity of yoga, regardless of the specific historical moment. Kuvalayananda and Sivananda represent two prominent examples of modern yogis whose early foregrounding of physical practices that could be easily interpreted through the lenses of bioscience and medicine was layered over deep assumptions about the centrality of Kuṇḍalinī, but this should not be taken as a universal trend. In fact, the relative invisibility of Kuṇḍalinī in today's postural yoga practice can at least partly be attributed to the ambivalence of another man of the very same generation, Tirumalai Krishnamacharya (1888–1989), a position mirrored by his globally renowned students.

Krishnamacharya developed the most influential iteration of his postural yoga (and taught it to his most prominent students) during his tenure as a chief preceptor of the physical culture program at the Jaganmohan Palace at Mysore.[45] The sources of Krishnamacharya's physical practice are complex and eclectic. But we know that, mystically, he claimed inspiration from the Āḻvār poet saints of the South Indian Śrī Vaiṣṇava tradition, the very tradition into which he was born and the one that colored his upbringing.[46] Simon Atkinson has shown that Krishnamacharya's position on Kuṇḍalinī was complex and not always consistent, but it can—with considerable effort—be squared with the Vaiṣṇava sources on which he and his native tradition would have drawn.[47] Here it is helpful to recall that Vaiṣṇava tantric and *haṭha* yogic texts, some of which we reviewed in chapter 1, tended to treat Kuṇḍalinī (if at all) as a blockage that must be overcome or removed. Of course, such a position would still afford a great measure of importance to Kuṇḍalinī (and thus to Kuṇḍalinī experience) as the blockage must be undone—often burned through—if yogic progress is to be made. Some elements of this view appear to have made it into Krishnamacharya's position, at least as extrapolated by his son and most faithful disciple T. K. V. Desikachar (1938–2016).[48] But a more straightforward position, and one more representative of his legacy, comes from an interview given around a half-decade before his death. "Kundalini is very simply physical," Krishnamacharya curtly states. "If a person controls a nadi, he controls Kundalini. This is not important. Kundalini yoga is not a yoga at all."[49]

Elizabeth De Michelis has made similar arguments concerning B. K. S. Iyengar (1918–2014), one of those famous students of Krishnamacharya. Iyengar, like his guru, was born into a highly respected family of Śrī Vaiṣṇava Brahmins in Karnataka. He likewise evoked Nāthamuni as a spiritual ancestor, and considered himself a Vedāntin, following the qualified nondual theism of the twelfth-century Śrī Vaiṣṇava philosopher Rāmānuja.[50] As De Michelis has argued, Iyengar's framing of *āsana* practice makes sense if examined in light of Rāmānuja's ultimately devotional approach to yoga,[51] an assertion that can be extended to Krishnamacharya as well as Krishnamacharya's other renowned student K. Pattabhi Jois (1915–2009).

However, Iyengar's position on Kuṇḍalinī does not seem to have come from Krishnamacharya—a notion that seems less surprising when one considers that their formal guru-disciple relationship lasted less than two years. Iyengar struck out on his own in 1937, but it was the popularity of his now-classic practice manual *Light on Yoga* (1966) that truly cemented his status as a global guru. And, in 1966, Iyengar's position on Kuṇḍalinī manifests in the same oblique references we saw in Sivananda's postural manual. Iyengar briefly mentions Kuṇḍalinī awakening as an effect of *padmāsana*, as described in the *Haṭha Pradīpikā*, but on this topic Iyengar advises the reader to consult Arthur Avalon's *The Serpent Power* and says no more.[52] Another such reference, again quoting from the *Haṭha*

Pradīpikā, appears in the section on *matsyendrāsana*.[53] We find the fullest treatment of Kuṇḍalinī in a short section on *prāṇāyāma* under the subheader "Bandhas, Nāḍis, and Chakras," which offers a very basic overview of these three concepts before concluding by speculating that Kuṇḍalinī is "perhaps an allegorical way of describing the tremendous vitality, especially sexual, which is obtained by the practice of Uḍḍīyāna and Mūla Bandhas described above. The arousing of Kuṇḍalinī and forcing it up is perhaps a symbolic way of describing the sublimation of sexual energy."[54]

That last reference is also our clearest hint that Iyengar's vagueness on Kuṇḍalinī is of a different brand than Sivananda's or Kuvalayananda's. It's not that Iyengar is bracketing off more specialized or deeper levels of practice; it's that he simply does not have much to say on the matter. In his *Light on Pranayama* (1981), where Iyengar is necessarily required to pay more attention to such *haṭha*-yogic aspects of breathwork, he is forced to refine his position a bit. But this does not lead to an integration of Kuṇḍalinī into his framework. Quite the opposite, he takes the stance that Kuṇḍalinī techniques are at best misguided and at worst dangerous. "Many people misconceive that bhastrikā prāṇāyāma awakens the kuṇḍalinī śakti," Iyengar notes. "The authoritative books have said the same regarding many Prāṇāyāmas and āsanas, but this is far from true. There is no doubt that bhastrikā and kapālabhāti refresh the brain and stir it to activity, but if people perform them because they believe that they awaken the kuṇḍalinī, disaster to body, nerves, and brain may result."[55]

This view reaches its full elaboration in Iyengar's *Light on the Yoga Sūtras of Patañjali* (1993). Here, Iyengar's position on Kuṇḍalinī gains both depth and coherence, and one particular passage is worth quoting at length. In a commentary on verse 3.6, dealing with *saṃyama* or the integrated application of Patañjali's meditative limbs (*dhāraṇa*, *dhyāna*, and *samādhi*), Iyengar states:

> There are many examples, even in modern literature, of people quite unexpectedly experiencing *saṁyama* even if they have been following no fixed path of yogic discipline. The Japanese refer to this sudden lifting of the curtain of ignorance as a "flash". This is undoubtedly a moment of grace, but it is not the same thing as enlightenment. . . . The modern fancy of "*kuṇḍalini* awakening" has probably arisen through these freakish experiences of "integration". Patañjali does not mention *kuṇḍalini* but speaks of the energy of nature flowing abundantly in a yogi (IV.2). *Kuṇḍalini* is a neologism. This energy of nature (*prakṛti shakti*) was originally known as *agni* or fire. Later yogis called this fire *kuṇḍalini* (the coiled one) as its conduit in the body is coiled 3 ½ times at the base of the spine. It is, however, clear that many who undergo an overwhelming experience of fusion with the universal consciousness reap, through their unpreparedness, more pain than benefit. To the lucky, healthy few such an experience can serve as a spur to begin a true spiritual search, but to many others it can bring severe physical and psychological disorders.[56]

Of course, the idea that Kuṇḍalinī is a new name for a somewhat older set of concepts (among them the idea of *agni* or fire, both in the natural bodily sense and as the cultivated fire of *tapas* or asceticism) is precisely the argument we made in chapter 1. And, in a sense, Iyengar's position on the nature of that fire is legitimately closer to the one common to Patañjali's own dualistic and asceticism-inflected context.

Is the consuming fire of nature something that must be overcome, or is it the channel for that very overcoming? Is nature the *other* thing (not us) that keeps us trapped? Or is it ultimately an aspect of us—just another refraction of the ultimate self? Does the Goddess deceive (being *māyā*), or does She liberate? We saw this tension in the medieval tantric literature where Kuṇḍalinī first appears, and we saw it in the Theosophical sources where the idea slips into modern global awareness.

It's also no coincidence that Iyengar articulates this ambivalent position in a commentary on Patañjali. Atkinson and De Michelis have both pointed to the prominence of Patañjali's framework (albeit with that devotional re-imagining of the later limbs) within Krishnamacharya's and Iyengar's systems, respectively. Jois went so far as to name his trademark system, Ashtanga Yoga, after the same rubric. Yet, despite the clear connection among the three men, the similarities of their positions are likely as much products of a general shared culture as a specific lineage. All three are Karnataka Brahmins, embedded in the Śri Vaiṣṇava tradition, and therefore in Rāmānuja's devotional brand of qualified nondual Vedānta. And, while all this would have also made them heirs to the tantric legacy of Pāñcarātra, such a framework would have looked very different than, say, the Śākta-flavored yogas of Bengal (to which we will turn in a moment).

For the time being, we might say that Kuṇḍalinī's disappearance from the landscape of modern postural yoga is perhaps less due to the serpent's inability to survive in a body-centric paradigm and more due to the disinterest of modern Indian yoga's most visible gurus. Western styles tend to draw on harmonial assumptions of tuning the strings that connect body, mind, and spirit. There, despite the efforts of all those Theosophists we met in chapter 3, we are more likely to find opened or, better yet, balanced *cakras* through which nothing needs to rise. The glaring exception to Kuṇḍalinī invisibility in this context is Yogi Bhajan's "Kundalini Yoga"—but this is a different, equally complex story, and one to which we will turn in chapter 6.

Yet it's also worth noting that, even in Krishnamacharya's and Iyengar's rather indifferent take on Kuṇḍalinī, the *experience* is still fire.

THE EVOLVING SERPENT OF METAPHYSICAL YOGA

And so, even when Kuṇḍalinī slips below the surface, Her presence often remains at the core of modern understandings of yoga. This is especially striking in those modern styles of yoga that, instead of expanding and foregrounding (and therefore modernizing) *āsana*, rather focus their innovations on what lies on the other side of *prāṇāyāma*—not the physical, but the metaphysical. Here, too, we see an emphasis on integrating traditional yogic frameworks with modern scientific theory. And the theory in question is usually evolution.

This trend, too, arguably starts with Vivekananda, though we would be remiss in not pointing to the spiritual evolution of the Theosophists as an important precedent. As he winds to the end of his commentary on the *Yoga Sūtras*, Vivekananda makes a rather interesting decision to translate a verse about transmigration as a verse about the change of one species into another. Something that might have traditionally been translated as "the changes [in bodily forms that take place] in other births" (*jātyantarapariṇāmaḥ*) becomes instead "the change into another species."[57] This, then, leads Vivekananda to get even more creative with the succeeding verse, where he renders a differentiation between the instrumental causes of *karma* and the fundamental causal nature of *prakṛti* (primordial matter) as a statement on ethics and biological evolution.[58] The translation is certainly novel—and not particularly supported by the commentarial tradition—but Vivekananda's resulting interpretation is nevertheless both interesting and influential. Vivekananda explains:

> Today the evolution theory of the ancient Yogis will be better understood in the light of modern research. And yet the theory

> of the Yogis is a better explanation. The two causes of evolution advanced by the moderns, viz., sexual selection and survival of the fittest, are inadequate. . . . The result of this theory is to furnish every oppressor with an argument to calm the qualms of conscience. Men are not lacking, who, posing as philosophers, want to kill out all wicked and incompetent persons, (they are, of course, the only judges of competency), and thus preserve the human race! But the great ancient evolutionist, Patanjali, declares that the true secret of evolution is the manifestation of the perfection which is already in every being; that this perfection has been barred, and the infinite tide behind is struggling to express itself. These struggles and competitions are but the results of our ignorance, because we do not know the proper way to unlock the gate and let the water in. This infinite tide behind must express itself; it is the cause of all manifestation.[59]

Leaving aside the ethical dimension, what we see here is a fairly standard model of progressive teleological evolution, not unlike the theories that preceded—and, for quite some time, competed with—Darwin's model of natural selection. The basic gist, of course, is that the evolutionary tree is not a map of the survival of the fittest, working itself out against the backdrop of random mutations. Instead, it is a story of progress toward increasingly advanced, more perfect forms of life, all the way up to—if we add a spiritual dimension—possible divinity.

Vivekananda himself does not make the explicit link to Kuṇḍalinī. But, given that he has already stated that Kuṇḍalinī awakening is the only path to perfection, the implications are clear. Kuṇḍalinī thus becomes the energizing principle of evolution. As such, She is perhaps less a thing and more a process—a metaphysical mechanism but also an experiential marker of the natural impulse toward perfection suffused into nature and accessible through yoga practice.

Reading Between the Lines of Paramahansa Yogananda

Born into a Bengali family as Mukundalal Ghosh in Gorakhpur, in the modern-day state of Uttar Pradesh, Paramahansa Yogananda (1893–1952) would spend much of his later childhood in Calcutta. The son of a prominent official of the Bengal-Nagpur Railway, Yogananda received a full education (despite his relative indifference to academic pursuits), culminating in a degree from the Scottish Church College of Calcutta. At the age of thirteen, he was initiated by his father into the *sādhana* of Kriya Yoga, the same lineage of practice to which his eventual guru, Swami Sri Yukteswar Giri, belonged.

Yogananda's Kriya Yoga is based on oral tradition, passed down through initiation from guru to disciple. The details of the practices involved, to say nothing of their interpretation, vary from one report to another even among today's teachers. And yet, though it is nearly impossible to map the system onto a specific textual source or tradition, the consistent core structure of the practice and its general correspondence with premodern systems of tantric *haṭha* yoga suggest that we are not dealing with a wholly novel modern synthesis. More than this, the system betrays clear Kaula undertones. Thus we have good reason to imagine that, despite the novel ways Yogananda portrays Kuṇḍalinī in his public work, a traditional framework of Kuṇḍalinī awakening was embedded in his lineage. In fact, it's the nature and structure of this practice that seems to tether Yogananda's otherwise eclectic forays into Neo-Vedānta, Christianity, and modern science.

Like the wider system of Kriya Yoga, it is somewhat difficult to reconstruct Yogananda's own spiritual convictions. Certainly, his exaltations of Jesus Christ should not be taken as insincere, a mere attempt to pander to his Christian audience. Yogananda's engagement with Christianity is both creative and profound, and it spans the entirety of his work. However, as much as his American writings (and his instructions to his disciples) consistently evoke a masculine God, it nevertheless seems significant that the earliest childhood moments of communion with the divine, as described in his *Autobiography of a Yogi* (1946), instead evoke the Divine Mother. Here we find the same maternal Kālī that held the devotion of Vivekananda's guru, Ramakrishna Paramahansa.

It's worth noting that Yogananda had a keen sense of Vivekananda's shadow. Born in the same year that Vivekananda embarked on his famous journey to the West, Yogananda would eventually find himself compelled to adopt the same trajectory. In his teenage years, Yogananda regularly frequented the Kālī temple in Dakshineswar and especially liked to meditate in Ramakrishna's favorite spots on the grounds. A book of advice attributed to the old mystic had a permanent place in his pocket.[60] This affinity, however, was also marked by a streak of ambition. One day, standing on the bank of the Ganga at Dakshineswar, across from the headquarters of the International Ramakrishna Mission and Math, the young Yogananda firmly declared: "I will make mine bigger than theirs."[61] Arguably, Yogananda succeeded. Today, his Self-Realization Fellowship (SRF) has over five hundred locations around the world, while the Ramakrishna Mission's number in the two hundreds.

As we will see, there is much in Yogananda's adoption of a modern scientific universalism that follows in the footsteps of his predecessor. But, in the end, Yogananda was not Vivekananda. Vivekananda led with philosophy, while Yogananda wove poetry. Vivekananda saw himself as a champion of India, while Yogananda spent most of his life in the West. Certainly, Yogananda held much more genuine affection for Christianity than Vivekananda ever betrayed. However, of the two, Yogananda was also far more firmly grounded in a traditional Indian lineage of yogic *sādhana*. And, though he was criticized by members of that lineage for going too far in adapting the practices for his Western students, the Kriya Yoga still taught by the SRF appears remarkably faithful to tradition.

In its outward form, Kriya Yoga is classical *haṭha* yoga. *Prāṇāyāma*, or breathwork, is a core feature of the practice and the individual *kriyās* (exercises) preserve a number of standard *bandhas* and *mudrās*.[62] However, reflecting that same model of the tantra-*haṭha* synthesis we find in the medieval literature, the core of the practice follows a deeper Kaula tantric logic. The *kriyās* culminate in the practitioner using *prāṇāyāma* techniques to break through the *mūlādhāra granthi* (root knot) and release Kuṇḍalinī.[63] The use of seed mantras and the focus on cultivating and perceiving the divine sounds (*nāda*) within the subtle body likewise hint at the precise kind of tantric scaffolding that we saw in the Kuṇḍalinī- (or Caṇḍalī-) centric Śaiva and Buddhist *laya* yoga (yoga of dissolution) schools we reviewed in chapter 1.

Yogananda's own language is inescapably eclectic. At first glance, we find Nature first and foremost as the illusory *māyā* of Advaita Vedānta (not the creative *śakti* of tantra). The serpent in the body is as much the deceiver of Eve—an event that Yogananda reads metaphorically to point to the conquest of feminine feeling over masculine reason—as it is the "life force"—suggestively like Kuṇḍalinī as the *prāṇakuṇḍalinī* envisioned by the nondual Kaula philosopher Abhinavagupta.[64] But when Yogananda, in his written instructions as they were mailed to his students, extols that we must draw this life current into the brain to rejoin God just as "Moses lifted up the serpent in the wilderness,"[65] it is perhaps not the Christian meaning that we should take as primary.

And so, if one digs beneath the words and considers how Yogananda actually uses them, as well as the full picture they form, both the Vedāntic and the Christian meanings succumb to something significantly more tantric. The world may be a manifestation of "Lady

Cosmic Dream" (Yogananda's colorful name for *māyā*), but it's also fundamentally real insofar as it's made up of divine effulgent light. Yogananda appeals to Einstein here, but one can't help but recall the nondual tantric notion of *prakāśa*, the undifferentiated luminous consciousness (identified with Śiva) that finds its reflection in the effervescent self-awareness of *vimarśa* (identified with Śakti), pulsing with creative vibration (*spanda*). Indeed, it is only in this light that we can make full sense of Yogananda's model of Kuṇḍalinī awakening:

> When the yogi withdraws the life force from material objects, sensory organs, and sensory-motor nerves and takes the concentrated life upward through the spiral passageway of *kundalini* (coiled energy) in the coccyx, he perceives, as he ascends, the various spinal centers with their petaled light-rays and sounds of life energy. When the yogi's consciousness reaches the medulla and the spiritual eye at the point between the eyebrows, he finds the doorway into the star-lotus of "a thousand" (innumerable) rays. He perceives the omnipresent light of God spreading over the sphere of eternity, and his body as a minuscule emanation of this light.
>
> In deepest ecstasy, the yogi perceives the cosmic light change into the vibrationless, ever-existing, ever-conscious, ever-new bliss of Spirit. It is this vibrationless Cosmic Consciousness that has become the one vibrating cosmic light. This light, projecting away from God, becomes shadowed with delusion, producing the cosmic motion picture of dream images, including the body of man.[66]

And yet, though the spiritual (and therefore metaphysical) dimensions of such a description can hardly be ignored, Yogananda is also very much talking about physics when he declares that "the essence of creation is light."[67] Because Yogananda's worldview is ultimately a nondual one, the scientific and the spiritual must be intimately entangled. Thus, spiritual perfection is a natural extension of biological evolution.

Quoting his guru, Sri Yukteswar, Yogananda declares, "*Kriya Yoga* is an instrument through which human evolution can be quickened." Specifically, he explains, "the *Kriya Yogi* mentally directs his life energy to revolve, upward and downward, around the six spinal centers (medullary, cervical, dorsal, lumbar, sacral, and coccygeal plexuses) which correspond to the twelve astral signs of the zodiac, the symbolic Cosmic Man. One-half minute of revolution of energy around the sensitive spinal cord of man effects subtle progress in his evolution; that half-minute of *Kriya* equals one year of natural spiritual unfoldment."[68] This same logic of microcosmic acceleration of cosmic rhythms within the body also shows up in the accounts of other teachers belonging to Yogananda's lineage,[69] indicating that there is something of a traditional framework at play here. Notably, though, they tend to frame this process in terms of purification of the *nāḍīs* rather than evolution, and the cosmic analogy is not the Zodiac but the lunar-solar cycle. This, of course, mirrors a *haṭha*-yogic framing of the *nāḍīs*, as well as older and more general Upaniṣadic understandings of the lifecycle, as we reviewed them in chapter 1. But the acceleration argument is actually a bit more complicated—after all, there's nothing in this framework that says time itself is enough to purify or otherwise perfect the yogi. The point of enacting this accelerated version of the temporal cycle is actually to burn through the cosmic cycle itself. According to traditional (specifically Purāṇic) Indian cosmology, we are currently in the final and darkest of the cyclical set of four ages of the cosmos, the Kali Yuga. By winding forward his internal clock, so to speak, the yogi is able to access spiritual virtues that only manifest in the other, superior *yugas*.

Yogananda, meanwhile, reinterprets this idea to accord with more literal models of biological evolution, albeit distinctly progressive ones. Thus, on the one hand, the ascent to spiritual perfection is the natural destiny of all beings, a kind of progressive model of biological-cum-spiritual evolution. In this sense, Yogananda departs from traditional understandings of spiritual perfection (*siddhi*) and liberation (*mokṣa*) as something that requires effort, whether in the form of practice or some other intervention. From this perspective, "the Science of Kriya Yoga," as Yogananda calls it, is not so much a reagent as it is a catalyst or simply an accelerant. That is, the practice is not a necessary condition without which this process of spiritual evolution would be impossible. Rather, it serves to significantly accelerate an already ongoing natural process. On the other hand, however, Kriya practice is also a bit like genetic engineering. Yogananda frames this idea in an analogy to the cultivation of plants, relying on the work of scientists like the Indian physicist-turned-botanist Jagadis Chandra Bose and the American botanist and horticulturalist Luther Burbank. In this sense, skillful manipulation can yield superior results, compared to natural processes alone.

And, although Yogananda's vision regarding the trajectory of this evolution extends well beyond the parameters of biology, it certainly features a physical dimension. Yogananda's framework allows for more "evolved" physical bodies, such as those belonging to self-realized human yogis whose bodies may show signs of incorruptibility or other perfections and who exhibit superhuman abilities in accordance with their degree of accomplishment. There are also, however, beings who inhabit "astral" bodies composed of something like *prāṇa* or, as Yogananda translates it, "lifetrons." These include "resurrected" bodies, which Yogananda treats as perfected forms willfully reconstituted from subtle elements. Such bodies may appear as gross matter but actually exist on a different sort of wavelength, if you will. Still higher are causal-bodied beings that exist beyond the "finer-than-atomic energies" of lifetrons in "the minutest particles of God-thought."[70] These bodies reflect the progressive stages of human physical and spiritual evolution. At the pinnacle of all this, we find beings that are somewhat a conflation of traditional concepts of *siddha* and *avatāra* (that is, ascended humans and descended gods)—completely free and therefore one with the cosmic ocean of light but choosing at times to manifest themselves and become embodied for a specific purpose. Babaji, the immortal mountain-dwelling sage who serves as the chief preceptor of the Kriya Yoga lineage, is precisely one such being.

So, where does Kuṇḍalinī fit into all of this? Because Yogananda does not use this term in describing the ladder to spiritual evolution, we are forced to be a bit speculative (or at least to read between the lines and make use of the transitive property, as we have been doing). Kriya Yoga is, at least in part, Kuṇḍalinī yoga. Kriya Yoga is also the method by which one races up the evolutionary ladder of perfection. How far up the ladder Kuṇḍalinī takes us depends on how we choose to interpret Yogananda's language. The most conservative understanding of his naming Kuṇḍalinī as the "life force" keeps things on the level of the physical body. Awakening Kuṇḍalinī is the physical key to accessing the astral body of lifetrons. But, of course, what is a "life force," if not "lifetrons?" And so, a more generous reading might see Yogananda's Kuṇḍalinī as the energy that comprises subtle reality itself. Would he have taken things higher still? Well, Yogananda always did love the Divine Mother.

Reimagining Tradition in Aurobindo Ghose

As much as Yogananda may have modeled his life and mission in the image of Vivekananda, Aurobindo Ghose (1872–1950) was arguably a man much more after Vivekananda's heart. Like the latter,

Aurobindo was an intellectual and a nationalist, and he harbored a distaste for the trappings of organized religion.

In fact, by his own account, Aurobindo had no interest in spiritual pursuits until he was roughly thirty-two. In 1904, he began a yogic practice. This he did without the aid of a guru, in a way that was "personal and apart." In 1908, he received some help from an unnamed "Maharatta yogi," which helped him firm up the foundations of his *sādhana*. Generally, however, Aurobindo resisted the notion that his eventual system was shaped by any external influence. He narrates:

My sadhana was not founded upon books but upon personal experiences that crowded on me from within. But in the jail I had the Gita and the Upanishads with me, practised the yoga of the Gita and meditated with the help of the Upanishads; these were the only books from which I found guidance; the Veda which I first began to read long afterward in Pondicherry rather confirmed what experiences I already had than was any guide to my sadhana. . . . It is a fact that I was hearing constantly the voice of Vivekananda speaking to me for a fortnight in the jail in my solitary meditation and felt his presence . . . The voice spoke only on a special and limited but very important field of spiritual experience and it ceased as soon as it had finished saying all that it had to say on that subject.[71]

And yet, despite the fact that his system was not founded upon books, Aurobindo seemed to have read a fair number of them. He would come to describe his yoga as embracing the truths of Veda and Vedānta, which he saw as prioritizing knowledge and the purity of divine consciousness, but also those of tantra, which he understood as the creative power of *śakti*. Yet it was important for him to assert that "our sadhana does not cleave to the knowledge given in the books, but only keeps to the central truth behind and realises it independently without any subjection to the old forms and symbols."[72] The truth of Aurobindo's statement is perhaps most fully reflected in the uniqueness of his practice. When he speaks of how the world is put together, one can certainly discern—as he himself admitted—strands of both Vedānta and tantra in that vision. But the *how* of it all was indeed a novel synthesis, and one deeply embedded in the complex layers and winding path of Aurobindo's own experience.

The system now called Integral Yoga does not prescribe an easily delineated and structured practice. In fact, as Ann Gleig and Charles Flores have suggested in their study of Aurobindo's influence on the modern yoga scene, it's possible that Aurobindo's system has failed to gain a broad global audience specifically because it was presented "not as a method but rather as a profound and challenging process of self-surrender and aspiration for the divine that was to be cultivated over a long period of time."[73] Aurobindo organized his approach into what he called the "Sapta Chatusthaya," or the seven tetrads. This system was a complex interplay of principles, incorporating domains ranging from perfections of the physical body to ways of engaging with the abstract principles of *brahman*. The unique complexity of the system derives from the fact that one could not simply progress linearly, moving on to the next tetrad after having perfected the previous. Instead, Aurobindo's *sādhana* involves a continuous process of return and reengagement between the levels of tetrads.[74]

And so, it is in this context that we need to place Aurobindo's understanding of Kuṇḍalinī. True to his position, Aurobindo accepts the "central truths" behind tantric models of Kuṇḍalinī, but not the specific practices. "The process of the Kundalini awakened rising through the centres as also the purification of the centres is a Tantrik knowledge," says Aurobindo. "In our Yoga there is no willed process of the purification and opening of the centres, no raising up of the Kundalini by a set process either. Another method is used, but still there is the ascent of the consciousness from and through the different levels to join the higher consciousness above; there is the opening of the centres and of the planes (mental, vital, physical) which these centres command; there is also the descent which is the main key of the spiritual transformation. Therefore there is, I have said, a Tantrik knowledge behind the process of transformation in this Yoga."[75] Because Aurobindo's method does not rely on that willed and systematic raising of Kuṇḍalinī through the progression of *cakras*, the experience of it is not easily pinned down. Kuṇḍalinī can be felt as a serpentine movement, coiling and pulsing, but it can also rise like a wave of ascending consciousness. It can be felt along the spine, in the centers of the *cakras*, or simply throughout the body in general.[76]

Notably, it's not that Aurobindo thinks the tantric method does not work; it's simply that this is not *his* method. One can systematically purify and open one's *cakras* and will Kuṇḍalinī to rise. In Aurobindo's method, however, this ascent happens spontaneously as a kind of emergent property of other processes. Kuṇḍalinī ascends, and then—more importantly—She *descends*. There is no willed opening of the *cakras* for Aurobindo because "they open of themselves by the descent of the Force,"[77] blossoming in reverse order.

It is this downward movement that Aurobindo views as unique to his system. At the very least, he claims, such a descent is not felt in "ordinary Yoga," presumably of the type recorded in the textual tradition. "Some may have had these things," Aurobindo allows, "but I don't know that they understood their nature, principle or place in a complete sadhana. At least I never heard of these things from others before I found them out in my own experience. The reason is that the old Yogins when they went above the spiritual mind passed into samadhi, which means that they did not attempt to be conscious in these higher planes—their aim being to pass away into the Superconscient and not to bring the Superconscient into the waking consciousness, which is that of my Yoga."[78]

Aurobindo uses the typically Vedāntic language of *brahman* to articulate something much more like a tantric cosmology. The infinite consciousness of *brahman* descends—or really "involves"—into matter, not because of ignorance or some other flaw, but "to trace the cycle of self-oblivion and self-discovery for the joy of which the Ignorance is assumed in Nature."[79] As in Yogananda's case, Aurobindo's reliance on the traditionally negative language of *māyā* (illusion) ultimately covers over a world-affirming vision. There is, certainly, an inferior type of illusion to our material world, which brings us no end but suffering. These are the illusory limitations of our mortal bodies and minds. But the true nature of *māyā* is the "Supermind," or the "power of infinite consciousness to comprehend, contain in itself and measure out, that is to say, to form—for form is delimitation—Name and Shape out of the vast illimitable Truth of infinite existence."[80]

Aurobindo's thinking also fuses traditional ideas of spiritual perfection with a modern understanding of biological evolution. He links the self's transmigration, conceived as a kind of karmic ladder to a human birth, to the historical development of increasingly complex species. But "evolution," he argues, "in its essence is not the development of a more and more organised body or a more and more efficient life—these are only its machinery and outward circumstance. Evolution is the strife of a Consciousness somnambulised in Matter to wake and be free and find and possess itself and all its possibilities to the very utmost and widest, to the very last and highest."[81] Man represents the highest reaches of natural physical evolution, evidenced by the fact that no more advanced species have emerged to walk the earth. However, in the grand scope of evolution, "man is a transitional being, he is not final; for in him and high beyond him ascend the radiant degrees which climb to a divine supermanhood. The step from man toward superman is the next approaching achievement in the earth's evolution. There lies our destiny and the liberating key to our aspiring, but troubled and limited human existence—inevitable because it is at once the intention of the inner Spirit and the logic of Nature's process."[82]

Thus, this next evolutionary step is as much spiritual as it is physical—though, it's important to note that it is that as well. Where Aurobindo's vision differs from certain traditional models, especially ascetic or Vedāntic ideals of spiritual liberation, is in his insistence on the experiential and therefore subjective dimensions of the "Supermind." Essentially, *brahman* involves itself in and into matter, so that it can evolve. Natural (that is, biological) evolution is part and parcel of this process, but a less advanced part because it happens unconsciously. It is only with the advent of the human mind that "evolution has now become conscious."[83] But, for Aurobindo, this conscious evolution results not in a return to the singularity of infinite and impersonal *brahman*, but in "divine supermanhood."

Thus, the ascent of Kuṇḍalinī becomes the unfoldment of this superhumanity. But as Aurobindo clarifies, again and again,

> in our Yoga it is not a specialised process, but a spontaneous uprush of the whole lower consciousness sometimes in currents or waves, sometimes in a less concrete motion, and on the other side a descent of the Divine Consciousness and its Force into the body. This descent is felt as a pouring in of calm and peace, of force and power, of light, of joy and ecstasy, of wideness and freedom and knowledge, of a Divine Being or a Presence—sometimes one of these, sometimes several of them or all together.[84]

And Aurobindo spends quite a bit of time dwelling on the nature of this descended divinity—the awakened Kuṇḍalinī—only She is not called by that name. She is "Divine Nature." She is "Divine Shakti." And, above all, she is "the Mother."

In the end, Aurobindo's vision is perhaps not quite as original as he had liked to imagine. Certainly, there are precedents in the medieval tantra and *haṭha* literature for the descent of Kuṇḍalinī, or at least of the flood of immortal nectar (*aṃrta*) that She releases into the practitioner's now-perfected body from the abode of Śiva in the cranial vault. And what is the ideal of *jīvanmukti* (embodied liberation) if not precisely the kind of enlightened waking consciousness that Aurobindo describes? Here it might help to remember Babaji. Of course, Aurobindo and Yogananda would agree on at least one thing—achieving such a state is a matter of evolution.

Tucked away amid the passages on the general topic of "Tantra" collected from Aurobindo's letters, there is an interesting fragment. Written in the third person—penned by Aurobindo's secretary, a footnote informs us—it offers regrets that Aurobindo as guru is not able to offer guidance to the unnamed enquirer. It is a lengthy letter, offering both reasoned explanation and some words of comfort, for the enquirer had written to Aurobindo in the midst of a most troubling experience. But this experience of Kuṇḍalinī, which made the writer fear for his very life, was not in accord with the path taught by Aurobindo, and Aurobindo could not guide a disciple along a path that he had not himself walked.[85]

The plea, as we will see, came from Gopi Krishna. And so, we know that Aurobindo was right. Gopi Krishna's Kuṇḍalinī experience was neither the willful raising of divine energy taught in the Tantras (and carried on by modern teachers like Yogananda) nor the spontaneous wave described by Aurobindo. And yet it was Gopi Krishna, more so than any of his predecessors, who would canonize in the public imagination Kuṇḍalinī as "the evolutionary energy in man."

5

WHEN THE SERPENT RISES

What Happened to Gopi Krishna?

I was not aware of the moment
when I first crossed the threshold of this life.

What was the power that made me open out into this vast mystery
like a bud in the forest at midnight!

When in the morning I looked upon the light
I felt in a moment that I was no stranger in this world,
that the inscrutable without name and form
had taken me in its arms in the form of my own mother.

Even so, in death the same unknown will appear as ever known to me.
And because I love this life,
I know I shall love death as well.

The child cries out
when from the right breast the mother takes it away,
in the very next moment to find in the left one its consolation.

—RABINDRANATH TAGORE, "THRESHOLD"

There is a guy in the bazaar, who writes poetry in languages he never knew. He is a Kashmiri Brahmin. I have an appointment with him. Do you care to come along?"[1] Those were the sort of words that commenced the chain of events launching Gopi Krishna (1903–1984) into the global spotlight, where he would hold discourse with the likes of Werner Heisenberg and become the uncontested touchstone of modern Kuṇḍalinī lore. The invitation was issued by James Hillman (1926–2011), then a twenty-five-year-old aspiring novelist, to his friend Frederik Jan (Tontyn) Hopman (1914–2016), a Dutch architect whose real passions lay in art and astrology. Hillman, American by birth, was in the midst of what we might today call a quarter-life crisis, and he and his future wife had set off on a period of spiritual wandering that in the spring of 1951 had led them to Srinagar, Kashmir.[2] Hillman would recall that it was actually Hopman who had introduced the idea of going to see the mysterious polyglot at the bazaar.[3] In any case, the meeting was nothing short of fateful.

Gopi Krishna would go on to author seventeen books on the topics of Kuṇḍalinī, consciousness and the brain, evolution, and the impending disasters (nuclear war, for one) that would result if humanity failed to heed the call of its natural impulse to evolve. Some of these books, like *The Riddle of Consciousness* (1976), are striking in that they are written entirely in rhyming couplets of iambic pentameter. But none would be quite so famous as the first: *Kundalini: The Evolutionary Energy in Man* (1967/1970), now published in edited form (and notably without Hillman's originally accompanying Jungian commentary) as *Living with Kundalini: The Autobiography of Gopi Krishna.*

That first book, which was likewise originally composed entirely in verse,[4] is effectively a memoir detailing the pivotal event of Gopi Krishna's life. An experience, beginning in the winter of 1937–38, that he would quickly identify as an awakening of Kuṇḍalinī. The text's massive popularity alone would guarantee its place in our account of Kuṇḍalinī's history. However, we devote this chapter to it for a more profound reason: Gopi Krishna's experience seems to shine light upon the central questions that have thus far occupied our analysis, even if it resists giving uncomplicated answers.

Can Kuṇḍalinī rise spontaneously, or does it require practice?

Both.

Is Kuṇḍalinī physical, psychological, or spiritual?

All of the above.

And what does it mean? When we experience Kuṇḍalinī, where is it taking us?

On this point, Gopi Krishna's answer is clear. Indeed, it's the subtitle of his book: Kuṇḍalinī is the "evolutionary energy in man." Although, this focus belies the reason behind the work's impact and popularity.

Gopi Krishna's metaphysical arguments—at least in the generic form they appear in his first book—are far from original. Their basic outlines can be found in the writings of any of the modern yogis who preceded him on the global stage over the previous century, perhaps most notably in Vivekananda's *Raja Yoga* (1896) and Yogananda's *Autobiography of a Yogi* (1946), as well as the work of Aurobindo. What is novel—indeed unique—about Gopi Krishna's book is the detail and immediacy of his experiential narration. Insofar as his metaphysical arguments present something beyond the scope of his predecessors, it is almost entirely because of the way that his lived experience grounds them in empirical, if subjective, reality.

Indeed, Gopi Krishna's experience forms the narrow point in the hourglass of this book.

His interpretation of his experience is clearly informed by the literature we have surveyed so far. Confronted with a dizzying diversity of descriptions, from the historical tantric to the Theosophical, he would come to distill his own experience into an evolutionary framework that seems to give embodied feeling to the writings of early modern spiritual innovators like Aurobindo. The ultimate popularity of Gopi Krishna's work, meanwhile, more or less guarantees that it informs nearly every subsequent interlocutor in Kuṇḍalinī's narrative web. To say nothing of the countless people who turned to his earnest account to make sense of their own—that is, to mold the fine lines of their experience based on his interpretation.

Gopi Krishna would also play a central role in the emerging fields of biofeedback experimentation and consciousness research, which (as we will see in chapter 7) represent one angle of approach to Kuṇḍalinī amid the cultural shifts of the 1960s and 1970s. However, Gopi Krishna's longstanding involvement with this scene and its cast of characters are now well documented in Teri Degler's biographical account, and so we will not dwell on them.[5] More than the historical details of Gopi Krishna's public work, what interests us here are the reasons why the people who would become his global collaborators found his private experience—and subsequently his ideas, which would support that public work—compelling. More so than the story of Gopi Krishna's life, then, this chapter is a story of his story.

WHO WAS GOPI KRISHNA?

Prior to the publication of Degler's biography in 2023, most of Gopi Krishna's life story came to the public by way of humble self-report. He was born into a Brahmin family in the small village of Gairoo, not far from Srinagar in the Himalayan Valley. When Gopi Krishna was barely two years old, his father retired from his well-paying government job and renounced the world, in the spirit of the ancient ideal of *vānaprastha*, secluding himself with his books and leaving the care of their household and their three children on the shoulders of his twenty-eight-year-old wife.[6] This must have had a deep effect on the young Gopi Krishna as, despite his clear interest in spiritual pursuits, he would go on to espouse an ideal quite different than the one valorized by his father. To the end of his days, Gopi Krishna firmly considered himself a householder and a man of the world.

Gopi Krishna's autobiographical accounts are littered with childhood anecdotes illustrating a handful of extraordinary events and various instances of precocious spirituality. In those accounts, he reports that he began meditating at seventeen,[7] though, in his letter to Aurobindo, he puts the marker at nineteen. Indeed, if we are looking to get an honest subjective account of the way Gopi Krishna saw himself prior to the decades-long ordeal that would irreversibly alter his life, the introduction he gives in that letter seems like as good a summary as any. Gopi Krishna writes:

> From the earliest age, the mystery of creation and of my own existence has been a subject of earnest enquiry on my part. When about 19, I was rather [of] an atheist bent of mind. Later on, I inclined towards "Vedanta" but doubts were ever present in my mind. I am somewhat of an idealist and have tried to lead a moral and a clean life, though on occasions I have fallen from my ideal. The utterance of great saints of all ages and climes like Sri Ram Krishan [Ramakrishna] Paramahamsa, Kabir, Shems Tabrez etc. have always evoked a response cord in me. I have a keen intellect and a critical mind. What I now proceed to state below is not a hallucination or a hysterical outburst, but a sober fact. I may say that I was never fully convinced by the writings of Theosophists or by other Yogic literature. I have never pursued "Hatha Yoga" methods. I did ordinary meditation from the age of nineteen regularly at first for about four years, then gave it up and practiced it at irregular intervals subsequently.[8]

Indeed, for all intents and purposes, it seems that until the winter of 1938, Gopi Krishna lived a perfectly ordinary life. After completing his college education in Lahore, Gopi Krishna returned to Kashmir to take a modest clerical position in the Public Works Department. He was married the following summer, at the age of twenty-three. Over the succeeding twelve years, he would hold a number of government positions, finally landing a role as a clerk in the director of education's office in Jammu.[9]

The lifelong arc of Gopi Krishna's spiritual interests and goals is clearly drawn out in his autobiography, penned more than two decades after the central chain of events it catalogs. One imagines the reality was messier, as it always is. It is clear that Gopi Krishna maintained some interest in spiritual pursuits throughout his young life, but both his practice and the extent of his knowledge appear to have been sporadic and unsystematic. For instance, his 1938 writings make it clear that he did not regard his meditation practice as "Yoga," though in his autobiography he uses this term frequently and freely. Thus, any sense of a coherent arc, much less a goal, emerges only in hindsight.

Still, it is clear that Gopi Krishna *did* have these spiritual interests. There is a famous impression of the man, drawn out in the introduction to his first book by the Stanford professor of religion Frederic Spiegelberg, that has served to buttress the raw authenticity of Gopi Krishna's Kuṇḍalinī experience in the modern imagination. The description runs as follows:

> Being exposed to Gopi Krishna's experiences is like meeting a space traveler who seemingly for no purpose has landed on a strange and unknown star without the standard equipment of the professional astronaut, and who simply reports about the bewildering landscape around him, colorfully, truthfully, without really knowing exactly what he has found. We have here, in

> this wholly unintellectual personality, a classical example of a simple man, uneducated in Yoga, who yet through intense labour and persistent enthusiasm, succeeds in achieving, if not Samadhi, yet some very high state in Yoga perfection, based entirely on his inner feeling development and not at all on ideas and traditions. Gopi Krishna is an extremely honest reporter, to the point of humbleness. Since he does not claim great powers and achievements, one is even more willing to accept his detailed descriptions of inner changes as exact reports. Thus, one of the consequences of his autonomous training is the aliveness of his account.[10]

Aspects of this do ring true to the experiences described in Gopi Krishna's letters, to which we will momentarily turn. To call the man a "wholly unintellectual personality," however, is quite a stretch. By the time he had written the book Spiegelberg is introducing, Gopi Krishna was clearly in command of the relevant literature on yoga and quite a few other subjects besides. This is no country peasant. What Gopi Krishna is, however, is an autodidact, and it is in this light that we must approach him.

Spiegelberg is correct about at least one thing, however. Gopi Krishna remains honest, earnest, and above all humble. His book is not filled with traditional yoga frameworks not because he does not know them at this stage in his life, but because after two decades he has not found them helpful. This does not mean that he did not try. Gopi Krishna's humbleness matters here specifically because it helps contextualize his reports of seeking help, from living gurus and from ancient texts alike. But the traditional theoretical frameworks prove to be of limited use when applied to the immediacy of his experience. Still, from an early point in his record of it, he does identify his experience as Kuṇḍalinī; in that sense, it seems incorrect to claim he doesn't know what he is experiencing. And, as we will see, his ultimate understanding of this experience does not evolve in a vacuum. Indeed, Gopi Krishna's vision of Kuṇḍalinī as an evolutionary principle comes incredibly close to the understanding espoused by one of the first teachers from whom he tried and failed to obtain help: Sri Aurobindo.

WHAT HAPPENED TO GOPI KRISHNA?

Experience is a tricky thing, and mystical experience perhaps most of all. An experience is an event—complex and subjective—but it is also a story, one we tell to ourselves as well as to others if we want to preserve the thing beyond the moment in which it occurs. Gopi Krishna's experience is significant because it has become a cultural touchstone for global understandings of Kuṇḍalinī. It is a story that has come to shape the stories of so many others who have come after. It is also a story that has been shaped, as all stories must be, by those who came before. But we place it here, at the heart of our book, because of a particular and rather rare feature: Gopi Krishna's dependable and guileless honesty coupled with a few accidents of history have given us a rare glimpse into how his particular story was written.

About three weeks after Gopi Krishna first experienced the stirrings of Kuṇḍalinī within his body, he wrote a lengthy letter to Aurobindo, seeking help. Curiously, he never references Aurobindo by name in his work. The only mention of this correspondence is the following passage:

> At last mustering my courage, I wrote to one of the best-known modern saints of India the author of many widely read books in English on Yoga, giving him full details of my extraordinary state and sought for guidance. I waited for his reply in trepidation, and

> when it failed to come for some days, I sent a telegram also. I was passing a very anxious time when the answer came. It said that there was no doubt that I had aroused Kundalini in the tantric manner and that the only way for me to seek guidance was to find a Yogi who had himself conducted the Shakti successfully to the Seventh Centre in the head. I was thankful for the reply which fully confirmed my own opinion, thereby raising my hopes and self-confidence. It was obvious that the symptoms mentioned by me had been recognised as those characterizing the awakening, thereby giving to my weird experience a certain appearance of normality. If I were passing through an abnormal condition, it was not an isolated instance nor was the abnormality peculiar to me alone, but must be a necessary corollary to the awakening of Kundalini, and with modifications suited to different temperaments must have occurred in almost all those in whom awakening had taken place. But where was I to find a Yogi who had raised the Shakti to the Seventh Centre?[11]

The utter earnestness of Gopi Krishna's letters to Aurobindo leaves no doubt that he really did try; though, as we noted above, the quest proved unsuccessful. Actually, Gopi Krishna sent to Aurobindo not one but two long letters. In the second of these, he unreservedly pleaded with Aurobindo to take him on as a disciple. Despite Aurobindo's rather cool reply, which Gopi Krishna references here with similarly cool detachment, Aurobindo's work (if not the man himself) must have played a central role in shaping Gopi Krishna's thought. In light of this connection, the similarities between their models of Kuṇḍalinī can hardly be a coincidence.

Just now, however, the most important thing about these letters (and the telegrams that followed) is that they afford us a rare instance of an experience being recorded as it is happening, or at least in very close proximity. Even more, they present us with a narrative of that extraordinary experience that is raw and uncontrived because it is colored by no motive other than to obtain help.

So, what happened to Gopi Krishna? What follows is what can be reconstructed from these correspondences.

January 16, 1938

Gopi Krishna feels "a curious lightness, a sort of intoxication while walking in a market." There is a "hazy sort of brightness" that surrounds objects in his field of vision. That evening, while sitting in meditation, he experiences the first instance of what he comes to understand as Kuṇḍalinī awakening. Gopi Krishna specifies that his ordinary meditation is to "concentrate on an imaginary lotus at the top of [his] head," but he has never practiced *prāṇāyāma*. He also relates that he subsequently described his condition to two unnamed *sādhus*, one of whom intimated that his experience was that of awakening Kuṇḍalinī. This makes it somewhat unclear whether Gopi Krishna himself would have named the experience as such at this stage—an ambiguity supported by the fact that he puts Kuṇḍalinī in scare quotes throughout his letter.

In any case, this section of the letter is worth quoting in full:

> I felt a curious sensation at the place where "Kundalini" is said to reside i.e. at the bottom of the spine. As I have said I have never given the system of Yoga any particular attention. Then there was a slight buzzing noise in my ears and I seemed to feel a sensation of light in my head. The sensation of the seat of "Kundalini" grew intense, diffusing a bliss over my whole system. A gentle warmth pervaded the spot and then began to rise up. The sensation of pleasure grew more and more intense and my attention was drawn and fixed on it. My consciousness seemed to expand

> and gave me an intense happiness. I cannot find words to define this state of my consciousness. It was inexpressible. My spinal column became hard and erect and a sensation of warmth and light seemed to pervade it also. So forcibly was my intention fixed in the contemplation of my consciousness that my breathing became rapid and irregular and my heart began to thump violently and painfully.

January 17–20

The sensations return, even more intensely, during Gopi Krishna's meditation the following day. Over the proceeding days, he reports a sense of calm and balance, a diminishing of sexual urges, and a repugnance toward meat. Overall, he appears to be thriving. He feels a great sense of health, "having an abundance of energy, fearless and in a state of exaltation." It seems that, during this period, he continues and even intensifies his regular meditation practice, keen as he is to recapture the "wonderful experience."

On the fifth day, he begins to feel a sense of detachment from his kin, and indeed from "all worldly ties." He is "listless and depressed." Now, the sensation of warmth at the base of the spine seems ever present, and any attempt to focus, regardless of the object, makes the sensation more pronounced. Attempting to focus also produces "a state of abstraction, in which bodily sensations were absent, though I could hear sounds quite well. When the condition was more pronounced, the sounds appeared remote." He reports further:

> While sitting, I had an ever present urge to detach my consciousness from the body. I at once fell into a state of abstraction, in which bodily sensations were absent, though I could hear sounds quite well. When the condition was more pronounced,

> the sounds appeared remote. When the feeling of abstraction came up, I seemed to feel a slight rocking motion as if the ground or bed under me had been removed without disturbing my equilibrium. I found it almost impossible to revert to my previous normal consciousness. So pronounced with the feeling of detachment and indifference that I seemed to think myself intoxicated or stupefied. This gave rise to acute anxiety in my mind.

This is accompanied by an occasional sense of discomfort in the regions of the heart, the navel, and the liver, and thus a feeling of fear.

January 21–February 6

Gopi Krishna tries to stop thinking about his experience and to return to his normal affairs. He struggles at first, and the physical condition of his organs is akin to the aftermath of an acute fever. He treats his physical symptoms by regulating his diet. He takes a course of laxatives and consumes only milk and fruit juice for about three days. After ten days of complete rest, his condition seems to normalize.

Some lingering effects persist, however. The feeling of detachment subsides, but he reports that other changes in his habits and temperament (presumably the calmness, reduced libido, and aversion to meat) persist. He has lost weight and feels an unspecified change in "the functional activities of [his] digestive system and urinary organs." He still feels an occasional surge of energy in different parts of his body, which increases if he allows himself to focus on it (which he does not). He has become incredibly sensitive to music. Most strikingly, the weakened sense of smell he's experienced since early childhood has been completely restored.

During this period, Gopi Krishna attempts to sit in meditation only twice. Of these attempts, he reports:

> I experienced in a lighter degree the same condition that I had experienced before. As soon as my attention got fixed in the contemplation of my consciousness the latter expands in ever widening circles, the light becomes more and more intense but so powerful in the emotional effect on me that my breathing becomes irregular and my heart thumps rapidly. I am aware of these two feelings in a dreamy sort of way. The sensation of body remains present, but the sensation is of a light etherial [*sic*] substance glowing with a pleasant sense of warmth. Sounds, though audible, convey no meaning. It takes me about 10 minutes to come down from this condition to my normal body consciousness. Brisk rubbing and walking help me to bring down my attention.

At the time of writing, Gopi Krishna assures, "I am as well as I was ever before and in complete possession of all my faculties." Yet, given all of the above, one gets the sense that his hold on this stability is tenuous at best. He admits to a persistent urge to sit in meditation so that he might recapture his "superconscious state."

The ultimate purpose of his letter is twofold. Firstly and most importantly, he seeks clarification regarding whether his condition "is really the result of the awakening of 'Kundalini.'" Secondly, and assuming that this is the case, he seeks advice on how he can bring himself back to normal consciousness after meditation.

February 7

Gopi Krishna sends his initial letter to Aurobindo.

February 8

The very next day, Gopi Krishna enters a period of crisis. He reports: "I was suddenly awakened in the morning by a feeling of pressure at my heart and the navel. I was terrified to find that I could distinctly feel the thumping of my heart and a motion as of a disk revolving at the site of my navel. . . . I found that my mind had become abnormally acute and I could distinctly feel the passing of the nerve currents not only between the heart and stomach centers but also in my back and at the site of the 'Kundalini.' " In subsequent days, he experiences a prolonged sensation of "red-hot needles" in the region between his stomach and bladder. His attention is strained.

February 14–19

Gopi Krishna sends a telegram to Aurobindo stating that the Kuṇḍalinī has grown uncontrollable, and he is experiencing incredible heat and is unable to sleep. Writing a few days later, he intimates, "The condition became unbearable and the presentment dawned on me that this was to be the end. . . . I prepared myself to die and in this condition remained on the bed suffering unutterable agony."

As his crisis peaks, he recalls a conversation he once had with his brother-in-law, whose guru had told him that "if the 'Kundalini' Shakti was aroused through the 'Pingala' Nadi, terrific heat was produced enough to consume a man." At this stage, Gopi Krishna seems to have adopted the working assumption that his experience is in fact Kuṇḍalinī, but his knowledge on the topic remains vague. "I had been told that the 'pingala' was on the right and the 'Ida' on the left side of the spine," he writes, "but as I have already explained I had never taken pains to go deeply into the subject." Thus, what comes next appears to be an act of desperate ingenuity and faith.

Gopi Krishna reports:

> At that time, my heart was beating at great speed at more than 130 beats per minute and my urinary organs were getting out of gear. I knew enough of my symptoms to feel positive that the end either of my life or of my sanity was not far off. I lay down on my bed and concentrated on the left side of the spine i.e. on the "Ida Nadi." Soon, I detected a cool current passing down my spine into my thigh. I concentrated on it with all my might, willing to drive the cool "Vayu" into my whole body. At that time a miracle happened. I distinctly felt a sensation of a connection snapping and a flash of light at the bottom of the spine. Instantly, the red-hot pinpoints that were searing my body ceased and a rush of energy neither warm nor cold rushed up my spine and held up the heart which was now fluttering violently, in a close embrace. Another rush cooled the burning fever of my brain. The energy circulated in all my vital organs, soothing my overwrought nerves and within fifteen minutes I was asleep after having passed six sleepless nights.

February 18

Aurobindo sends a telegram to Gopi Krishna, assuring him that his experience is normal and that the unpleasantness has arisen due to "wrong mental reactions." He instructs Gopi Krishna to stop meditating or to find a competent guru.

February 20

Gopi Krishna sends a second letter to Aurobindo, thanking him for his telegram and elaborating on the crisis referenced in his own telegram. He describes the means he used to bring himself back from the brink by concentrating on the *iḍā nāḍī*. Interestingly, Gopi Krishna explains that this experience has led him to believe that Kuṇḍalinī awakened in him and took this incorrect path through the *piṅgalā* six or seven years prior, while he was not meditating at all. Since this time, "the hot element" has predominated in his body.

In any case, at the time of writing, Gopi Krishna claims to have once more returned to normal health. The day after his intervention, he awoke to find himself weak, but with his mind clear and his body free of pain. "The energy continued to work all through the next day," he reports, "sometimes caressing my heart, sometimes my digestive organs and steadying my thoughts." Indeed, it seems that Kuṇḍalinī has integrated Herself permanently into his organism. The heat at the bottom of the spine is replaced by a gentle warmth. "I could actually feel energy being drawn up from my thighs, buttocks and occasionally from the organs of generation," writes Gopi Krishna. "This sensation appears to me like a gentle bombardment of myriads of tiny particles or the creeping of small insects." Kuṇḍalinī now appears to be at his implicit disposal—the energy "only works when it is actually needed"—rising to the head when he is engaged in mental labor; aiding his stomach and bowels when they are obstructed.

Gopi Krishna states that he has ceased to meditate and is proceeding, in all aspects of his life, with extreme care. He closes his letter with a lengthy and heart-wrenching plea for guidance, expressing the strength of his commitment and the depth of his earnestness, humbly begging Aurobindo to accept him as a disciple.

March 10

Gopi Krishna sends a telegram to Aurobindo reporting that *śakti* is still active in his vital organs and he is experiencing some continuing digestive symptoms and changes in mood (chiefly "abstraction" and occasionally fear), and he is unable to find a guide. Aurobindo sends a reply urging Krishna to remain calm and seek help, and promising to write at greater length.

March 11

Gopi Krishna sends another telegram to Aurobindo reporting that Kuṇḍalinī is still active, leading to changes in his body and mind. He seems to report a transfer of the burning he previously experienced to the brain and the top of his head and is concerned about a growing tendency toward "abstraction," being unable to perform his duties and care for his family. Aurobindo replies that he can add no more via telegram and asks Gopi Krishna to await his letter.

March 12

One final telegram is sent to Aurobindo, possibly by Gopi Krishna's brother-in-law on his behalf, reporting the same complaint of "abstraction" and the sensation that his brain is "melting away."

After . . .

Aurobindo's full letter to Gopi Krishna must have arrived sometime after March 12. In light of all the preceding correspondence, the reply, though eminently kind, is actually quite heartbreaking. Written in the third person by Aurobindo's assistant, the letter offers some clarifications and advice but cordially declines to take Gopi Krishna on as a disciple. The communications between Gopi Krishna and Aurobindo end here, and so we must turn to Gopi Krishna's official account, written some two decades later, to fill in the rest of the story.

In his autobiography, Gopi Krishna reports no further acute crises immediately following the episode described in his second letter. He does speak of an ongoing vibrating luminous glow in his head,[12] which might perhaps be what he means in his telegrams when he speaks of a burning sensation in his head, and his brain "melting away." However, following this, he does appear to generally recover.

He speaks to "several scholars and Sadhus" but is disappointed to receive only a "parrotlike repetition of information gathered from books," which they often admitted were difficult to interpret, and no guidance based on practical experience.[13] The results of his information-gathering are perhaps best summed up by the following:

> I consulted other holy men and sought for guidance from many reputed quarters without coming across a single individual who could boldly assert that he actually possessed intimate personal knowledge of the condition and could confidently answer my questions. Those who talked with dignified reserve looking very wise and deep, ultimately turned out to be as wanting in accurate information about the mysterious power rampant in me as those of a more unassuming nature who unbosomed themselves completely on the very first occasion without in the least pretending to know any more than they really did. And thus in the great country which had given birth to the lofty science of Kundalini thousands of years ago and whose very soil is permeated with its fragrance and whose rich religious lore is full of references to it from cover to cover, I found no one able to help me.[14]

Around 1939, his office is moved from Jammu to Srinagar. Sometime roughly two years later, Gopi Krishna experiences a permanent shift in his vision, which renders everything "lit with a brilliant silvery lustre that lent a beauty and a glory to [the scene] and created a marvellous light and shade effect impossible to describe."[15] As the years pass, he finds his mental and physical health restored, though the luster flooding his vision only increases. He observes in himself a heightened metabolic activity.[16] He recounts:

> Often at night for years, when lying awake in bed waiting for sleep to come, I felt the powerful new life energy sweep like a tempest in the abdominal and thoracic regions as well as the brain with a roaring noise in the ears; a scintillating shower in the brain, and a feverish movement in the sexual region and its neighbourhood around the base of the spine, both in front and behind, as if an all-out effort were being made to fight an emergency caused by some poison or obstruction in the organism threatening the supersensitive and extremely delicate condition of the cerebro-spinal system.[17]

However, besides this perceived flow of energy, he notices no other higher mental or spiritual development and begins to doubt his experience, wondering whether he has perhaps been found unworthy of reaching the highest stages.[18]

In 1943, renewed meditation practice brings on another crisis, the physical pain of which nearly drives Gopi Krishna to suicide. The cure comes through an extremely disciplined control of diet.[19] Justifiably cowed by his experience, Gopi Krishna throws himself into worldly affairs. In 1946, he devotes himself to his community, focusing on economic reform.[20] He makes no more effort to meditate, but does find himself sinking within himself, absorbed in his now luminous and expansive consciousness. Toward the end of 1949, this tendency becomes more pronounced and frequent. In December, he finds himself suddenly compelled to write verse—which, at last, seems to materialize before him, drawn out in light upon the air—first in Kashmiri, then English, then Urdu, and then Punjabi. These languages—Gopi Krishna knew. But then the poetry begins to flow in Persian, then German, and French, and Italian. Of the latter three languages, Gopi Krishna had absolutely no knowledge. Eventually come Sanskrit and Arabic.[21]

The news spreads. Crowds begin to gather.

Gopi Krishna's breakthrough happened on the day that the first Kashmiri verses appeared to him, while crossing Tawi Bridge in Jammu. Afterwards, he came home, sat down to dinner and entered a state that most would probably call *samādhi*. "Without any effort on my part and while seated comfortably on a chair," he writes, "I had gradually passed off, without becoming aware of it, into a condition of exaltation and self-expansion similar to that which I had experienced on the very first occasion, in December 1937, with the modification that in place of a roaring noise in my ears there was now a cadence like the humming of a swarm of bees, enchanting and melodious and the encircling glow was replaced by a penetrating silvery radiance, already a feature of my being within and without."[22] Of course, if one goes by the original description of his experience—not the posited one on December 1937 (more on that in a moment), but the January 16, 1938 event described in his letter—perhaps the beginning and the end are closer in kind than they appear. But, however it began, it seems that in the waning days of 1949, Gopi Krishna finally settled into a new "normal." Gopi Krishna was no "superman"—not in the physical sense, anyway. He admitted that, if anything, his constitution had emerged from the ordeal more sensitive than average. In the end, he summed up his situation like this:

> I feel utterly lost between the two worlds in which I live . . . the incomprehensible and infinitely marvellous universe within and the colossal but familiar world without. When I look within I am

> lifted beyond the oppressive weight of the material cosmos, beyond the confines of time and space, in tune with a majestic, all-conscious existence, which mocks at fear and laughs at death, compared to which seas and mountains, suns and planets, appear no more than flimsy rack riding across a blazing sky; an existence which is in all and yet absolutely removed from everything, an endless inexpressible wonder that can onlv be experienced and not described. But when I look outside I am what I was, an ordinary mortal in no way different from the millions who inhabit the earth, a common man pressed by necessity and driven by circumstances, a little chastened and humbled—that is all.[23]

If one links up the timelines, Hillman and Hopman would have met Gopi Krishna in 1952, just a couple of years after the final resolution of his Kuṇḍalinī experience into this newly stable (albeit radically transformed) consciousness. It would take another decade for him to complete his manuscript, with Hopman's assistance.

EVOLVING NARRATIVE

Not surprisingly, there are some differences between the account conveyed in Gopi Krishna's letters and the one that appears, over two decades later, in his published work. First and foremost, it is worth emphasizing that our memories naturally tend to shift over time, especially when trauma is involved, as we process, contextualize, and recontextualize the messy tangle of bodily sensations and external events that constitute raw experience. Thus, perhaps what is *most* remarkable is how consistent Gopi Krishna's account of those harrowing weeks in the winter of 1938 remains between his original reports and the publication of his book all those years later. That said, let us get the most glaring inconsistencies out of the way.

In writing to Aurobindo, Gopi Krishna locates the start of the experience during a rather mundane stroll through the market on January 16, 1938, with the sensation distinctly named as Kuṇḍalinī occurring later that evening. The book, on the other hand, opens with a breakthrough visionary experience that overtakes Gopi Krishna during a morning meditation around Christmas 1937. It seems unlikely that Gopi Krishna got the date wrong in his original letter (especially given that he correctly identifies the day of the week as Sunday). Did he simply forget?

Here is the full opening to the book:

> One morning during the Christmas of 1937 I sat cross-legged in a small room in a little house on the outskirts of the town of Jammu, the winter capital of the Jammu and Kashmir State in Northern India, I was meditating with my face toward the window on the east through which the first grey streaks of the slowly brightening dawn fell into the room. Long practice had accustomed me to sit in the same posture for hours at a time without the least discomfort, and I sat breathing slowly and rhythmically, my attention drawn toward the crown of my head, contemplating: an imaginary lotus in full bloom, radiating light.
>
> I sat steadily, unmoving and erect, my thoughts uninterruptedly centered on the shining lotus, intent on keeping my attention from wandering and bringing it back again and again whenever it moved in any other direction. The intensity of concentration interrupted my breathing; gradually it slowed down to such an extent that at times it was barely perceptible. My whole being was so engrossed in the contemplation of the lotus that for several minutes at a time I lost touch with my body and surroundings. During such intervals I used to feel as if I were poised in mid-air, without any feeling of a body around me. The only object of which I was aware was a lotus of brilliant colour,

> emitting rays of light. This experience has happened to many people who practise meditation in any form regularly for a sufficient length of time but what followed on that fateful morning in my case, changing the whole course of my life and outlook, has happened to few.

Let us take a momentary step back and consider the realities of publishing. This reads like a standard literary hook. What better way to set the scene for a life-altering flash of transcendence than the image of a quiet Christmas morning, the pale winter light filtering through the windows? Mid-January is still close enough to the Christmas season, after all.

The experience that follows is a close match to descriptions found in Gopi Krishna's letters, though the language becomes sharper, more lyrical, more attuned to the conventions of mystical literature. This too is hardly surprising—again, Gopi Krishna is now writing a book, not a letter of inquiry. The chief difference is that we seem to skip the five-day "honeymoon" during which Gopi Krishna's experiences intensify but bring only exhilaration and a desire for more. Instead, as he comes back down to normal consciousness, he is shaken, exhausted, and immediately moody. He has lost his appetite. He goes to work (not something he would have done on a Sunday, perhaps) and is plagued by feelings of detachment. He has trouble sleeping and, when he attempts to summon the experience again the next day, it comes back weaker. In other words, this is exactly where Gopi Krishna reported being by around January 21. It seems he has simply taken some narrative license.

It is nevertheless worth examining how that narrative license, especially when it comes to the nature and intensity of Gopi Krishna's descriptive language, impacts our understanding of his experience. Let's consider the initial experience of Kuṇḍalinī awakening as it appears in the opening pages of the book:

> Suddenly, with a roar like that of a waterfall, I felt a stream of liquid light entering my brain through the spinal cord. . . . The illumination grew brighter and brighter, the roaring louder. I experienced a rocking sensation and then felt myself slipping out of my body, entirely enveloped in a halo of light.
>
> It is impossible to describe the experience accurately. I felt the point of consciousness that was myself growing wider, surrounded by waves of light. It grew wider and wider, spreading outward while the body, normally the immediate object of its perception, appeared to have receded into the distance until I became entirely unconscious of it. I was now all consciousness, without any outline, without any idea of a corporeal appendage, without any feeling or sensation coming from the senses, immersed in a sea of light simultaneously conscious and aware of every point, spread out, as it were, in all directions without any barrier or material obstruction.
>
> I was no longer myself, or to be more accurate, no longer as I knew myself to be, a small point of awareness confined in a body, but instead was a vast circle of consciousness in which the body was but a point, bathed in light and in a state of exaltation and happiness impossible to describe.

Several things are of note here. In addition to the timing of the experience, the details have not only sharpened but heightened. Rather than a "slight buzzing noise in my ears," a "sensation of light in my head," and a rising "gentle warmth," Gopi Krishna now recounts: "With a roar like that of a waterfall, I felt a stream of liquid light entering my brain through the spinal cord." Gopi Krishna is now able to express the feeling of warmth and light and the indefinable state of consciousness as the complete loss of self—a feeling of unconfined consciousness bathed in a "sea of light." Whereas previously he framed the former only as happiness and expansion. Similar shifts in descriptive language characterize the rest of the narrative.

And just as there is no honeymoon period, there is no reprieve to reflect the time that Gopi Krishna first wrote to Aurobindo, having felt himself return to some sense of normalcy. Instead, he expressly states that "there was no remission in the current rising from the seat of Kundalini."[24] Nearly from the very first moment, Gopi Krishna describes being immediately launched into a living nightmare. At night, he reports, "a large tongue of flame sped across the spine into the interior of my head . . . the stream of living light continuously rushing through the spinal cord into the cranium gathered greater speed and volume during the hours of darkness."[25] Kuṇḍalinī is ever present in his spine as "a jet of molten copper,"[26] filling him with "a vast internal glow, disquieting and threatening at times, always in rapid motion, as if the particles of an ethereal luminous stuff crossed and recrossed each other, resembling the ceaseless movement of wildly leaping lustrous clouds of spray rising from a waterfall which, lighted by the sun, rushes down foaming into a seething pool."[27] The other sensations on which his original reports dwelled, localized in the heart or around the digestive organs, are still occasionally present, but appear as mere epiphenomena. The picture is now clear: a fiery current flows from the seat of Kuṇḍalinī and up through the spinal column, toward the brain.

So, how much of this is a function of imperfect memory, how much is the natural evolution of an interpretation, and how much is owed to the nature of formal narrative? In some places, it does appear that Gopi Krishna genuinely conflates the times that he entered particularly intense periods of crisis. For example, he places the *iḍā nāḍī* exercise as happening around "the holy festival of Shivaratri . . . towards the end of February"—in 1938, the date of Mahāśivarātri would have been March 1—but we know that this would have happened sometime between February 14 and 20, based on the date of Gopi Krishna's letter to Aurobindo.[28] And yet the published account, though more elaborate, comports incredibly closely with the contents of that letter. In fact, the only notable differences once again arise in the specificity of the language and imagery used. Here is the core of the account as it appears in the book:

> With my mind reeling and senses deadened with pain, but with all the willpower left at my command, I brought my attention to bear on the left side of the seat of kundalini and tried to force an imaginary cold current upward through the middle of the spinal cord. In that extraordinarily extended, agonized, and exhausted state of consciousness, I distinctly felt the location of the nerve and strained hard mentally to divert its flow into the central channel. Then, as if waiting for the destined moment, a miracle happened.
>
> There was a sound like a nerve thread snapping and instantaneously a silvery streak passed zigzag through the spinal cord, exactly like the sinuous movement of a white serpent in rapid flight, pouring an effulgent, cascading shower of brilliant vital energy into my brain, filling my head with a blissful luster in place of the flame that had been tormenting me for the last three hours. . . . Tortured and exhausted almost to the point of collapse by the agony I had suffered during the terrible interval, I immediately fell asleep, bathed in light, and for the first time after weeks of anguish felt the sweet embrace of restful sleep.[29]

Actually, the account is strikingly similar to the one in Gopi Krishna's letter, with two notable exceptions. In the earlier account, he describes a "rush of energy neither warm nor cold" that rises up the spine to wrap around his heart, and then a second rush that cools his brain. Here, there is a single rush that goes straight to the brain, while the heart is no longer mentioned. This is consistent with the overall reframing of Gopi Krishna's descriptions which now focus much more on the imagery of a current flowing from the bottom of the spine into the brain, while the heart (or any other part of the torso) is rarely mentioned. The second notable feature, of course, is the form this energy takes. It's a serpent and it travels in a zigzag. Indeed, serpents are never mentioned in Gopi Krishna's letters; this image appears only in the later account.

At this point, it is important to note that we are not suggesting that Gopi Krishna somehow inaccurately reinterpreted or embellished the facts of his original experience. In the end, we cannot say whether the objective (if there is such a thing, when it comes to experience) sound in Gopi Krishna's head was closer to a buzz or a roar. Instead, what we are highlighting are the ways Gopi Krishna's experience *of* his experience develops through framing and language. These are both a function of external "information gathering" as well as internal self-examination for Gopi Krishna. However, the implications of this process mirror the wider dynamic of how experiential narratives evolve through framing and transmission. Gopi Krishna's coupling of research and self-reflection affects his individual "internal" narrative of Kuṇḍalinī, but also the "external" informational substrate available to each new practitioner (that is, experiencer) who comes across his narrative.

GOPI KRISHNA'S INTERPRETATION

It's tempting to say that because Gopi Krishna was an autodidact who experienced Kuṇḍalinī awakening more or less spontaneously and endured it without the guidance of a guru, he was operating outside the confines of tradition. (This, in a sense, is what Spiegelberg claims in his introductory statements). But of course the very fact that Gopi Krishna referred to his experience as Kuṇḍalinī at all means that he was not immune to the influence of tradition. The difference is that Gopi Krishna did not approach Kuṇḍalinī through a structured set of practices located within and passed to him through the framework of a specific lineage. Instead, he encountered Kuṇḍalinī the way that a modern—and indeed, especially a Western—student would. He read about it in books and tried to form a coherent picture.

We see this explicitly as Gopi Krishna narrows the wider constellation of his physical symptoms (which is apparent in his letters) down to what he now understands to be the core phenomenon. This he describes as "the most extraordinary sensation at the base of the spine followed by the flow of a radiant current through the spinal column into the head," and he notes that "this part of the strange experience tallied with the phenomena associated with the awakening of Kundalini, and hence I could not be mistaken in supposing that I had unknowingly aroused the coiled serpent and that the serious disturbance in my nervous system as well as the extraordinary but most awful state I was in [was in] some way occasioned by it."[30]

It seems that Gopi Krishna arrived at the initial conclusion gradually—it is still half-formed in his second letter to Aurobindo—and that he drew on a variety of sources to do so. In his autobiography, he relates a conversation with his brother-in-law and the subsequent advice, a consultation with at least one "learned ascetic from Kashmir" (presumably one of the two *sādhus* he had mentioned to Aurobindo), and then advice from an unnamed person encouraging him to consult "a couple of books on Kundalini Yoga, translations in English of ancient Sanskrit texts."[31] Elsewhere, Gopi Krishna refers to "popular books on Yoga"—he claims to have read these in the years before his experience, but, if true, we can assume he paid careful heed to their contents only in the years after. Some of these, presumably, were the types of popular manuals we surveyed in chapter 4, of which Gopi Krishna states "the learned authors confined themselves to the description of various postures and methods, all borrowed from the ancient writings on the subject," with only the occasional "passing reference to Kundalini Yoga."[32] Others, focusing more on the tantric frameworks of Kuṇḍalinī as a divine power that ascends to meet her spouse Shiva in the crown of the head, sound an awful lot like Arthur Avalon's *The Serpent Power*.

In fact, Gopi Krishna admits to going down a sort of Kuṇḍalinī research rabbit hole as he attempts to make sense of his experience once the most acute symptoms have subsided. He recounts:

> With the restoration of my faculties and the growing clarity of mind I began to speculate about my condition. I read all that came my way pertaining to Kundalini and Yoga, but did not come across any account of a similar phenomenon. The darting warm and cold currents, the effulgence in the head, the unearthly sounds in the ears, and the gripping fear were all mentioned, but there was no sign in me of clairvoyance or of ecstasy or of communication with disembodied spirits or of any other extraordinary psychic gift, all considered to be the distinctive characteristics of an awakened Kundalini from the earliest times. On the contrary, I was undergoing the ordeal with a shaken physical frame and had only now begun to think coherently and act with confidence after months of uncertainty and travail.[33]

Note the ongoing skepticism as he attempts to cross-reference his lingering symptoms with the traditional literature. Gopi Krishna seems troubled by the relatively ordinary physicality of his experience, which seems to show "no sign" of the spiritual wonders promised by the texts he is reading. He feels this way despite reporting ongoing visual and auditory phenomena—lights, sounds, distorted faces, and twisting shapes—that are far from mundane. Perhaps we should read a bit more into Gopi Krishna's confusion than that to which he himself admits. What he means is he does not develop superpowers (*siddhis*) as the traditional texts imply he should.

Historian of religion Joseph Alter framed this difficulty of comparing subjective experience with the canon, faced by many a modern student, aptly when he wrote, "Unless one can, with complete honesty—and that is the rub—claim to be a perfected immortal and immune from all diseases or to have achieved a state of consciousness wherein one's continued state of being is just a reflection of the will to help others transcend the entanglement of reality, which is the existential if not essential heaviness of the guru's burden, it is difficult to know how to read the medieval literature."[34] On the one hand, it seems impossible to doubt the extraordinary nature of Gopi Krishna's experience. On the other hand, Gopi Krishna himself continuously doubts it because he doesn't appear to be living out the precise verses of the *Ṣaṭcakra Nirūpaṇa*.

Ultimately, however, Gopi Krishna's experience is his primary guide. Thus, it is precisely on experiential grounds that he finally proceeds to contest some features of the traditional literature. For example, because he understands Kuṇḍalinī to be a perfectly natural and biologically grounded phenomenon, he cannot square it with the objective reality of certain features of the tantric texts, such as the elaborate descriptions of the *cakras*. "I did not come across any in the course of my own long adventure, not even a vestige of one in any part of the cerebrospinal system," he says, before further adding that "to assume their existence even for an instant in these days of physiological knowledge and research would mean nothing short of an insult to intelligence."[35] Gopi Krishna admits that had he been trained in and practiced the traditional tantric methods of visualization he may well have experienced the *cakras* as instructed in those texts. However, this makes them mentally constructed imaginal features, used as tools and for symbolic purposes. At most, he allows, "the idea of Chakras and lotuses must have been suggested to the mind of the ancient teachers by the singular resemblance which, in the awakened state, the lustrous nerve centres bear to a luminous revolving disc, studded with lights, or to a lotus flower in full bloom glistening in the rays of the sun."[36] (This, as the reader might recall, is exactly the kind of logic advanced by the Theosophist Charles Leadbeater to explain why his descriptions of the *cakras* don't comport with traditional sources.)

This does not mean that Gopi Krishna dismisses as imaginal and unscientific all traditional features of Kuṇḍalinī frameworks. For instance, he relies heavily on the traditional physiology of *bindu*, albeit in an updated form. He does this because it seems to accord with his experience. Let us consider his explanation at length:

> There was no doubt an extraordinary change in my nervous equipment, and a new type of force was now racing through my system connected unmistakably with the sexual parts, which also seemed to have developed a new kind of activity not perceptible before. The nerves lining the parts and the surrounding region were all in a state of intense ferment, as if forced by an invisible mechanism to produce the vital seed in abnormal abundance to be sucked up by the network of nerves at the base of the spine for transmission into the brain through the spinal cord. The sublimated seed formed an integral part of the radiant energy which was causing me such bewilderment and about which I was as yet unable to speculate with any degree of assurance. I could readily perceive the transmutation of the vital seed into radiation and the unusual activity of the reproductive organs for supplying the raw material for transformation in the mysterious laboratory at the lowest plexus, or muladhara chakra, as the yogis name it, into that extremely subtle and ordinarily imperceptible stuff we call nervous energy, on which the entire mechanism of the body depends, with the difference that the energy now generated possessed luminosity and was of a quality allowing detection of its rapid passage through the nerves and tissues, not only by its radiance but also by the sensations it caused with its movement.[37]

The sublimation of sexual fluids is a fairly typical feature of the Kaula tantric frameworks that foreground Kuṇḍalinī. However, Gopi Krishna's Western commentators—both of the illustrious men (one a Jungian psychologist, the other a physicist) whose reputations lend legitimacy to his first two books—struggle to make sense of this claim. Both of them can read it only figuratively and symbolically, just as Gopi Krishna reads the *cakras*. Indeed, as we will see, neither man, to whose framings of Gopi Krishna's work we'll turn shortly, picks up his positing of Kuṇḍalinī as evolutionary. However, in Gopi Krishna's view, the physicality of Kuṇḍalinī's function within the body is a crucial feature of its participation in the evolutionary process, which for him is as biological as it is spiritual.

As we've mentioned, this evolutionary understanding of Kuṇḍalinī was likely inspired by Gopi Krishna's engagement with Aurobindo's work. Indeed, there are physical aspects to much of the latter, including the perfecting of the seven tetrads that make up Aurobindo's Integral Yoga (though Aurobindo does not spend much time dwelling on them). Gopi Krishna, however, brings not only a physical but imminently physiological dimension to Aurobindo's theory of spiritual evolution. He understands the ongoing symptoms manifesting in his own body—the increased metabolism, the unusual activity of the sexual organs, the heightened sensitivity to diet and changes in the processes of elimination—as Kuṇḍalinī acting to purify and perfect his internal bodily processes. In effect, he finds that his body is essentially being rewired on a metabolic and therefore energetic level.

It is an important aspect of Gopi Krishna's thought that this process is not only natural but inevitable, like the general progress of evolution. Like Aurobindo, and others before him, Gopi Krishna's understanding of evolution is teleological, but its ends are the birthright of all humanity. Kuṇḍalinī awakening is not, therefore, an individual spiritual attainment afforded to a select few, but the natural trajectory of human evolution. We all stand on the brink of the next step. Even the attainment of *samādhi* becomes, in this framing, not the highest goal—the final attainment of ultimate reality, "complete and whole"—but simply the next rung on the evolutionary ladder.[38] Having analyzed the processes occurring inside his body, Gopi Krishna sums up the physical features of this model as follows:

> On the strength of these and other facts I gradually came to the conclusion, which it shall rest with future investigators to confirm or disapprove, that by virtue of the evolutionary processes still going on in the human body, a high-powered conscious centre is being evolved by nature in the human brain at a place near the crown of the head built of exceptionally sensitive brain tissue. The location of the centre allows it to command all parts of the brain and the entire nervous system with a direct connection with the reproductive organs through the spinal canal. In the common man the budding centre draws its nourishment from the concentrated nerve food present in the seed in such extremely limited measure so as not to interfere with the normal reproductive function of the parts. When completely built the centre in evolved individuals is designed to function in place of the existing conscious centre, using for its activity a more powerful vital fuel extracted by nerve fibres from the body tissues in extremely minute quantities connected and rushed through the spinal tube into the brain.[39]

In light of this physicality, it follows, Gopi Krishna says, that various purificatory techniques and other means of disciplining and developing the body have historically been required by forms of yoga geared at awakening Kuṇḍalinī. But these systems do not have a monopoly on Kuṇḍalinī's effects. Rather, Kuṇḍalinī is the single force responsible for the special talents of mystics of all stripes—from renunciates to mediums—but also for the special talents of "men of genius," as Gopi Krishna continuously calls them, poets and scientists alike.

Here, then, is the vision of Kuṇḍalinī at which Gopi Krishna arrives after his two-and-a-half decades of searching:

> In the human body there exists an extremely subtle and intricate mechanism located in the sexual region which while active in the normal man in the naturally restricted form tends to develop the body generation after generation, subject of course to the vicissitudes of life, for the expression of a higher personality at the end; but when roused to rapid activity, it reacts strongly on the parent organism, effecting in course of time subject again to numerous factors, a marvellous transformation of the nervous system and the brain, resulting in the manifestation of a superior type of consciousness, which will be the common inheritance of man in the distant future. This mechanism, known as Kundalini, is the real cause of all genuine spiritual and psychic phenomena, the biological basis of evolution and development of personality, the secret origin of all esoteric and occult doctrines, the master key to the unsolved mystery of creation, the inexhaustible source of philosophy, art and science, and the fountainhead of all religious faiths, past, present and future.[40]

GOPI KRISHNA ON THE GLOBAL STAGE

One wonders what would have become of Gopi Krishna's story if he had not met the young James Hillman. Gopi Krishna, after all, never strove to become a guru. Would he have remained "a guy in the bazaar?" Or would his story have found some other way to weave itself into the web of Kuṇḍalinī lore on which it was already pulling, by virtue of his own striving toward understanding?

Hillman begins his commentary, which appears appended to the chapters of the original editions of *Kundalini: The Evolutionary Energy in Man*, with the following personal confession:

> On a hot day in the early summer of 1952, I remember going to the house of Gopi Krishna in Srinagar with my wife and two friends, Gerald Hanley and F.J. Hopman who has done so much to see that this book finally reached the public. We were all living in Kashmir and had come upon the work of Gopi Krishna at a local fair where a pamphlet of his poetry with a brief account of his experiences was distributed by one of his followers. I went on the visit out of curiosity, sceptically, critically, expecting a mountebank, ready to argue, disprove, and later perhaps laugh.
>
> I recall the heat, the flies, and my shirt stuck with sweat to the back of an old leather arm-chair. He sat on a cot, reposed, round-bodied, in white, smiling. The look of his skin seemed different from others I had met during the past year in Kashmir; then I thought he looked healthy, now I might say he glowed. I remember the simplicity in which our conversation took place. Above all, I remember the eyes of the man: friendly, luminous, huge, softly focussed. They attracted and held my attention and somehow convinced me that what was happening in this room and with this man was genuine. I visited him several times for talks before we left on a pony-trek to Shishnag and then the return to Europe. Because one or two unusual events occurred to me in the high mountains after meeting with Gopi Krishna, I tend to regard him as an initiator and a signal person in my life. Our meeting went deeper than I then realized. His eyes first led me to trust my own sight, my own convictions, beyond my

> trained sceptical Western mind. This was itself an initiation into actual psychological work which I only later took up.
>
> So it is with reverence to him and to the culture from which he has risen that I add these short comments as an act of gratitude. It is my intention neither to explain nor defend what Gopi Krishna has written, but only to relate where I am able some of his experiences to Western depth psychology, especially to the process of individuation as described in the Analytical Psychology of C. G. Jung.[41]

This highlights the personal and, indeed, the spiritually involved aspect of Hillman's contribution. Hillman's background, his experiences, and ultimately his model of Kuṇḍalinī are of a different world than those of Gopi Krishna. Yet the marriage (or, perhaps more accurately, respectful cohabitation) of their perspectives in that book is a striking example of the complex and at times contradictory state of modern understandings of Kuṇḍalinī.

Hillman's psychological commentary does indeed draw heavily on Jungian analysis. This makes for an interesting juxtaposition because it causes Hillman to almost entirely disregard the bodily dimension of Gopi Krishna's symptomology. It also leads to an interesting reinterpretation of the traditional cultural logics on which Gopi Krishna is himself drawing. For instance, Hillman makes interpretive moves like applying Western alchemical symbolism to Gopi Krishna's manipulation of the *iḍā* channel, evoking the gentle and cooling influence of the feminine moon. But of course, in Indian alchemy, the logics of which traditional formulations of Kuṇḍalinī generally follow, the moon is the repository of *bindu*, firmly connected to the masculine principle (as well as sexual fluid). "We would call this redemptive cooling grace of Ida the first appearance in our text of the archetypal effects of the anima," says Hillman.[42] Does this gendering matter? How much does it inflect how we interpret the experience? Certainly, it throws a wrench into the coherence of Gopi Krishna's own interpretation, given how much significance he ultimately places on the transmutation of seminal fluid.

Of course, Hillman's interpretation of the experience as one of Jungian individuation also diverges in the grander scheme from Gopi Krishna's own evolutionary explanation. One is psychological and symbolic; the other is biological and irrefutably physical. The book thus appears to the public as a juxtaposition of two distinctly modern (and, in their own ways, hybridized) but competing systems. One wonders what Gopi Krishna thought of this, given his later criticisms that he found Jung so "entirely preoccupied with his own theories about the unconscious" that he is able to find in his Asian sources "only material for the corroboration of his own ideas, and nothing beyond that."[43]

Both Gopi Krishna and his commentator, however, despite their other differences in interpretation, at least maintain the uncontested assumption that the body experiencing Kuṇḍalinī is male. This breaks down in the introduction to Gopi Krishna's second book, *The Biological Basis of Religion and Genius* (1972), penned by the German physicist Carl Friedrich Freiherr von Weizsäcker (1912–2007). Weizsäcker is also somewhat at a loss of what to do with Gopi Krishna's *bindu*-based argument. He half-heartedly tries to frame it in Freudian terms, before abandoning the effort to name and leave dangling the central difficulty. He writes:

> Gopi Krishna presents the sexual substance as nourishment of consciousness and not as its essence. His image of these phenomena is physiological and makes the claim of openness to physiological examination. It is a constantly recurring thought in his writings that no natural scientist will doubt the reality of these phenomena once he has observed and measured them. But does

> not the conflict here become finally inevitable and irreconcilable? What can physiology make of the thesis that the seminal substance wanders along the nerve paths to the brain? And how are we to account for the physiological difference between male and female sexuality here?[44]

And yet, Weizsäcker's introduction to Gopi Krishna's book is generous, and composed with great attention, charity, and care—not only toward the man who authored it, but the ideas contained within. Weizsäcker, a well-respected and highly accomplished physicist, was at an age as well as a stage in his career where he would be forgiven no small amount of eccentricity. He had by this time already turned his attention squarely to philosophical questions. Still, Weizsäcker's introduction makes it clear that he consented to put his name to the book not because he agreed with the thrust of every interpretation of science contained therein, but because he "would like to contribute to its understanding and its effect."[45]

Weizsäcker may not have agreed with Gopi Krishna's points about semen but, in the broad thrust of his evolutionary argument, the physicist-turned-philosopher found something that resonated with his own sense, based in quantum theory, of "probability amplitude" as a kind of "moving potency" or "the quantified expression of that toward which the 'flow of time' is pressing to evolve."[46] If Hillman's commentary represents one major direction that the marriage of mysticism and science has taken, Weizsäcker's introduction represents the other. Hillman's Jungian approach reads the subjective experience of the individual as a personal journey made legible through signs and symbols. Weizsäcker's use of quantum theory attempts to break down the barrier between subject and object.

Gopi Krishna would later comment that Weizsäcker's introduction to his book was "a landmark in [his] career as a writer," and that "it was this introduction that made many Western readers, more so the learned class, accept [his] works as something deserving attention."[47] Weizsäcker's contribution, notably, came after "Spiegelberg's preface and Hillman's commentary had broken the ice and affixed the seal of credibility to [Gopi Krishna's] first work."[48] Why does this matter? Well, at this stage, it would be difficult to imagine that it was the specifics of Gopi Krishna's interpretation—the evolutionary framing—that compelled these men to lend the credibility of their names and reputations to disseminating Gopi Krishna's work. In all cases, they appear to have been charmed by the man himself. Weizsäcker, like Hillman, reports entering his first meeting with Gopi Krishna with skepticism, only to be immediately overcome with his presence. Weizsäcker recounts:

> When the announced guest entered my room, I felt in the fraction of a second: This man is genuine. He was unassuming and sure of himself, a man who did not show his almost seventy years, who looked his partner firmly in the eyes, was dressed in the native clothing of a Brahman from Kashmir . . . he answered precise questions precisely, in a sometimes surprising way and with a deeply human sincerity which was often enhanced by a smile. His presence was good for me, and I could feel within me the traces of his simple and good emanations for as long as a month afterwards.

One feels the same fondness in Spiegelberg's preface. Gopi Krishna's presence is such that even his writing carries the imprint of it. This brings us to the other reason behind Hillman's and Weizsäcker's endorsements, which is the very same reason that Gopi Krishna's account has become a cornerstone of Kuṇḍalinī literature: there is a quality in his raw narration of experience that speaks to the experiences of others, even when they are not precisely the same.

Here it is helpful to return to Hillman. Hillman would later recall listening to Gopi Krishna's account of his Kuṇḍalinī awakening when they first met in 1952. The connection was not immediate, it seemed. As Gopi Krishna began to speak about spirit, Hillman found himself arguing that spirit and mind were both simply products of the body. "More or less squeezed out of the brain," he later puts it, as he reflects on this instance of what he calls "your basic Western, material, scientific thinking." Gopi Krishna, apparently, did not appreciate this. After he recovered from his initial shock, he proceeded to explain to Hillman the theory that would weave itself through all his subsequent work: that spirit, which he referred to as Kuṇḍalinī, was surely a biological mechanism, but it did not emerge from the body, and that it lay at the root of all genius and all mysticism, all religion, and quite a few brands of madness. Hillman would later identify this as an intellectual turning point—"a fantastic idea, revelatory," he writes. "This was a big moment for me, that somebody could think the opposite of the Western approach. Not that I'm choosing between two points of view, but it was an important relativization of my point of view, which I had simply assumed. And this actually turned out to be so close to the theory of neo-Platonism in Ficino [a Renaissance philosopher] that it did in fact still bear upon my later thinking. It was as if it rang a bell that was in my own philosophy, but hadn't been awakened."[49] Hillman would return to this point of resonance in his commentary, where he speaks of "the flow into the head of a living liquid light . . . called in Greek, Arabic, and medieval thought the 'breath,' 'the animal spirits,' or 'spirits of the soul.' "[50]

Much could be said about the foreign layers of meaning Hillman's commentary imposes onto Gopi Krishna's experience. The fixation on gender archetypes seems especially striking, in light of their distance from (and indeed occasional clash with) the tropes of Gopi Krishna's own tradition. But these impositions are fascinating, too—at least, if we take Hillman not as an impartial scholarly analyst, but as he introduces himself: an initiate and an experiencer. Decades later, Hillman would share the transformative event that befell him high in the Himalayan mountains. It was not the voice of God, as he had hoped. And no, nor was it Kuṇḍalinī. Not exactly. It was a dream—a nightmare, Hillman calls it, though there is nothing objectively terrifying in it—so simple that it seemed "embarrassing." Hillman saw his mother and grandmother sleeping in bunk beds. That was it. But his reaction was "horror and descent. As if to say, this is no holy place for me."[51] We could, of course, use our own framework to sit back in the proverbial armchair and psychoanalyze Hillman, just as he psychoanalyzes Gopi Krishna, using frameworks that are foreign to his experience. But perhaps it is enough to point out that, in the mountains of India, the feminine has rarely worn the face of "weakness, sensitivity and physical limitations," as Hillman paints it in his commentary.[52] After all, this was the land of Kaula tantra. Perhaps it was *not* the place for Hillman.

Hillman's Kuṇḍalinī experience, incidentally, would happen some months later, on the eve of his wedding, as he and his bride were lying in bed, discussing her feelings for her Anthroposophist ex-boyfriend.[53] "Suddenly, I felt lifted off the bed," Hillman would recall later. "I had the sensation of extreme heat in the sacrum. Starting from the base of the spine came an upward movement, all the way up the back of my neck to the scalp. My voice shot up high, my scalp stiffened and rolled back, pulling my eyes up, lifting the eye sockets. It almost knocked me out. I was terrified."[54] It was arguably this experience, which Hillman found he scarcely wanted to repeat, that led him the following year to begin his studies at the C. G. Jung Institute in Zürich.[55]

About a decade after their meeting, Gopi Krishna sent Hillman the manuscript of his book. Their now-mutual friend Hopman, who in those intervening years had had his own Kuṇḍalinī experience, had spent many years helping Gopi Krishna edit and publish the volume. Hillman, impressed with the manuscript, wrote to Aldous Huxley in 1963: "It is the honest report of the spontaneous appearance of

Kundalini, continuous (off and on) over many years . . . described in more detail than anything I have ever read. As a document of psychological interest I believe it should be published. I had the feeling that you might find the manuscript of interest, and might like writing an introduction."[56] Huxley was forced to decline due to ill health, and the task passed instead to Frederic Spiegelberg, who had just helped found the Esalen Institute some couple of years prior, and who no doubt found himself intrigued by the offer not only due to his interest in Indian religions but because he had attended Jung's 1932 seminars on Kuṇḍalinī.[57]

These connections, woven of resonances both cultural and personal, would launch Gopi Krishna and his story onto the global stage. And, once there, his story would not only be read by "the learned class," as Gopi Krishna called them—the countercultural movers and shakers, though they would read it also—but by regular practitioners and experiencers. Like Hillman, each of them would impose their own meaning upon it, and often one that was remote from the meaning it held to Gopi Krishna himself. But the story would change them too. The story would change Kuṇḍalinī.

6

THE SERPENT IN THE MARKETPLACE

Global Gurus Make Their Mark

I cannot be satisfied until I speak with angels
I require to behold the eye of god
to cast my own being into the cosmos as bait for miracles
to breathe air and spew visions
to unlock that door which stands already open and enter into the presence
of that which I cannot imagine

I require answers for which I have not yet learned the questions

I demand the access of enlightenment, the permutation into the miraculous
the presence of the unendurable light

perhaps in the same way that caterpillars demand their lepidoptera wings
or tadpoles demand their froghood
or the child of man demands his exit
from the safe warm womb

—LENORE KANDEL, "AGE OF CONSENT"

It would be false to say that Gopi Krishna opened the floodgates to Kuṇḍalinī moving into the West. As we've seen, accounts of Kuṇḍalinī had been slinking their way into the Western imagination for over a century by the time *Kundalini: The Evolutionary Energy in Man* hit the shelves in 1967. And the movement of ideas had hardly been one-directional, as Gopi Krishna's own work clearly shows. Still, a number of historical and cultural factors—including the countercultural revolution in the West and a crucial shift in immigration policy in the United States—combined to produce a new wave of South Asian gurus who began presenting their versions of Kuṇḍalinī to interested seekers across the world.

In this chapter, we will focus particularly on the concepts, stories, and approaches to practice constructed by some of the most famous of these teachers. In later chapters, however, we will also return to their legacies, including the teachings of their students, the centers they established, and the general ways that they have added nodes to the web of Kuṇḍalinī. The time period addressed in this chapter represents a sort of inflection point. Though it is not the beginning of Kuṇḍalinī's "popularization," it marks a juncture where, in the popular imagination, Kuṇḍalinī becomes inextricably bound to the idea of yoga. This connection does not come out of nowhere. As we saw in chapter 1, yogic methods were among a range of practices that have historically been used to raise Kuṇḍalinī. Such links persist among early modernizers of yoga, like those we examined in chapter 4. However, in this instance, the "bundling" of Kuṇḍalinī and yoga also becomes a "marketing tactic" in a way that reflects contemporary social and economic realities.

In the second half of the twentieth century, global gurus increasingly encountered audiences who knew what Kuṇḍalinī was, or at least they thought they did. A standard model was beginning to form, driven in large part by the popularly available written sources we have surveyed over the preceding chapters. Part of any guru's project, therefore, would have been to respond to this set of preconceptions, often by disagreeing with crucial parts of it. A common target—if only because it was an easy one—was the "master narrative" of the "Serpent Power." The serpent image was never literal, of course; not even in the Western sources that have their roots in Gnostic claims that the serpentine shape of the intestines betrays the mark of the serpent in the human body. But in the curious refusal of late twentieth-century gurus to identify Kuṇḍalinī as a serpent, we can glimpse the inner workings of what it meant to define yourself as a purveyor of Kuṇḍalinī in an increasingly crowded marketplace. Taking the Serpent Power literally is a rather obvious oversimplification, and so it would be tempting to see the avoidance of doing so as a move by gurus grounded in traditional lineages (a sticky notion in and of itself) resisting a "watering down" of authentic concepts and practices. This is certainly part of the story. However, we also see gurus taking jabs at one another's approaches, essentially trying to one-up each other for authenticity as they build their own "brands" of the best way to awaken Kuṇḍalinī.

Kuṇḍalinī as the Serpent Power may have been a compelling concept, but energy is difficult to package. Yoga, on the other hand, had by this point already become a known commodity. Packaging the two together, even if in name only, lent Kuṇḍalinī an air of concreteness. And so, even teachers like Swami Muktananda, whose "method" was not overly technical but consisted for the most part of simple devotion to the guru, adopted labels like "Siddha Yoga" to represent their teachings as an approachable brand.

This sort of capitalist approach to Kuṇḍalinī might strike the reader as being itself pessimistic at best and inauthentic at worst. We often think of the most famous gurus of the twentieth century—both those belonging to the first pre-World War II wave, with Vivekananda as their de facto leader, and to the second wave of the post-War hippie counterculture—as bringing traditional Indian wisdom to a spiritually starved West. However, as Andrea Jain has pointed out, Indian culture has not been exempt from either modernity or capitalism.[1] These are global phenomena. The gurus discussed in this chapter all first developed their followings in India. Their brands were already well formed when they made their way into the West. (The exception here is perhaps Amrit Desai, though we need only shift the focus to his own guru, Kripalvananda, popularly known as Bapuji, to make the generalization sound again.) Such trends were surely buttressed by an influx of spiritual tourism from Westerners, yet they are also not without domestic precedent. As market-savvy capitalists, modern gurus are a product of their time, both in India and abroad. And yet, we cannot ignore how the figure of the modern global guru—for better and for worse—continues a trend already woven into centuries (if not millennia) of South Asian history.

THE GRAVITY OF GURUS

To understand this continuity, we need to talk about gurus more generally. The oral quality of South Asian traditions has made the student–teacher relationship a key feature of the historical transmission of knowledge. This is all the more true of traditions that rely on embodied and especially esoteric practices, such as those involving Kuṇḍalinī. In the original Sanskrit, *guru* means literally "heavy," and it is one of several terms that one might use to address a teacher (some others being *ācārya* or *śāstrin*, both of which translate more or less as "teacher"). Traditionally, such terms are in fact titles that are granted to very advanced individuals through an established system of hierarchy. For instance, within the Southern Indian Śaiva Siddhānta and Vaiṣṇava Pāñcarātra tantric traditions, the *ācārya* is the highest of four possible stages in a hierarchy of initiated practitioners and the only one who has the authority to initiate others.

The very nature of the word "guru" is meant to signify the weighty and authoritative character of the role it represents. The traditional relationship between guru and disciple is indeed intensely hierarchical, requiring absolute commitment, obedience, and surrender. In other words, the relationship between a disciple and a guru is ultimately not so different from the relationship between a devotee and their god—over time, it becomes understood as *bhakti*: absolute interpenetrating dependence and devotion.

Though there is much precedent for it in earlier traditions, the role of the guru as a figure of religious authority matures into its prime during India's early medieval period (500–1200 CE). In contrast to the preceding age of sprawling empires, this historical period was characterized by smaller regional kingdoms vying for power. Rulers invested in building up rich cultural networks of architects, artists, scholars, and religious specialists, all of whom sought to elevate their particular kingdom and position it at the center of the civilized world.[2] In this context, individual holy men who could be directly accessible to their disciples—including their royal disciples-cum-patrons—became the chief preceptors of religion.[3]

Such a direct relationship is especially crucial in tantric traditions, which usually require the practitioner to be initiated into the secret ritual knowledge of their particular sect. Because tantric practice often works on the premise of transforming and perfecting the human body—rooted in the idea that to worship the divine you must first become divine yourself—the initiation is not a matter of simple intellectual teaching.[4] Instead, it is an embodied ritual in which the guru spiritually penetrates and enters the body of the disciple, clearing it of impurities and imbuing it with the divine cosmic energy (*śakti*) that his status allows him to wield.[5] In such a framework, it becomes all the more reasonable that the student should approach the guru (who is, after all, the most accomplished kind of practitioner) as a god in human form.

This aspect of the guru's power has been popularized on the modern global scene as *śaktipāt*, a "casting down of energy," touted as the quickest and most direct way to awaken Kuṇḍalinī. Because *śaktipāt* is an act of grace, bestowed by the guru upon a receptive disciple, it is perhaps the strongest example we have of the complete surrender and dependence that a traditional guru–disciple relationship would have entailed. The intimate connection embodied by the experience of *śaktipāt* lies at the heart of the communities of followers built by modern global gurus. However, as a means to an end—the end being an awakening of Kuṇḍalinī—*śaktipāt* also lends itself to easy commodification. It is literally something the guru can *give*.

The chief popularizer of this approach to Kuṇḍalinī was Swami Muktananda. His own experience of receiving *śaktipāt* from his guru was foundational to Muktananda's spiritual life. He therefore sought to offer this same experience to others, first at his ashram at Ganeshpuri and then through a series of weekend "Intensives," which he would conduct during his global tours. This, in Andrea Jain's words, made "the bestowal of *śaktipāt* to hundreds—and today, thousands—of people at a time efficient, cost-effective, and available for immediate consumption."[6] Muktananda would make his way around the room, tapping seekers with a bundle of peacock feathers. The spectrum of reported experiences ranged from blissful to terrifying.[7]

The shortcoming of such an approach, of course, is that it requires some form of direct contact with the guru. (Gurumayi Chidvilasananda, Muktananda's successor, has been known to give *śaktipāt* over webcast—it's not clear, however, whether such an experience is commensurate with the in-person version.[8]) Other gurus, such as Yogi Bhajan, privileged instead an easily transmissible method, encapsulated in a set of specific techniques that could be taught by anyone to anyone. Still others, such as Amrit Desai and Osho, sought to strike a balance between the unique personal touch of the guru and a reproducible technique that puts control in the hands of the individual practitioner.

It is easy to take a pessimistic perspective on the "commodification" of Kuṇḍalinī experience or of spirituality in general as some corruption wrought by the scourge of modern capitalism.[9] This is all the more true when we are dealing with concepts and practices that have their roots at least partially in non-Western cultures, which evoke the additional specters of colonialism and cultural appropriation. Without dismissing such concerns, we hope that the preceding chapters have been enough to show that things are in fact quite complicated when it comes to the latter charges. And, on this count, if commodification is a problem (which is itself a question we may want to consider with some care), then we need to ask who is doing the commodifying. Ultimately, it would be a mistake to dismiss the individual agency—and indeed the ambition—of the gurus themselves. One need only remember the young Paramahansa Yogananda standing on the bank of the Ganga at Dakshineswar, across from the headquarters of the International Ramakrishna Mission and Math, as he declared, "I will make mine bigger than theirs."[10] And, as we'll see in this chapter, popularizing gurus were quite comfortable with playing to their audiences' worldly interests. Even Muktananda, who encouraged a fairly traditional attitude of temperance and even celibacy from his devotees, spoke of Kuṇḍalinī awakening as a sort of prosperity gospel. "Kundalini is the wish-fulfilling tree," he said. "She will bring you whatever you want in this world."[11]

Finally, one cannot speak of global gurus without addressing the scandals (usually involving abuse of power, sexual impropriety, or both) that have, perhaps inevitably, erupted around every one of them. We question neither the truth of the reports—most of the modern cases are extremely well documented and supported by large numbers of witness and survivor accounts—nor the seriousness of the transgressions nor even, perhaps, the problematic nature of a "guru" as such. These accounts and the ethical conclusions that might be drawn from them have been extensively treated elsewhere and so we will not rehash them here. There is undoubtedly something to be said for the ways in which the potential for abuse present in any hierarchical system of authority is exacerbated by the deep intimacy, vulnerability, and unconditional surrender required by the traditional guru–disciple relationship. Amanda Lucia has suggested that the problem lies not only in the transgressions of individual gurus but in the very nature of the framework where they happen. The power attributed to the guru, his personal presence, and especially his touch create, in Lucia's words, "conditions wherein physical contact with the guru becomes a sacred opportunity, but also the high spiritual value placed on physical proximity to the guru has social ramifications. Special audiences, private meetings, and unconventional intimacies between guru and disciple are communally lauded as sacred. Such events are communally envisioned as a blessing for any devotee, and to reject an offering of proximity to the guru constitutes a radical social breech."[12]

In the wake of scandal, there is often an attempt within the affected community to separate the practice from the person transmitting it. And yet, the deeply intimate and experiential nature of Kuṇḍalinī muddies the waters here perhaps more so than anywhere else. It is one thing to accept that a set of teachings can retain its value even after we have lost faith in the teacher. This move mirrors Roland Barthes's notion of "the Death of the Author." Practices are what we make of them. But it is understandably more difficult to come to terms with the idea that an imperfect—even a deeply flawed and indeed violent—human being can make those he touches experience the divine.

And yet, if we are to take Kuṇḍalinī experiences seriously, this might be unavoidable. How else to make sense of the reports of disciples and practitioners? Perhaps we can get there by making the

Death of the Author (or, in this case, the Teacher) not simply epistemological—that is, dealing with how we make sense of a thing—but ontological. If we want to treat Kuṇḍalinī experience as a potentially genuine point of contact with some larger-than-human reality, then the human teacher quickly loses relevance. As Jeffrey J. Kripal has put it, "there simply is no necessary relationship between many forms of mystical, ecstatic, and visionary experience and a particular set of ethical norms and social values. They are certainly both true, but they are true in fundamentally different ways: they are functions of entirely different levels of the human being—one ultimate and one conventional, as a Buddhist philosopher might say."[13] On the topic of gurus, in particular, Kripal reminds us that approaching reality in this doubled fashion also "implies an appreciation for charismatic spiritual teachers, however imperfect or even abusive they might be as human persons. After all, by affirming the Human as Two, one can freely acknowledge and even honor mystical experiences on an ontological level without accepting, even condemning the moral behavior or political beliefs of a particular charismatic teacher on a moral or social level. An abusive jerk can be enlightened (and often is). An asshole can know himself as God (and often does)."[14]

To bring things full circle, we can extend this argument to the dynamics of capitalism as well. Just because an experience has been packaged and sold does not nullify that it was also experienced—and that, in being experienced, it touched something real and radically transformational.

KUṆḌALINĪ YOGA AS TAUGHT BY YOGI BHAJAN™

If there is one single name that is today associated with the practice of Kuṇḍalinī in the marketplace of popular spirituality, it is Yogi

Bhajan (1929–2004). Born Harbhajan Singh Puri to a Punjabi Sikh family, Yogi Bhajan arrived in North America in 1968 and quickly established himself as a teacher of yoga. The myth behind the man tells of Yogi Bhajan's tutelage, as a young boy, under a Sikh spiritual master named Sant Hazara Singh, who, through strict discipline and instruction so stern it bordered on brutal, inducted his student into the martial art of *gatakā* as well as the spiritual disciplines of "White Tantric Yoga" and "Kundalini Yoga." The discipleship reached its conclusion when the young Harbhajan was only sixteen, at which point Hazara Singh confirmed him a master of Kuṇḍalinī and declared that student and teacher were not to meet again. This made Yogi Bhajan the last link in the "Golden Chain" of an esoteric lineage of Kuṇḍalinī practice, stretching back to time immemorial.[15]

However, as Philip Deslippe has shown, the claims to lineage and antiquity made by Yogi Bhajan and canonized by his disciples are historically questionable at best.[16] This is not a unique fault. Any guru on the landscape of modern yoga who has tried to evoke ancient tradition to prop up their method of postural yoga has done so on shaky ground. The fact of the matter is that modern postural yoga—like modern *anything*—is simply not that old a formulation. This, in our view, does not invalidate the methods themselves. But we should perhaps be wary of the ways that claims to a lineage of ancient wisdom buttress claims to authority and authenticity.

There is an earlier version of Yogi Bhajan's origin story, which traces his enlightenment to a touch on the forehead by a different teacher, Maharaj Virsa Singh, a Sikh teacher living in New Delhi to whom he was introduced by his wife (Virsa Singh's original devotee) in the late 1960s when he was working as a customs officer at the Delhi airport. In his early days in Los Angeles, Yogi Bhajan claimed that it was Virsa Singh who had sent him to the West after ceremonially presenting him with his sandals,[17] a mark of the guru's grace. Deslippe has demonstrated that this, too, is only partially historically verifiable and—at best—not the full story. The physical elements of what would become Yogi Bhajan's hallmark "Kundalini Yoga" practice, which is indeed quite distinct from other popular forms of modern postural yoga, likely came from a Hindu yogi and physical trainer named Swami Dhirendra Brahmachari.[18] Dhirendra Brahmachari's system fused elements of *haṭha* yoga with an indigenous system of physical exercises often used by wrestlers known as *vyāyāma* (which indeed translates to something like "exercise") to produce what he called "Sūkṣma Vyāyāma" (Subtle Exercise).

As multiple scholars of modern yoga, including Joseph Alter, Jerome Armstrong, Mark Singleton, and Jason Birch, have demonstrated, such remixing of *haṭha* yoga methods with other forms of physical development, including *vyāyāma*,[19] was a common feature of Indian physical culture going at least as far back as the eighteenth century. The rhythmic swinging and rotating motions that appear so distinctive to Yogi Bhajan's "Kundalini Yoga," and which he refers to as *kriyās*, can also be found in the "Energization Exercises" that preface Paramahansa Yogananda's "Kriya Yoga" as the method still taught by his organization, the Self-Realization Fellowship. To formulate these (at least three decades before Yogi Bhajan or, indeed, Dhirendra Brahmachari), Yogananda likely drew on European forms of physical culture as much as on indigenous Indian ones.[20] Yogananda's Kriya Yoga is, of course, a method of raising Kuṇḍalinī (and indeed one that far more closely resembles the older medieval fusion of tantric Śaiva-Śakta *laya* and *haṭha* techniques). However, Yogananda viewed the calisthenic Energization Exercises as largely preparatory to Kriya Yoga; indeed, he never referred to them as "yoga" proper, nor as *kriyās* more specifically. This, to be clear, does not mean one cannot do so. Tradition is an evolving thing. But such areas of overlap between innovators also make one wonder how the current "market share" on Kuṇḍalini, *kriyā* practice, and yoga at large might have been shaped differently.

Yogi Bhajan's presence as a preceptor of Kuṇḍalinī is chiefly embodied by the Healthy, Happy, Holy Organization, commonly known as 3HO, as well as the Kundalini Research Institute. There is also Sikh Dharma International, founded in 1973 as the Sikh Dharma Brotherhood and later called Sikh Dharma for the Western Hemisphere, which represents the more overtly religious face of Yogi Bhajan's guru persona. Besides these, Yogi Bhajan left behind a veritable juggernaut of capitalist ventures, assembled under the name of Khalsa International Industries and Trades. All in all, the man had a hand in creating seventeen businesses, ranging from beauty products to a security firm.[21] One of these was the American tea brand, found today on the shelves of nearly every mainstream supermarket, known as Yogi Tea. The tags attached to its tea bags still feature select words of wisdom attributed to Yogi Bhajan. These facts may seem like unrelated trivia, but they are actually crucial to understanding the cultural impact of "Kundalini Yoga as taught by Yogi Bhajan." To Yogi Bhajan, Kuṇḍalinī was a brand, and it was one he went about developing with all the acumen of a businessman, keeping a strategic eye on image and competition.

Yogi Bhajan's devotees, and so, therefore, many of the top teachers of his Kundalini Yoga, are instantly recognizable. They are turbaned men and women—the latter being unusual if not wholly unprecedented from an ethnically Punjabi Sikh standpoint—dressed all in white (also culturally idiosyncratic). Teachers who place themselves in Yogi Bhajan's lineage are careful to specify that what they are representing is Kuṇḍalinī yoga "as taught by Yogi Bhajan." On the one hand, of course, this implicitly allows for the existence of many different types of yoga and methods of engaging with Kuṇḍalinī. On the other hand, however, it serves to further reinforce the link between the otherwise generic notion of Kuṇḍalinī yoga, and the specific "brand" associated with Yogi Bhajan's name.

Perhaps more so than any other figure mentioned in this chapter, Yogi Bhajan represents the split between a guru as the charismatic leader of a community—the tightknit body of devotees that creates the social conditions rife for abuse and enough whispers of "cult" to inevitably yield a documentary exposé once the dust has settled—and the popularizing brand mascot. And Kundalini Yoga as taught by Yogi Bhajan has outgrown the tarnished legacy of its founder enough that it seems likely to survive regardless of what happens to the community that first supported it. Its relatively simple rhythmic movements, which become challenging due to the length at which one must repeat them, combined with the shallow and rapid diaphragmatic breathing known as *bhastrikā* (sometimes also known as "bellows breathing," but named "Breath of Fire" by Yogi Bhajan) are distinctive among popular varieties of things called "yoga" today.[22] Again, this is not to say that they are entirely original or wholly unprecedented on the yoga scene, but they have become a recognizable part of the brand. Moreover, the identification of Yogi Bhajan's brand with Kuṇḍalinī practice in general is likely to act as a continuous lifeline, despite the fact that the method diverges from most other current forms of Kuṇḍalinī-oriented practice.

This is the ingenious key to Yogi Bhajan's approach. From the start, it billed itself as generic even as it was highly specific. "You may have heard of transcendental meditation and integral meditation; there are many labels," says Yogi Bhajan. "Just as there are for mustard seed: yellow mustard seed, sunflower mustard seed, Sun Valley mustard seed, California mustard seed, Wisconsin mustard seed, New York Mustard seed; mustard seed is mustard seed. Similarly, different techniques of yoga have been given different names. Hatha yoga has the same end. Bhakti, shakti, gian [i.e. *jñāna*], karma yoga—all have the same end. To raise the dormant power of infinity in the man; that's all."[23]

Of course, to assert that all yogas lead to Kuṇḍalinī awakening is a move we have seen before. This was the position taken by Vivekananda, Sivananda, and even (in his own way) Aurobindo. It is also, as we will soon see, very much like the stance of Muktananda with regard to his Siddha Yoga. However, while Yogi Bhajan explicitly acknowledges the multiplicity of methods, his teachings (and, not unsurprisingly, the arguments of his disciples) imply again and again that it is his method that is superior and his understanding that is correct. For example, the 3HO contribution to *Kundalini: Evolution and Enlightenment*, a collection of available sources on Kuṇḍalinī edited by John White and published in 1979, is incredibly strategic in its framing and subject matter. The piece, aptly titled "Exploring the Myths and Misconceptions of Kundalini," begins with an introduction by disciple Gurucharan Singh Khalsa that offers a laundry list of condemnations: Gopi Krishna, Vasant Rele, Arthur Avalon, Joseph Campbell, Ram Dass—all of them got Kuṇḍalinī wrong. (Swami Vivekananda, interestingly, gets a pass, as does Sivananda.) Since he began teaching in the United States in January of 1969, Gurucharan writes, Yogi Bhajan "was, and still is, the only recognized master of kundalini yoga."[24]

The appended "Question and Answer" session with Yogi Bhajan does not go so far as to name names, but likewise implicitly addresses popular contemporary understandings of Kuṇḍalinī, including those represented by competing gurus. "Does a student of the kundalini yoga have to be celibate?"[25] (For example, as Muktananda's disciples commonly were.) No. "When the kundalini rises, do you go into trance or become rigid?"[26] (As most available accounts of Kuṇḍalinī experience would have reported.) No. "What about people who have great visions and psychic experiences, or whose bodies jerk and tremble after meditation? Is this the Kundalini rising?"[27] (Likewise as commonly reported, especially by disciples of contemporary *śaktipāt*-bestowing gurus, including Muktananda and Amrit Desai).

Also no. Or at least, this is not Kuṇḍalinī awakening itself but only "glitter at the bottom of the ladder."[28] Indeed, Yogi Bhajan also rejects the usefulness of *śaktipāt* itself, stating that "kundalini can be stimulated directly by a teacher. But that teacher is not much of a teacher! The students should be prepared, then given a technology to raise in themselves. Why should they wait at the feet of that teacher like puppies? They should go through the experience, then share the techniques with others."[29]

While Yogi Bhajan's teachings draw heavily on ideas and practices originating in Hindu (especially Śaiva-Śākta) traditions, he has also consistently mixed these elements both with Western spirituality as well as logics rooted in his native Sikh background. One clear example of this is his stance on not cutting one's hair (a traditional Sikh practice), which he not only reinterprets but indeed uses to, in turn, reinterpret the very definition of Kuṇḍalinī. When asked whether it is necessary to grow one's hair in order to practice his Kundalini Yoga, as most of his students do, Yogi Bhajan replies:

> No. You can practice with any length hair, but the hair was the first technique to raise the kundalini energy. When the hair is at its natural full length and coiled over the anterior fontenelle for men or the posterior fontenelle [*sic*] for women, it draws pranic energy into the spine. The force of this downward positive energy causes the kundalini energy to rise for balance. This is why you always find grace and calmness in a person with uncut hair from birth if they keep it well. Actually the hair was so important that the word consciousness, kundalini, actually derives from "kundal" which means "a coil of the beloved's hair."[30]

Such claims, of course, no more mirror the understandings of mainstream Sikhs than they do those of practitioners of Hindu tantra. The theory is a novel remixing of a Sikh practice (not cutting the hair) with a Hindu tantric concept (Kuṇḍalinī as a coiled energy associated with the spine) and a Western esoteric logic (likely the harmonial understanding of spiritual influx).[31]

Indeed, scholars who have looked at 3HO and Yogi Bhajan's Sikh Dharma, such as Constance Waeber Elsberg and Doris Jacobs,[32] have repeatedly noted tensions between Yogi Bhajan and his white followers on the one hand and ethnically Punjabi Sikhs on the other. In particular, Elsberg has suggested that Yogi Bhajan's desire to gain the approval of traditional Sikh organizations, who took issue with his teaching of tantric practices as well as the liberal behaviors of his disciples, was at least partially responsible for his restrictive treatment of women.[33]

This blending of tradition(s) and social interests is also key to Yogi Bhajan's understanding of the very thing he named his method after: Kuṇḍalinī Herself. This understanding, interestingly, though perhaps not surprisingly, is rather amorphous since it is not grounded in a single specific religious or conceptual background. At one point he says, drawing on the same syncretic symbolism of hair: "The fundamental awareness is the fundamental uncoiling of oneself, the kundalini. What is kundalini? It is not a serpent power. Kundalini means kundal. Kundal means lock of the beloved's hair. Uncoiling the coil within yourself, that is what kundalini means—the energy to be uncoiled."[34] Elsewhere, he takes on a more physiologically grounded approach reminiscent of the innate evolutionary models of teachers like Vivekananda, Aurobindo, and Gopi Krishna:

> What is kundalini? The energy of the glandular system combines with the nervous system to become more sensitive so that the totality of the brain perceives signals and interprets them, so that the effect of the sequence of the cause becomes clear to the man. In other words, man becomes totally, wholesomely aware. That

> is why we call it the yoga of awareness. As the rivers end up in the same ocean, all yoga ends up by raising kundalini in the man. What is the kundalini? The creative potential of the man.[35]

In its general public-facing version, Kundalini Yoga as taught by Yogi Bhajan has tamed Kuṇḍalinī into a sort of optimized state for the organism. It explicitly rejects the disorienting, the extreme, and the numinous. "Hallucinations, psychism and nerve weaknesses mean nothing," says Yogi Bhajan.[36] Instead, "a raised Kundalini will give you grace of motion. Life fills every cell, so you're able to move smoothly with an awareness of the rhythm and music of all your environments. The Kundalini makes you alive and graceful, not rigid like some kind of death."[37] This is yoga for the ordinary "householder," to make them "healthy, happy, and holy."

In this sense, we might propose that Kundalini Yoga as taught by Yogi Bhajan has grown in popularity in part by routinizing Kuṇḍalinī and de-emphasizing the kinds of radically transformational states that other sources and teachers have associated with Kuṇḍalinī awakening. A successful brand, after all, attempts to capture as broad a demographic as possible.

BY THE GRACE OF THE GURU: *ŚAKTIPĀT* AND MUKTANANDA'S SIDDHA YOGA

If Yogi Bhajan's legacy as a celebrity guru is primarily method-driven, then his opposite pole might be found in someone like Muktananda, the paradigmatic "*śaktipāt* guru."[38] *Śaktipāt* and Kuṇḍalinī are certainly related terms, but they are not identical, and so we would do well to differentiate how they have been understood both by the gurus who wield them and by the practitioners who have reported experiencing them.

Most typically tied to nondual Śaiva-Śākta traditions, *śaktipāt* is a phenomenon in which the guru's *śakti* (that is, his awakened divine energy) enters into and activates the subtle body of the disciple. Effectively, it is a kind of intentional energetic contagion, and it is usually understood as the first step to Kuṇḍalinī awakening, if not the awakening itself. This phenomenon of "energetic possession" by the guru has historically been referred to using a number of terms, including *vedha dīkṣā* (initiation by piercing) and *samāveśa* (co-penetration),[39] and it would have traditionally signified a formal act of initiation by the guru bestowing it. In this sense, gurus who offered *śaktipāt* to large groups of people they had never met at retreats, or at weekend "Intensives" occasionally staged in a suburban living room,[40] were not doing something traditional. And, for the very same reason, they can be thought of as popularizers in the truest sense of the word.

The key here is that *śaktipāt* is not a technique that can be taught, like a set of exercises. It is an act of the guru as a conduit of the divine in which the recipient is utterly passive. As Muktananda liked to say, quoting the *Śivasūtravimarśinī* of Kṣemarāja, "the Guru is the grace-bestowing power of God."[41] In *śaktipāt*, you do not awaken your Kuṇḍalinī; your Kuṇḍalinī awakens you.

Muktananda (1908–1982) was born as Krishna Rai in Karnataka. After a long period of spiritual exploration, he became the disciple of a man named Nityananda (1897–1961) at an ashram in Ganeshpuri, and it was from Nityananda that he received his *śaktipāt* initiation on the morning of August 15, 1947.[42] Because *śaktipāt* experiences are context-specific and rely on a layered narrative of setting, mental state, emotional response, and insights that literally transcend language, they are very difficult to excerpt succinctly, much less summarize. For this reason, we will be relying on some fairly lengthy quoted passages in this section, so that we stand some chance of conveying how and why those who experience *śaktipāt* find it transformational. Muktananda's account, which appears in his spiritual autobiography, *Play of Consciousness* (1974), is the first of these, and it goes like this:

> The sun had risen slightly in the sky, and the atmosphere was tranquil. I was standing in the corner, to the east, contemplating my Guru. In the opposite corner stood Monappa, Gurudev's cook. In the meditation hall, Gurudev was making little humming sounds in his throat, indicating he was about to get up from his meditation on the Self, and in a little while he came out. He looked a little different than usual; in fact, I had never seen him looking like this before. He had on a beautiful pair of wooden sandals, and as he walked to and fro, to and fro, he was smiling. At one point he went into a corner and began to chant some secret mantras. Then he came in front of me and smiled again. He began to sing. He was wearing a white shawl, and underneath it only a loincloth and the sandals on his feet. He kept coming and standing in front of me, making his familiar noise of endearment. An hour passed like this.
>
> Then he came near me and touched my body with his. My body was stunned with this new wonder. I stood facing west. Gurudev, his body close to mine, stood opposite. I opened my eyes, and saw Gurudev gazing directly at me, his eyes merging with mine, in the *shambhavi mudrā*. My body became numb. I couldn't shut my eyes; I no longer had the power to open or close them. The divine splendor of his eyes completely stilled my own eyes. We stayed like this for a while. Then I heard the divine sound of Gurudev's "hunh." He stepped back a couple of paces, and I partially regained my consciousness. He said, "Take these sandals, put them on." Then he asked, "You'll wear my sandals?" I was amazed, but replied reverently and firmly, "Gurudev, these sandals are not to be worn by my feet. Babaji, they are for me to

> worship all my life. I'll spread my shawl, and then please be so gracious as to put your feet on it and leave your sandals there."
>
> Gurudev agreed. Making the same humming sounds, he lifted his left foot, and its sandal, and placed it on the edge of my outspread shawl. Then he put his foot down, raised his right foot, and placed the other sandal on the shawl. He stood directly in front of me. He looked into my eyes once more. I watched him very attentively. A ray of light was coming from his pupils, and going right inside me. Its touch was searing, red hot, and its brilliance dazzled my eyes like a high-powered bulb. As this ray flowed from Bhagawan Nityananda's eyes into my own, the very hair on my body rose in wonder, awe, ecstasy, and fear. I went on repeating his mantra *Guru Om*, watching the colors of this ray. It was an unbroken stream of divine radiance. Sometimes it was the color of molten gold, sometimes saffron, sometimes a deep blue, more lustrous than a shining star. I stood there, stunned, watching the brilliant rays passing into me. My body was completely motionless. Then Gurudev moved a little and again made his "hunh, hunh." I became conscious again. I bowed my head upon the sandals, wrapped them in the shawl, and prostrated myself on the ground. Then I got up, full of joy.[43]

At least a few things are immediately of note here. The first is the relative ordinariness of the event, at least from the outside. This is not a formal ritual setting. In fact, an external observer might not have noted what had happened at all, aside from the fact that the interaction between the two men had been a little strange. The second is the intimacy of the encounter, as well as the physicality. Throughout, Muktananda is acutely aware of his guru's body as well as his own. The most tangible vehicle of the exchange is Nityananda's sandals (recall, here, Yogi Bhajan's ceremonial gift from his own teacher). The third is the ultimately ineffable quality of the transcendent experience. We are told of the physical sensation ("searing, red hot") and Muktananda's emotional state ("wonder, awe, ecstasy, and fear," and later, finally "joy"), but the content of the thing itself can only be described as an iridescent stream of light.

An account by an anonymous scholar-practitioner who received *śaktipāt* from Muktananda at a weekend Intensive in Florida in 1975 attempts to assign more explicit meaning to the insight gained, but it does so with great caution:

> Then, at last, I almost jumped when the peacock feathers, firmly but with a soft weightiness, hit me repeatedly on my head, and then gently brushed my face as Swamiji, with a quiet rumbling in the back of his throat, powerfully pressed one of his fingers into my forehead, at a spot located just between my eyebrows . . . Here's where I feel like I need to begin to step very carefully. I'm honestly somewhat reluctant to write about what happened next because I know that whatever I say will inevitably diminish it, will make it sound as if it were just another "powerful experience." This was not an experience. This was THE event of my spiritual life. This was full awakening. This wasn't "knowing" anything, because you only know something that is separate from you. This was being: the Ultimate—a fountain of Light, a dancing, ever-new Source. Utter freedom, utter joy, swirling with unfettered delight at the center of it all, the Heart of the cosmos, pouring out everything from my own Self, yet always having More. Completely fulfilled, completely whole, no limits to my power and love and light. The Lord of the Universe. This was my true nature. Eternally. Always. I never have been anything different than this, ever, not even in a dream. Not even when I forget.[44]

Another published account by poet and literary critic Paul Zweig (1935–1984) speaks in similar terms of a meeting that likely happened sometime in the late 1970s at a temporary "ashram" in New York. Unlike the anonymous young man from the previous account, who had already had a previous experience of insight and was searching for more, Zweig came in as a skeptic. He had been invited by a friend he had not seen in some time, who had gone to India to "shop around for a guru" and ended up spending three and a half years in Muktananda's ashram. At the session Zweig attended in New York, Muktananda did not make the rounds with his wand of peacock feathers; he simply answered questions. In fact, Muktananda never touched Zweig at all; and yet, the account is strikingly similar in its spirit:

> I found myself paying attention suddenly, not so much to what the woman said as to a feeling of vulnerability in her voice. When she meditated, the experience of a silvery light was intense, but then nightmarish forms came between her and the light, and she was frightened. Her voice became increasingly tenuous as she talked, and then it broke. I could tell she was crying. She had lifted up a hand, as if to describe the nightmares, and I saw that it was shaking. And suddenly I was shaking too. I felt as if I were rooted to the floor, trembling with intense feeling. I became aware that I had to make an effort not to cry, yet it wasn't simply crying, for my body had become buoyant and warm. I stared at the woman's hand sketching a movement in the air: it was pale, delicate. Even after the hand was tucked away in her lap, and Muktananda's voice had begun to speak an answer, I went on staring. My eyes seemed to be peering out of a deep, silvery tunnel, while the forms and colors of the room glided across their surface like paper cutouts.

> The words, "afloat in tears," repeated themselves over and over in my mind. With no transition I seemed to be seeing my life from a new angle. An overwhelming idea had seized hold of me: all of us did our best against suffering and useless pain. Those nightmarish forms the woman had talked about were the element of my life, and everyone's life. All of us sitting in this room were on the point of crying out, for we existed far from the light. I had accomplished all sorts of things in my life. I had a position in the world; I wrote books; I was a discriminating person who cringed from the naïve self-importance of these "kids." Yet nothing I had done meant a thing from the viewpoint of that light. I too was defenseless, full of longing; and we were equal, because we were human. Great clots seemed to be floating loose in my mind. Shapes so old they had come to seem part of the landscape were breaking up, and through the cracks in their ruin tears poured, like an imprisoned element suddenly set free.
>
> As I stared at Muktananda's quick aimless movements, I was aware that my mouth was hanging open, but I couldn't seem to close it. For some reason I wasn't frightened; I was even pleased, though I wouldn't say why. Muktananda had done this, but what had he done, and how? We hadn't talked much, and he had hardly looked at me. He was not especially charismatic: no great gestures or fixed, piercing glances. He moved around a lot, and played with his fingers. All the while I was holding back my tears by an effort of subtle attention. The tears seeped onto my face anyway, a few at a time.[45]

Interestingly, Zweig's experience is actually prompted by the experience of another—not Muktananda—and yet he is certain that it was Muktananda who did *this* to him. Interesting, too, is Zweig's observation that Muktananda's presence was not of the sort we normally associate with charisma. He was not particularly impressive, physically. It was nothing about his voice or demeanor. And yet, it was there. Something happened, and it was Muktananda who did it.

Following the Kaula tradition, Muktananda understood Kuṇḍalinī in its strongest sense, as the divine essence of the cosmos. Though he did use the term "Kuṇḍalinī," even more frequently he referred to "Chiti" (Sanskrit: *citi*), which he translated as "consciousness." This was the light he experienced radiating from Nityananda's eyes, which he came to refer to as the "Blue Pearl," or "Neeleshwari, the Blue Goddess, who is all in all—Chiti, Kundalini, Parashakti, the Absolute, God, the Guru, Soul, the Abode of Supreme Peace. . . . the self-luminous Chitshakti, playing in the form of the universe."[46] His method would come to be known as Siddha Yoga, after the "Perfected Ones," the quasi-mythic tantric adepts who had started out as human but became gods.

According to Muktananda, the guru can bestow *śaktipāt* in four ways: touch, an enlivened mantra, a look, and mere thought.[47] This is the special province of the guru. "Only a doctor is qualified to give medicine, a lawyer to practice law, a teacher to teach. Similarly, only a Guru can activate Kundalini,"[48] he would say. For Muktananda, the guru and Kuṇḍalinī are so closely intwined as to be one. Both embody, in their essence, the divine power of grace. He explains:

> When the disciple is initiated, the Guru's Shakti enters him. As a tree exists in the form of a seed, so the Shakti exists in the form of the Guru, and entering the disciple, it induces many types of yogic movements. As the seeker, remembering his beloved Guru, sits for meditation, identifying himself with the Guru and repeating the Guru's mantra, then the Guru in the form of the mantra becomes active within him. These movements, or kriyas, are not meaningless or fruitless. It is the Guru's Shakti which works

> inside in the form of these kriyas, producing many different contortions of the body, many kinds of yogic postures, pranayama, dances, mantras, and mudras. If anybody were to see these from the outside, they would look very strange and frightening, but the seeker is not afraid. He experiences from these movements a kind of intoxication, an ecstasy, a lightness of the limbs, a sturdiness of the body. Some of the kriyas are a part of Raja Yoga, some of Hatha Yoga, some of Mantra Yoga, and some of Bhakti Yoga, for when the power of the Guru enters the disciple, all these yogas occur spontaneously according to the disciple's needs.[49]

Śaktipāt initiates the practitioner into—or, more accurately, it induces—the process of Siddha Yoga, which Muktananda translates as the "perfect yoga." He also calls it "Maha Yoga" or the "great yoga." This is because it effectively contains all the other yogas within it.[50] When Kuṇḍalinī is awakened by the grace of the guru, the *haṭha*-yogic *kriyās*, such as various forms of *prāṇāyāma*, *āsanas*, *bandhas*, and *mudrās*, begin to manifest in the body spontaneously, says Muktananda.[51] Techniques that might otherwise take years to learn and perfect come naturally, whether the practitioner knows them or not. And, while this may seem like an unfair shortcut, Muktananda explains that it is better than doing it the hard way. Because Kuṇḍalinī is a sentient force, She knows precisely what the practitioner's particular organism requires. Effectively, Kuṇḍalinī is the will of the guru, which is also the will of the divine, working within the disciple.

While Siddha Yoga is a method, the technique of it is basically devotional. For instance, chanting is a core practice. One can chant the names of God, or a longer text such as the *Guru Gītā*, or simply "Guru Om," as Muktananda did. Ultimately, the method does not depend on anything the practitioner does. The method is grace.

A METHOD FOR GRACE DEFERRED: THE CASE OF AMRIT DESAI

However, this is not to say that the logics of *śaktipāt*, which depend on the autonomous force of the divine, are incompatible with a more intentional method of practice. A good case in point here is Amrit Desai (1932–), the founder of Kripalu Yoga as well as the Kripalu Center for Yoga and Health, which persists today—albeit without Desai's involvement, following a series of scandals—as one of the largest spiritual retreat centers in North America.[52]

Desai met his guru seemingly by chance at the age of fifteen. He had been occupied with teaching himself yoga *āsana* from wall posters at a local exercise center in Halol, Gujarat, when he happened upon Swami Kripalvananda who had been using a room in the building for his daily meditation while visiting the city. From this time onward, Desai's family maintained close ties with the swami.[53]

Desai first came to the United States to study at the Philadelphia College of Art, pursuing an existing interest not out of character with his somewhat eclectic background. To make ends meet he washed dishes at the college, worked nights at a paper bag company, and on the weekends he would teach yoga and fashion design classes at an adult education center. Desai continued to pursue his interest in art after graduating from the college in 1964, but it must have eventually become apparent that teaching yoga held far more promise. When Desai saw Kripalvananda on a return visit to India in 1966, he walked away from the meeting with an initiation, a set of instructions, and a blessing. More such meetings would follow.[54] Ultimately, Desai would name both his method and his yoga center "Kripalu," in honor of his guru.

This is where things take an interesting turn. Desai's relationship with Kripalvananda was clearly an important part of his journey as both a practitioner and a teacher. However, Desai's *śaktipāt* experience actualized itself not as he was staring into the eyes of his guru, but while he was practicing *āsana*, and he found that he could return to that extraordinary state of consciousness at will though postural practice. This combination would become foundational to the five-stage practice he would formalize as "Kripalu Yoga." Desai describes further:

> One morning in 1970 I was performing my daily routine of yoga postures in the meditation room of my home in Philadelphia. . . . A tape recording of yogic chanting by my guru, Swami Shri Kripalvanandji, played in the background. The intonations of his voice and the gentle background accompaniment of the drum stirred feelings of love and deep reverence within me that led me to perform my daily routine with special concentration that morning. As I continued to move, I became absorbed in the rhythm of the chants. Gradually I became more and more relaxed and absorbed, even while my body continued to move. My movements flowed with the chanting.
>
> Suddenly, like an unexpected spring downpour, bliss flooded throughout my entire being, and I felt myself being irresistibly drawn to another level of consciousness. As my mind was drawn more and more inward, and the external surroundings dissolved far into the background, I began to feel that I was no longer the performer of the exercises; they were being performed through me.
>
> A new flow of energy coursed throughout my system, and with no conscious effort on my part, my body spontaneously began to twist and turn on its own, flowing smoothly from one posture to the next. The movements were effortless and free, a command and a gift from a newly opened, higher dimension of my inner being. My body became extraordinarily elastic and stretched smoothly and easily beyond its previous limits. I was

> moving in perfect rhythm with the whole universe. I was not aware of giving any direction to the movements. Thoughts continued to come, but now they passed through my mind in slow motion, seemingly disconnected from my body's activity. I realized that if I wished, I could stop this experience, and yet I had no desire to do so. . . . One after another the postures flowed. Some of them were traditional yoga exercises; others were movements which I had never seen before. Gradually, I became more and more absorbed in my experience. At the end of this flow of postures, my body naturally entered the lotus position, and a deep stillness, so deep that it penetrated every level of my being. Then a second explosion of ecstasy spread through me, and I became engulfed, overwhelmed, by a state of complete inner bliss.[55]

Desai's wife Urmila, as well as two of his students, had been practicing in the room with him. From their external vantage point, they, too, had felt whatever had happened to Desai. It was a comment from Urmila that ultimately helped Desai make sense of his experience. She called his movements "automatic." It was then that Desai remembered the only other time when he had seen someone move automatically. When Desai was seventeen, his guru had allowed him the special privilege of joining him in his meditation room; this was how Desai had seen Kripalvananda move.[56] Still not quite believing the logical conclusion, Desai wrote to his guru for confirmation. It was in his reply that Kripalvananda revealed that during Desai's last visit to India the prior year, the guru had bestowed a mild *śaktipāt* upon his unknowing disciple. The ensuing experience was the flowering of that seed, fed by Desai's diligent practice.[57] On his next visit, Desai received a formal *śaktipāt* initiation from his guru, as well as a blessing to bestow *śaktipāt* upon others.[58]

Notably, Kripalvananda differentiated (and Desai continued to differentiate) between what happened to Desai and "full" Kuṇḍalinī awakening. The former was the awakening of *prāṇa* (or, more literally, the "raising of *prāṇa*," *prāṇotthāna*), understood as a precursor to the awakening of Kuṇḍalinī.[59] To some extent, this is a technical distinction that proves to be more of semantics than of substance, once one digs into it. Desai's explanation of *prāṇa* closely mirrors the three-Kuṇḍalinī model of tenth-century nondual Śaiva philosopher Abhinavagupta, who speaks of *prāṇakuṇḍalinī* as associated with life force, *śaktikuṇḍalinī* as the power of creation, and *parākuṇḍalinī*, who is the supreme Goddess.[60] Given that Kripalvananda traced his lineage through the medieval Siddha tradition, including the Nāths who produced much of the medieval *haṭha* literature combining visionary (and Kuṇḍalinī-centric) Kaula tantra with physical techniques, all the way back to the ancient Śaiva Pāśupata sect,[61] slotting Desai into this framework is not a stretch. But it is perhaps significant that this distinction meant that Desai did not speak of his method, which he referred to as "Meditation-in-Motion" or "Kripalu Yoga," as Kuṇḍalinī yoga, or even as a method to raise Kuṇḍalinī more generally.

Basic yoga practice (which Desai ambiguously refers to as "Ashtang yoga," likely an oblique reference to Patañjali) is willful; it is the mind doing the work. In Kuṇḍalinī yoga, meanwhile, the mind is fully surrendered to the autonomous working of the *prāṇa*. Kripalu Yoga is a middle path between the two.[62] Through physical relaxation, deep rhythmic breathing, and focused attention on internal experience, the postures—and this is key: Kripalu Yoga is *postural* yoga—become "effortless and spontaneous." "In this state," says Desai, "the innate intelligence of prana, the wisdom of the body, takes over and the mind becomes merely a choiceless witness. The body is then able to respond to its own needs and chooses with extraordinary intelligence whatever sequences of postures, pranayama, kriyas, mudras, meditations, resting periods may be necessary to remove the energy blocks and tensions which create weakness and disease in the body-mind."[63] This, of course, sounds quite a bit like Muktananda's discussion of how *śaktipāt* induces the body to spontaneously perform whatever *kriyās* the individual student's constitution requires. However, Desai's way of talking about the phenomenon stops at the level of *prāṇa*, leaving the practice's relationship to Kuṇḍalinī somewhat ambiguous. Ironically, this means that the only "Kundalini Yoga" taught at the Kripalu center today is of the Yogi Bhajan variety.

Consequently, neither Desai nor Kripalu are very firmly associated with Kuṇḍalinī in the public imagination, despite Desai's fame as a *śaktipāt* guru. And yet, when students of Desai speak of their experience, they reliably fall back on what, by the second half of the twentieth century, has become the standard tropes of Kuṇḍalinī. For example, Kripalu practitioner Stephen Cope, who is a continuing scholar-in-residence at the Kripalu Center, writes of his experience while watching Desai demonstrate his Meditation-in-Motion:

> As Amrit entered deeper into the dance, the entire room seemed to be pulled down by a deep undertow of absorption. We were lost with him in the dance of energy. . . . I noticed a change in my perception. Colors had become brighter, bolder. The blue and gold tiles behind the altar were fairly pulsing with flashing hues. Light itself had become a palpable golden presence. At moments the whole room dissolved into waves of light, particles of energy. And all the while, I felt the whole room breathing together and somehow moving together, pulsing and expanding and contracting. At one point, I had an experience of energy rushing up and down my spine, as I'd had when he'd touch me, a tingling at the crown of my head, my whole body suffused with an intense heat.[64]

In general, the accounts of *śaktipāt* reported in Desai's presence prove every bit as intense as those attributed to Muktananda.

THE GURU OF RADICAL AUTHENTICITY

Before Osho (1931–1990) was Osho (as he rebranded himself toward the end of his life),[65] he was Bhagwan Shree Rajneesh, and before that he was Rajneesh Chandra Mohan, born into a wealthy Jain family in a village in Madhya Pradesh. As an adult, he received a master's degree and for nine years taught philosophy at the University of Jabalpur. However, having achieved a state of self-proclaimed full enlightenment by age twenty-one, in 1967 Rajneesh decided that the time had come to spread his wisdom to the community. In the early 1970s, he began calling himself Bhagwan (from *bhagavān*, or "blessed one," an epithet for God) and built an ashram in Pune. By 1981, however, legal and financial trouble forced him and his devotees to flee India. He ultimately settled at a large ranch in Oregon. Under the leadership of senior administrators, Rajneeshpuram ("Rajneesh's Town"), as the community dubbed itself, evolved into a highly authoritarian institution. What's more, their large numbers allowed them to orchestrate a virtual political takeover of the neighboring town's local government. By 1986, a laundry list of criminal charges resulted in Rajneesh's deportation from the United States, upon which he returned to Pune.[66] Not to be undone, he became Osho, cosmic trickster and "spiritually incorrect mystic." He spent the final four years of his life preaching what he called a universal message, grounded in a variety of neo-esoteric techniques, and the center he founded only continued to grow in popularity following his death.[67]

As a guru, Osho taught a religion of antireligion, rejecting every norm, every boundary, and every metanarrative. He took explicit inspiration from tantric traditions but reinterpreted them into his own brand of "Neo-Tantra," glorifying transgression, personal (including material and sexual) gratification, and absolute individualism all premised on the innate divinity and perfection of human (and, indeed, of all) nature.[68] In practice, for Osho and his community, this looked like group sex and a fleet of ninety-three Rolls Royces. Unlike nearly every other guru whose saintly legacy has been tarnished by revelations of scandal, Osho never claimed immaculate purity. Instead, his methodology has been shock tactics in every sense of the phrase.

Hugh Urban has described Osho's radically subversive and ever-shifting teachings as a "postmodern pastiche" stitched together from "a remarkable range of sources, from Plato to Śaṅkara to Lao Tzu to Sartre," with "a special fondness for the more radical figures such as Nietzche, Gurdjieff, and Crowley."[69] Upon close inspection, Urban's analysis is true not only of Osho's thought in general, but of his practical methods in particular. As Urban has pointed out, the "catharsis" stage of Osho's Dynamic Meditation evokes scream therapy, popularized around the same time and clearly linked to Arthur Janov's *The Primal Scream* (1970).[70] And, when it comes to the "freeze" stage, Osho explicitly credits the early twentieth-century Armenian mystic Geogiy Gurdjieff.[71] And yet, there is something of a traditional *haṭha*-yogic logic to Osho's method, as well. His explanation of the "Hoo!" mantra, for example, very much resembles earlier ideas of striking at the root *cakra* (or nerve plexus, depending on the time period and the source).

All of this casts an interesting light on Osho as a node in the narrative of Kuṇḍalinī. Taking what is now a common relativism and an emphasis on personal experience to their logical extreme, Osho declares that things like *cakras* and Kuṇḍalinī are real (though they do not exist in the physical anatomy, where they only correspond to certain points), but they are not experienced in a standard way from one practitioner to another. This, according to Osho, is why historical traditions will talk about different numbers of *cakras*. And, for this same reason, it is best not to worry about tradition at all. According to Osho, "no theoretical knowledge is helpful. When you have some theoretical knowledge, you begin to impose it on yourself. You begin to visualize things to be the way you have been taught, but they may not correspond to your individual situation. Then much confusion is created."[72]

This is the crux of Osho's argument and his chief claim to superiority over competing methods and teachers. Kuṇḍalinī awakening is based on feeling, rather than knowing. In fact, externally imposed, "theoretical" knowledge can actually be harmful because it muddles and even disrupts the natural internal intuition that must guide any true engagement with Kuṇḍalinī. "The more knowledge gained," Osho says, "the less the possibility of feeling the real, the authentic, things."[73] Instead, as the practitioner visualizes a theoretical experience—a constructed subtle body reality that may not correspond to their authentic individual reality—the mind will actually begin to produce an internal imaginary reality that will reify this externally imposed knowledge. But this will not be a true experience; rather, it will be something more like a dream or an illusion. "The world that is without is illusory, but not so illusory as the one you can create inside," Osho explains. "All that is within is not necessarily real or true because imagination is also within, dreams are also within. The mind has a faculty—a very powerful faculty—to dream, to create illusions, to project."[74] For this same reason, Osho explicitly insists that it is not helpful to think of the feeling of Kuṇḍalinī as a serpent, because the serpent is only a symbol, and such a symbol only has meaning to people who have a direct and daily familiarity with serpents (which, presumably, most in the modern West do not).[75] The key, once again, is to feel something. Then "the symbol comes automatically, and the moment the symbol comes, the force is molded into that particular symbol . . . because you cannot feel an abstraction."[76] So, you might feel Kuṇḍalinī as a snake, but the snake must come from inside you.

Osho's signature method—the one most commonly practiced at his centers and associated with his name today—is called "Dynamic

Meditation" or "Chaotic Meditation." This is a five-step exercise that runs as follows:

1. Ten minutes of deep, rapid, chaotic breathing. Originally this was preceded by ten minutes of deep, rapid, regular breathing.
2. Ten minutes of "catharsis" to release the energy generated by the breathing through chaotic, intuitive movement intended as a total letting go. "Laugh, shout, scream, jump, shake—whatever you feel to do, do it! Just be a witness to whatever is happening within you," say Osho's original 1978 published instructions.[77] Today, his organization's website encourages the practitioner, "Hold nothing back; keep your whole body moving. A little acting often helps to get you started. Never allow your mind to interfere with what is happening. Consciously go mad. Be total."[78]
3. Ten minutes of gutturally shouting "Hoo!" while jumping with the arms raised above the head and landing hard on the soles of the feet. This activates the "sex center." One should exhaust oneself completely.
4. Fifteen (originally ten) minutes of freezing completely in whatever position one lands so that the energy can work internally.
5. Ten to fifteen minutes of celebration.

Osho had prescribed—as his centers continue to do—a number of other such exercises that incorporate actions such as swaying, shaking, speaking in gibberish, dancing, and laughing. However, all of these have key features in common: they are primarily based on natural and intuitive but intentionally chaotic actions, and they are meant to reorient the practitioner into something other than their normal state of being.

Despite being called "meditations," Osho's methods, in terms of the action-oriented techniques popularized in his published materials, are not to be understood as meditation itself. "The Chaotic Meditation, or the Kundalini, or the Nadabrahma," he says,

> are not really meditations. You are just getting in tune. It is like . . . if you have seen Indian classical musicians playing. For half an hour, or sometimes even more, they simply go on fixing their instruments. They will move their knobs, they will make the strings tight or loose, and the drum player will go on checking his drum—whether it is perfect or not. For half an hour they go on doing this. This is not music, this is just preparation.
>
> Kundalini is not really meditation. It is just preparation. You are preparing your instrument. When it is ready, then you stand in silence, then meditation starts. Then you are utterly there. You have woken yourself up by jumping, by dancing, by breathing, by shouting—these are all devices to make you a little more alert than you ordinarily are. Once you are alert, then the waiting.
>
> Waiting is meditation. Waiting with full awareness. And then it comes, it descends on you, it surrounds you, it plays around you, it dances around you, it cleanses you, it purifies you, it transforms you.[79]

The goal of such methods, then, is to create the proper conditions within the organism to induce a break with reality as it is normally experienced. Essentially, the goal is to jar the practitioner into "waking up."

And so, the practice can be anything, provided that it accomplishes this goal. In fact, "practice" is perhaps the wrong word here, since it implies a kind of disciplined habit, the repetition of which is like honing a skill. For Osho, spiritual insight comes in moments of crisis, when our habits fail us and so the ordinary way of experiencing the world cracks open. He explains:

> Then what is the technique to jump into meditation? I have talked about two: fasting and dancing. All techniques of meditation are to push you to the verge where you can take the jump, but the jump, itself, can be taken only through a very simple, very nonmethodical method. If you can *be aware* at the very moment when fasting has led you to the precipice of death, if you can *be aware* at the moment when death is going to set in, if you can *be aware*, then there is no death. And not only is there no death this time. Then there is no death forever. You have jumped! When the moment is so intense that you know in one second it will be beyond you, when you know that should a second be lost, you will not be able to come back again, *be aware* . . . and then jump![80]

Because the practice must be authentic—that is, born of the individual and their immediate experience—it cannot be taught, it can only be induced. Thus we arrive at a kind of paradox. An effective practice cannot be practiced. Breaking through to the divine requires an element of surprise. This is because, according to Osho, "you can only be aware in emergencies, in sudden emergencies. Someone puts a gun on your chest. You can be aware because it is a situation that you have never practiced."[81] So, if you have practiced fasting, then fasting will not help. Dancing only creates an emergency if you have never danced before. "But if you are an expert dancer," says Osho, then even "Sufi dervish dancing will not do. It will not do at all because you are so perfect, so efficient, and efficiency means that the thing is now being done by the nonvoluntary part of the mind. Efficiency always means that."[82] And so, the concept of a structured, repeated practice is antithetical to Osho's understanding of *sādhana*.

The only "method" is to be aware when you are thrown into the deep end of the pool of consciousness.

Still, Osho does not altogether eschew theory, just as he does not eschew some level of structure when it comes to practice. In fact, a theory of the subtle body is essential to making sense of his method. In his framework, there are seven bodies altogether: (1) the physical; (2) the etheric; (3) the astral; (4) the mental; (5) the spiritual; (6) the cosmic; and (7) the nirvanic.[83] Methods that involve Kuṇḍalinī are expedient because they work on the second (etheric) body, which is closest to, and therefore can be accessed through, the first, physical body with which we are generally familiar and which we know how to manipulate. And so, Osho's fairly compartmentalized understanding of methods corresponds to a circumscribed understanding of Kuṇḍalinī. "Kundalini," he says, "is not, itself, a life force. Rather, it is a particular passage for the life force, a way. But the life force can take other ways also, so it is not necessary to pass through kundalini. It is possible that one may reach enlightenment without passing through kundalini—but kundalini is the easiest passage, the shortest one."[84] Thus, there are many ways—the methods of other yogas, but also the methods of other religious traditions entirely. These, according to Osho, do not rely on Kuṇḍalinī. Only *haṭha* yoga does. To be clear, this does not mean that Osho considered his method of Dynamic Meditation or his other exercises to be *haṭha* yoga. In his understanding, *haṭha* yoga is a specific historical method (and a primitive one at that) that has been used to train the physical body and manipulate the etheric body. His method, which he fully recognizes to be a novel and synthetic one—meaning, no appeal to ancient tradition here—also does this and it does so in ways that are most effective in meeting his students where they are as individuals, so that their authentic experiences may emerge naturally.

Indeed, according to Osho, it is not even necessary to actually "experience" Kuṇḍalinī (that is, to *feel* it) in order to reap the benefits. Kuṇḍalinī is only felt when the life force encounters blockages in its passage and thus encounters resistance.[85] This is what the *cakras* are there to resolve, and this is why there is no standard number of *cakras*. One person's issues are not another's. If there is no resistance, then there is no sensation of Kuṇḍalinī. This is why, Osho says, neither the Buddha nor Mahāvīra (the founder of Jainism, the tradition Osho was born into) ever mentioned it.

The etheric body speaks the language of love and hate, or, more generically, attraction and repulsion, and so in the human body it is linked to the sexual impulse. The goal, therefore, is to reverse the normal flow of this energy from down-and-out to in-and-up. Just as blood flows through the circulatory system of the physical body, so Kuṇḍalinī is the medium of circulation for the etheric body. As such, it is nonvoluntary. "Even a hatha yogi," says Osho, "cannot do anything with it voluntarily."[86]

On this point, Osho is in agreement with the *śaktipāt* gurus. Kuṇḍalinī is an autonomous phenomenon that is not subject to the practiced, conscious control of the individual. And, for this reason, though it is ultimately the authentic experience of the individual that takes center stage, a guru still has a crucial role to play. Only a guru can teach—but again, really guide or help to induce—the kind of practice that can create a breakthrough from the first body into the second. And so, ironically (and likely intentionally so), despite producing literally dozens of books, Osho declared them to be more or less useless. "A living guru is needed, not a dead book," he declared. "A book cannot know what type of individual you are. . . . No book can know the individual. Books are meant for no one in particular; they are meant for everyone. And when a method is to be given, your individuality has to be taken into account, very, very exactly, scientifically."[87] This is why secrecy is essential to spiritual practice. Because the experience of truth that is real for one person may not be real for another, it cannot be communicated without leading the other astray, and even into danger. Only a guru can teach the truth, because a guru is one who has ceased to be a specific self—an individual someone—and so has become potentially everyone.[88]

Ultimately, then, although a number of the second-wave gurus of the 1960s and 1970s agree on the centrality of Kuṇḍalinī to spiritual advancement, they differ both on what Kuṇḍalinī actually is as well as on the best methods of access. For Osho, Kuṇḍalinī was only the specific passage that the life force might take if it were to be raised through the second of his seven bodies. Even then, it was not essential to actually "experience" Kuṇḍalinī at all—at least not as such. If your etheric body contained no blockages, then there would be no energetic experience, only the raising of consciousness. In the case of Yogi Bhajan, Kuṇḍalinī was conceived in a grander sense as ultimate human potential, but he nevertheless de-emphasized the more anomalous aspects of it. For Muktananda, to experience Kuṇḍalinī was to touch the divine.

For Muktananda, then, *śaktipāt* was the purest conduit not only of Kuṇḍalinī but of ultimate reality itself. Yogi Bhajan, on the contrary, dismissed the usefulness of *śaktipāt*, and Osho, if we can use his published discourses as a gauge, was at best ambivalent.[89] This is not to say that their followers did not find them charismatic—hence why we should differentiate between *śaktipāt* and common understandings of charisma—or did not report extraordinary experiences in the presence of their gurus. However, like Kuṇḍalinī itself, *śaktipāt* is just as much a matter of framing, narrative, and interpretation as it is of immediate experience. Desai did not "feel" Kripalvananda's *śaktipāt*, at least not in the moment. He felt the awakening of *prāṇa* mediated by his *āsana* practice.

Yet, it is likely no coincidence that in the case of the gurus we've discussed in this chapter who have prescribed specific methods of practice (rather than relying on the dynamics of *śaktipāt*), those methods are primarily physical, and they are undeniably intense. On Osho's Dynamic Meditation, Urban comments, "I have personally practiced Dynamic Meditation during my own visits to the Pune center. Leaving aside whatever spiritual, psychological, and emotional benefits that have been claimed for the technique (which I would not dismiss), there is one fact about the practice that is undeniable: it is a tremendous physical workout. The initial phase of chaotic breathing alone is physically very demanding, and when combined with the 'freak out' stage, jumping up and down and then holding a frozen position for ten minutes (possibly the hardest part of all), it is actually a very rigorous aerobic and muscular workout."[90] Following Urban's lead, one of the present book's authors (Anya Foxen) would add that, having personally experienced Kundalini Yoga as taught by Yogi Bhajan (or at least by one of his more famous students), the takeaway is very much the same. The *bhastrikā* breathing used throughout is physically demanding in a similar way to Osho's chaotic breathing. The repetitive motions of most of the *kriyās* involve moving a limb but often also holding it aloft for significant periods of time, and so in some ways they combine the demands of Osho's "freak out" and "freeze" stages. There are important differences as well. Where Yogi Bhajan uses repetitive order, Osho calls upon chaos. However, the physical exertion and the concomitant alteration of consciousness produced by both methods surely have some overlap. Desai presents an interesting middle between the two, but he, too, understood that intensity was a key aspect of an "effective" practice. This was why he invited Bikram Choudhury, the (in)famous Hot Yoga guru, to serve as a consulting teacher at his Kripalu Center in the early 1990s.[91]

Though this is somewhat more difficult to do with *śaktipāt* gurus like Muktananda, it's helpful to differentiate between gurus as charismatic community builders, and producers of popularly available written works, group classes, and other materials that are meant to reach a wider audience beyond their devoted followers. The impact of the latter is arguably much greater—if also more difficult to track—than the former. And even Muktananda had his weekend Intensives. All of these approaches would find ready consumers in the counterculture of the 1960s and 1970s. Evolutionary approaches to Kuṇḍalinī would become especially attractive to the nascent Human Potential Movement. None of this is precisely new. We can see the same dynamic happening between Vivekananda and the Boston Brahmins of the 1890s, or with Yogananda as he set up shop in Los Angeles right at the peak of Hollywood's Golden Age. But tangles have a way of getting bigger, and serpents have a way of growing more heads.

7

THE SERPENT IN THE MELTING POT

Kuṇḍalinī in North American Counterculture

The woman with her body
in the sea—The frog who
never moves & thunders, sharsh
—The snake with his body
under the sand—The dog
with the light on his nose,
supine, with shoulders so
enormous they reach back to
rain crack—The leaves hasten
to the sea—We let them
hasten to be wetted & give
em that old salt change, a
nuder think will make you see
they originate from the We Sea
anyway—No dooming booms
on Sunday afternoons—We
run thru the core of cliffs,
blam up caves, disengage no
jelly or jellied pendant
thinkers—

—JACK KEROUAC, "SEA"

If there is one artifact that captures the state of Kuṇḍalinī amid the mass cultural ferment of the 1960s and 1970s, it is a book edited by John White and titled, *Kundalini: Evolution and Enlightenment*. The first edition appeared in 1979, and another edition was issued just shy of two decades later in 1998. Both covers are variations on the same theme: a serpent weaving its way through seven *cakras* that are bursting with the colors of the rainbow.

The chapters are more or less evenly split between South Asian and Euro-American authors. They range from defining Kuṇḍalinī, to offering personal experiences, to speculating on possibilities for clinical research. And they agree on very little. This is true to tradition, of course. And, in its own way, the list of contributors tells the story of a continuing tradition—an evolving canon—the textual web of Kuṇḍalinī's tale, woven back and forth upon a century of modernity. The canonical names whose words don't appear in the volume are inevitably referenced—Vivekananda, Rele, and especially Avalon.

In his introduction, White proposes Kuṇḍalinī as a kind of "common denominator" of extraordinary experience and the answer to modern spiritual malaise. He also offers what has by now become a standard definition: "The Sanskrit word kundalini means 'coiled up' like a snake or spring. It implies latent power or untapped potential—the possibility within each person of attaining a new and more fulfilling condition of life. . . . Kundalini is traditionally symbolized in yogic texts as a sleeping serpent coiled at the base of the human spine. This indicates its close connection with the reproductive organs and life force."[1] On an individual level, tapping into this latent potential brings spiritual enlightenment. But a critical mass of enlightened individuals would signal something else: evolution. White echoes Gopi Krishna in claiming that Kuṇḍalinī is responsible for a broad range of extraordinary human mentality, from scientific and artistic genius, to psychopathy, to psychic powers. Perhaps most importantly of all, because Kuṇḍalinī is in part a biophysical phenomenon, it is subject to scientific verification. Nothing has to be taken on faith alone.

White's model is also grounded in a now-standard universalism. "Although the word kundalini comes from the yogic tradition," he writes, "nearly all the world's major religions, spiritual paths, and genuine occult traditions see something akin to the kundalini experience as having significance in 'divinizing' a person. The word itself may not appear in the traditions, but the concept is there nevertheless, wearing a different name yet recognizable as a key to attaining godlike stature."[2] Kuṇḍalinī, according to White, is the "personal" aspect of a universal life force common to nearly every culture. This is the *prāṇa* of South Asian tradition, the *ch'i* and *ki* of Chinese and Japanese thought, the Holy Spirit of Christianity, and so on. At this point, White reiterates: "Kundalini, often referred to as the 'serpent power' because it is symbolized by a coiled snake, can be concentrated and channeled through the spine into the brain."[3] But there is something very curious about this universalism. Though a life force and other extraordinary states of consciousness tied to mystical experience and practice (being, in the end, rather generic things) are indeed common to many traditions across the world, the idea of a serpentine energy rising up the spine, from base to brain, is not. Indeed, as we've seen, even yogic traditions don't agree on anything so standard, historically speaking.

As we pass the halfway mark of the twentieth century, the image of Kuṇḍalinī as a serpent rising up the spine has now become ubiquitous. And yet, the singularity of this image belies an ever-growing diversity. The serpent is more like a many-headed Hydra, or else the primordial Śeṣa himself. And, in true Hydra-like fashion, any attempt to prune back the wild tangle of what qualifies as Kuṇḍalinī to, let's say, the explanatory framework of a single tradition, has been unsuccessful.

As we've seen, this diversity is hardly new. But now, the core question begins to coalesce: Is there one Kuṇḍalinī of which there are many experiences? Or are there in fact many Kuṇḍalinīs?

Moving into the 1960s, the textual substratum (historical and modern alike) that has come to inform Kuṇḍalinī experience is enlivened by global contact with living South Asian gurus, or at least by a new range of experience-based narratives that their movements spawned. As we saw in the previous chapter, the models offered by these gurus were far from uniform. For every attempt to reframe Kuṇḍalinī in "traditional terms" with reference to tantra, there is a parallel attempt to connect it to modern psychotherapy. Indeed, sometimes these moves are made by the same teacher in the span of a single presentation, as evidenced by Swami Rama's contribution to White's volume.[4] Nearly every Hindu guru, at one time or another, can be found making appeals to the ecstasies of Christian mystics. Universalism, in other words, is a powerful trope.

In some ways, it almost seems that the explosion of different experiences we witness during this time itself creates (or at least reinforces) a counter-push to fit them into a single model—the fiery serpentine energy rising up the spine, root to crown. The stakeholders in this push-and-pull of stories and paradigms are many. There are, of course, the highly visible global gurus we have already discussed. But we also increasingly find Westerners who take on the mantle of "guru," and who have their own interests and their own stories to tell. There are the visionaries of the Human Potential Movement, inspired by the evolutionary spirituality of teachers like Aurobindo and encouraged by the empiricism of those like Gopi Krishna. There are the psychiatric professionals seeking to make sense of extreme embodied experiences through lenses less reductive than simple pathology, even while fears of the dangers of Kuṇḍalinī awakening reach peak intensity as experience narratives proliferate. And then, of course, there are all the experiencers . . .

GURUS, THE NEXT GENERATION

Scholars have tended to talk about global gurus in waves.[5] The first wave washed ashore in North America beginning in the late nineteenth century, bringing Vivekananda and other Ramakrishna Mission swamis, Paramahansa Yogananda, and any number of other lesser-known figures. This wave was ultimately stymied by the reactionary immigration bans that went into effect in the United States during the 1920s. The second wave, then, came after the repeal of these restrictions in the 1960s, and so we got the likes of Yogi Bhajan, Muktananda, Desai, and Osho. Of course, this model only makes sense if one is interested in tracking movement over seas. Unsurprisingly, Indian gurus continued to thrive in India in the intervening years. And, though their numbers posed no contest to the droves of questing Westerners that would be driven to South Asia by hippie counterculture, there were still quite a few Europeans and North Americans that made the long trek to see them. Thus, the third wave, which chronologically overlapped with the second, originated on Western shores. Euro-American students of Indian gurus eventually became gurus in their own right. And, though they largely saw themselves as carrying on the Indian lineages of their teachers, it matters that their starting point lay in Western concepts and practices.

Though there is any number of figures we could discuss, even just in the realm of Kuṇḍalinī-oriented practice, we will limit ourselves to two examples. The first is Swami Sivananda Radha, the German-Canadian disciple of Swami Sivananda Saraswati. The second is the American nondual guru Adi Da. We chose these two figures because they seem, at first glance, to inhabit opposite sides of nearly every spectrum on which one tries to place them. Sivananda Radha's traditionalist ethic and dutiful evocations of monastic lineage stand in stark contrast to Adi Da's eclectic and irreverent style. This is perhaps true—but not exactly in the way one would expect—and yet, upon closer examination, the similarities are at least as compelling as the differences.

Sivananda Radha (1911–1995) was born Sylvia Demitz in Germany, where she was a concert dancer until the world fell apart. Having lost her parents and her husband in World War II, then a second husband (the composer Albert Hellman) a year after their marriage in 1947, she immigrated to Canada in 1951 and thence soon departed to India. There she studied with Swami Sivananda, in Rishikesh, who initiated her into *sannyāsa* and officially gave her the title of "Swami." Because of visa restrictions, Sivananda Radha had only six months with her guru. The brief discipleship was nevertheless intense, and Sivananda Radha would speak of it continuously for the rest of her life.[6] While such a claim to monastic lineage would have certainly had other benefits as Sivananda Radha worked to establish herself as an authoritative teacher upon her return to Canada, and even more so as she began to build up her Yasodhara Ashram, there is no reason to doubt the earnestness of her experience. And yet, if we want to understand her role as a teacher of Kuṇḍalinī, it seems significant that after returning from her sojourn with Sivananda, she proceeded to order a full set of John Woodroffe's (that is, Arthur Avalon's) works.[7]

Indeed, little of Sivananda's fairly traditional *haṭha*-oriented imprint is felt in the outward form of Sivananda Radha's Kuṇḍalinī yoga, even if it is impossible to fully speak to its spirit. Her first book, *Kundalini Yoga for the West* (1978), remains arguably her most famous work to date. What *is* felt in the book is Sivananda Radha's diligent study of Avalon, as she begins every chapter with an elaborate list of the Indian symbols associated with each *cakra*. Perhaps the most traditionally Indian element of the Kuṇḍalinī "map" that Sivananda Radha charts out is the way it follows an ascent pattern through the *tattvas* (elements), associating them with the senses, and with levels of consciousness. The actual practice, however, more closely resembles contemporary self-help and related psychological methods as the practitioner is encouraged to reflect upon their relationship to their possessions, to their actions, and ultimately to themselves. It is essentially self-analysis.

Sivananda Radha presents her method without dwelling on its exact sources, but in her second major work, *Hatha Yoga: The Hidden Language* (1987), she makes clear her debt to Abraham Maslow and Joseph Campbell. Though Carl Jung never makes an explicit appearance, his spirit looms heavy. Sivananda Radha explains, "To blend East and West, we can take what is valuable in the West and put it together with yogic philosophy and methods. Western psychology, particularly Transpersonal Psychology, is a stepping-stone to the analysis that is done by the Easterner through the application of Yoga Psychology."[8] She thus argues that symbolism, which is ultimately transcultural, can be used to delve into hidden recesses of the mind. That's where Kuṇḍalinī dwells.

Then, there is Adi Da (1939–2008), an American guru more in the Osho mold. This is despite the fact that Adi Da was never actually involved with Osho. Instead, he is most closely tied to the lineage of Muktananda, having studied with Swami Rudrananda (or "Rudi," born Albert Rudolph, a disciple of Muktananda) and then Muktananda himself, from whom Adi Da received *śaktipāt* initiation. Born Franklin Jones in Long Island, New York, Adi Da went through a deluge of names, including Bubba Free John, Heart-Master Da, Da Free John, Avadhoota Da Love-Ananda, Da Kalki, Da Avabhasa, Adi Da, Ruchira Buddha, and Avatar Adi Da Samraj.[9] Like Osho, Adi Da had a quasi-academic background. (Osho's MA was in philosophy, while Adi Da's was in literature, but the overall thrust was, perhaps, the same.) Like Osho, Adi Da drew on a variety of teachers and sources, Asian and Western alike. And, like Osho, his method owed much to shock tactics of "crazy wisdom" that were irreverent and at times salacious.[10] Adi Da, likewise, never claimed celibate spiritual purity.

In some ways, Adi Da took Osho's message of authentic experience and carried it to its natural conclusion. The only truly authentic experience is that of absolute truth, and any experience that is born of the body–mind complex can never actually transcend itself. As laid out in Adi Da's most infamous work *Garbage and the Goddess* (1974), extraordinary experiences are just so much "garbage," totally superfluous to the truth that always already is. And such a truth, it turns out, is nearly impossible to communicate, especially when extraordinary experiences like Kuṇḍalinī are on the table. People insist on mistaking the garbage for the Goddess. Such, ironically, was the fate of the book, which detailed the vibrant, bizarre, and often bawdy life of Adi Da's community. But, in doing so, it achieved the opposite of its larger goal, as people came flocking to the community's doors, looking for parties and paranormal experiences. In the end, the community itself pulled the book from the market and burned every copy they could get their hands on.[11] Thus, when it came to Kuṇḍalinī, Adi Da had the following to say:

> The lust for the kundalini in the brain core is exactly the same as the lust for the kundalini in the sex center. It is using that mechanism in a different direction. But neither direction is toward God . . . Attachment to the brain through the inversion of attention in the kundalini, or the Life-Current, is traditionally promoted as the way to God. This is an error that has crept into the spiritual traditions. The way to God is not via the kundalini. The awakening of the kundalini and becoming absorbed in the brain core is not God-realization. It has nothing to do with God-realization. It is simply a way of tuning into an extraordinary evolutionary mechanism. The way to God-realization is the one by which that mechanism is understood and transcended completely.[12]

This was the position that Lee Sannella, one of the leading figures in clinical Kuṇḍalinī research, would eventually come to adopt as he became Adi Da's student.

Interestingly, with both Sivananda Radha and Adi Da, we see an attempt to sublimate the "hype" of Kuṇḍalinī experience—the fascination with the fiery serpent power as felt in the physical body—into something far more abstract. Sivananda Radha, for all her evocations of Sivananda's legacy, is a much more comfortable fit for the lineage of Jung. Her background as a dancer more or less guarantees that she was steeped from an early age in the harmonial logics of Western aesthetics.[13] In terms of her interests and angle of approach, she was both a product of and a contributor to the strains of transpersonal psychology and "human potential" ideas laced through the intellectual currents of contemporary counterculture. As for Adi Da, it would be historically inaccurate to call him a descendant of Osho, no matter how compelling the parallels. But it seems similarly meaningless to place him in the lineage of Muktananda. In the end, he too was a product of Western esoteric thought and both a child of and a player in the counterculture. Adi Da's intellectual background was firmly rooted in the likes of Blavatsky, Gurjieff, and Jung.[14] Some of his first mystical experiences were born of experimentation with hallucinogenic drugs.[15] And yet, his philosophy easily places him alongside some of the most radical South Asian nondualists, including those who regard Kuṇḍalinī as Goddess, not garbage.

SCIENTIFIC KUṆḌALINĪ, TAKE TWO

Just as some Americans took on the guru mantle, others took up the project pioneered by empirically inclined Indian yogis like Swami Kuvalayananda nearly a half-century prior (though, it seems, without much knowledge of their legacy). Here, in addition to Gopi Krishna, whose global connections led to the launch of several research initiatives, the major place of honor goes to Itzhak Bentov (1923–1979), an Israeli-American biomechanical engineer and consciousness researcher whose model would become the standard for clinical explorations of Kuṇḍalinī experience.

Bentov identified a "sensory-motor cortex syndrome" or a "physio-kundalini syndrome," which he viewed as a mechanism of evolution in the nervous system. Technically speaking, this amounts to a "stress-release mechanism" by virtue of which the nervous system is able to clear itself of accumulated stress and thus enter a state of greater maturity allowing for a higher (and vaster) functioning of consciousness.[16] Even more technically speaking, Bentov postulated that this mechanism manifests itself in a rhythmic motion that develops in the aorta, the body's main artery, which runs from the left ventricle of the heart and passes along the front of the spine through the chest and abdominal cavities to terminate in the pelvis. This is caused by a specific interaction of the heart rate, the respiratory rate, and the motion of the diaphragm, which can be achieved during meditation but also "accidentally" due to exposure to certain mechanical vibrations, electromagnetic waves, and even sounds. (Bentov suggests the mechanism can be activated by a car ride or an air conditioning duct, provided that they produce frequencies in the required range.)[17] Essentially, the aorta becomes a simple harmonic oscillator, which then activates a number of other resonant vibratory motions within the body, producing sensory phenomena like internal sounds and ultimately creating a pulsating magnetic field around the brain. At this point, we might remark that Bentov's model sounds like an updated version of Vasant Rele's.

Unlike Rele and his purely speculative theory, however, Bentov supported his conjectures with data collected through the use of a specially modified ballistocardiograph, an instrument that can detect micromovements within the body produced by the ejection of blood from the heart. He also attempted to substantiate the postulated magnetic field. However, Bentov's conclusions necessarily relied on subjective reporting from his subjects. Because the mechanism is ultimately geared at releasing stress, it is only keenly felt when stress is encountered. And so, Bentov suggests, a relatively relaxed person may not feel much at all. Moreover, symptoms can manifest sporadically over the course of months and even years, which makes them difficult to record. Nevertheless, Bentov suggests that the typical "syndrome" progresses like this:

> Its complete presentation usually begins as a transient paresthesia of the toes or ankle with numbness and tingling. Occasionally, there is diminished sensitivity to touch or pain, or even partial paralysis of the foot or leg. The process most frequently begins on the left side and ascends in a sequential manner from foot, leg, hip, to involve completely the left side of the body, including the face. Once the hip is involved, it is not uncommon to experience an intermittent throbbing or rhythmic rumbling-like sensation in the lower lumbar and sacral spine. This is followed by an ascending sensation which rises along the spine to the cervical and occipital regions of the head.
>
> At these latter areas, severe pressure-caused occipital headaches and cervical neck aches may be experienced at times. These pressures, usually transient but occasionally persistent, may also be felt anywhere along the spine, right or left side of chest, different parts of the head and the eyes. Some individuals will notice tingling sensations descending along the face to the laryngeal areas. The tracheolaryngeal region may also be felt as a sudden rushing of air to and fro. Respiration may become spasmodic with involuntarily occurring maximum expirations.

> Various auditory tones have been noted, from constant low-pitched hums to high-pitched ringing. Visual aberrations and temporary decrease or loss of vision has been observed. The sequence of symptoms continues later down into the lower abdominal region.[18]

Bentov notes that regular meditators whose experience follows this pattern may in fact have lighter symptoms. However, when the syndrome occurs spontaneously (that is, activated by something other than an intentional practice), it is associated with much more trauma, and frequently leads to hospitalization and a diagnosis of schizophrenia.[19] This, according to Bentov, is obviously far from ideal, since it not only fails to properly interpret the symptoms and therefore trigger the appropriate care for the patient, but it also tamps down the potential of the mechanism's inherently spiritual dimensions.

Notably, while Bentov clarified that he was primarily addressing the physiological dimensions of Kuṇḍalinī, his larger project sets its sights higher. He speculated that once the mechanism had completed its circuit, the nervous system would be more finely attuned to energies flowing in and out of the body, including electromagnetic fields associated with our planet and with the Sun, but also to beings that exist at higher states of consciousness.[20] Bentov's work on Kuṇḍalinī would ultimately be published as part of his book *Stalking the Wild Pendulum: On the Mechanics of Consciousness* (1977), which explores the manifestations of consciousness within the body, but also within the universe at large. However, it first appeared one year earlier, as an appendix to a different book: Lee Sannella's *Kundalini: Psychosis or Transcendence?* (1976).

Sannella (1916–2010) began his medical career as an ophthalmologist, but he subsequently went on to study and practice psychiatry. He ran a psychiatric clinic in Berkeley, California, from 1962 until

1972. In 1974, he cofounded the Kundalini Clinic in San Francisco.[21] Building on Bentov's model as well as observations made in his own clinical practice, Sannella proposed what he called a "physio-kundalini cycle." By "physio-kundalini" Sannella meant approximately the same thing as Bentov, that is "those aspects of kundalini awakening, both physiological and psychological, which can be accounted for by a purely physiological mechanism."[22] However, due to his perspective as a psychiatrist, his model included some additional cognitive dimensions that Bentov did not delve into. Clearly working in close contact with Bentov, as well as sharing his interests, Sannella also devoted some attention to exploring the ways that these symptom patterns are different from diagnosable conditions such as, for instance, schizophrenia.

Sannella identifies four basic categories of "signs and symptoms" characteristic of Kuṇḍalinī awakening:

1. Motor: any manifestation that can be physically observed and measured, including bodily movement and abnormal breathing patterns.
2. Sensory: inner perceptions such as bodily sensations (tingling, vibrating, itching, orgasm, and so on); sensations of hot and cold; lights or visions, and sounds.
3. Interpretive: mental processes that interpret experience such as extreme emotions, distorted thought processes, and detachment or dissociation.
4. Non-physiological: phenomena that have no currently accepted physical explanation (that is, basically, paranormal phenomena) such as out-of-body experiences or psychic perceptions.[23]

Most of these, he explains, can be accorded with Bentov's physiological model, though some (even stopping short of the "non-physiological") remain outside the scope of that causal framework. Overall, Sannella's explanation of the nature and function of Kuṇḍalinī likewise agrees with Bentov's. The ascent of Kuṇḍalinī essentially "causes the nervous system to throw off stress." Acting "on its own volition, engaging in a self-directed, self-limited process," the energy spreads out through the body's physio-psychological system to clear away blocks wherever it encounters them.[24]

This explanation also more or less agrees with the "classical model"—that is, the one found in South Asian traditions—at least as Sannella understands it. "Classically," Sannella says, "the energy awakens at the base of the spine, travels straight up the spinal canal, and has completed its journey when it reaches the top of the head. Along this route, however, there are said to be several chakras, or psychic energy centers, which the kundalini must pass through to reach its goal. These chakras contain impurities that kundalini must remove before it can continue its upward course."[25] And yet, once Sannella gets into the weeds of his explanation, it turns out that the correspondence is not so neat after all. Sannella's archive of case studies was substantial (by 1989, the total would reach nearly a thousand),[26] so there is good reason to take seriously the empirically supported patterns he outlines. Consequently, there is also good reason to take seriously the way these patterns diverge from the "standard" Kuṇḍalinī narrative. "Most notably," writes Sannella, in describing these differences, "we observe, and several traditions report, that the energy or sensation rises up the feet and legs, the body, back and spine to the head, but then passes down over the face, and through the throat, finally terminating in the abdomen. This is entirely in accord with predictions from Bentov's model, but somewhat at variance with the reports of Muktananda, Gopi Krishna and classic yoga scriptures."[27]

Of course, the "classic" yogic model of Kuṇḍalinī to which Sannella refers at this stage of his work is something like a straw man.

If we really wanted to accord Sannella's clinical findings with the South Asian textual tradition, we might point not only to the baseline diversity across Kuṇḍalinī models—starting locations, points of interest along the ascent, even the nature of Kuṇḍalinī itself—but also to the relative commonality of Kuṇḍalinī's return, as She bathes the body in immortal nectar. However, having now traced the history of the "standard" (which is effectively Sannella's "classic") model nearly to its culmination, it is worth remarking on this divergence. After all, Sannella's model is "standard" in its own way. It is a common profile distilled from a large amount of otherwise diverse empirical data. More importantly, it is drawn from data collected from his patients for the most part either while they were still in the midst of their Kuṇḍalinī experience, or shortly thereafter. Here we might think back to the evolution of Gopi Krishna's narrative: the way that a chaotic constellation of sensations gradually becomes interpreted in light of an external framework. Is Sannella's empirical "standard" more objectively accurate than the other model, distilled not from direct experience, but rather from layers of cultural tropes, symbols, philosophies, and visionary constructs? Is experience (including the experience of Sannella's patients) anything other than a heap of all these things?

A version of this question—the cultural relativity of not only experiences but practices—enters into Sannella's discussion in a fascinating way. At the outset of his book, he identifies the Kuṇḍalinī experience with a common cross-cultural phenomenon of spiritual rebirth. This rebirth process, according to Sannella, has been relatively rare in the West (though, at this stage, he does not elaborate on why), but now it appears to be happening more frequently (also for reasons he does not specify). While many, if not all, world spiritual traditions have their own models for this process, most focus only on the internal subjective dimensions, while treating the objective external ones as peripheral at best. Sannella thus sees the Kuṇḍalinī model as unique in allowing access to a physiological dimension, insofar as it speaks of an energy rising from the base of the spine to the crown of the head.[28] However, he presents a number of cross-cultural analogs, from the ecstasies of Christian mystics to the *n/um* dances of the !Kung tradition of Botswana. Implicitly, these are all examples of the same phenomenon as Kuṇḍalinī.

And so, we are back to the same question we have asked so many times now: Is Kuṇḍalinī a discrete and limited phenomenon associated with a culturally specific set of practices (even if these practices travel, evolve over time, and blend across cultures), or is it something universal, manifesting in common patterns regardless of what cultural frameworks and practices are applied? To point to a more circumscribed example, many of Sannella's subjects were practitioners of Transcendental Meditation (TM), even though this tradition's model does not technically center on or even include Kuṇḍalinī. Popularized by Maharishi Mahesh Yogi, TM is a form of *mantra* meditation, which Maharishi originally explained in a tantric (though not Kuṇḍalinī-oriented) manner as harnessing the power of divine beings, but he ultimately framed TM in light of nondual Vedānta. Sannella, in fact, seems aware of this difference, and he recommends TM as well as Zen meditation (or else "spontaneous awakening by the direct influence of an enlightened Guru, such as Muktananda") to those suffering from troubles connected to Kuṇḍalinī.[29] Sannella even speculates that it's possible "the Zen method discourages the experience of the rise of kundalini by its open-eye meditation, which encourages the meditator to flow with the external, as well as with the internal world."[30] In the end, he goes so far as to state, "We especially want to caution that, methods designed specifically to hasten kundalini arousal, such as the yogic breath-control exercises known as pranayama, should be considered hazardous, unless practiced directly under the guidance of a teacher, or Guru, who is fully realized."[31]

We thus find ourselves in the curious situation where it seems not only that nearly any spiritual practice (or, indeed, nothing at all) can prompt Kuṇḍalinī awakening, but that it is perhaps best to stay away from methods that purport to deal with Kuṇḍalinī directly. Later in his career, Sannella would walk this back and refine his framing. In the decade following the initial publication of his book, his understanding of the world's mystical traditions would grow both broader and deeper.

At this stage, however, Sannella's background and thus his angle of approach was not that of a scholar of religion, but of a medical professional. In light of this, his most immediate concern was with better understanding and supporting his patients. Thus, whatever else his book may have accomplished, its primary thesis was this: the spiritual rebirth of Kuṇḍalinī only appears pathological if one misinterprets what it is. This, Sannella says, would be the same for physical birth if it were examined only in terms of its "symptoms"—emergence, in short, is a gruesome process. All the more important, then, that it be understood properly.

A STATE OF SPIRITUAL EMERGENCY

This was the precise attitude of Christina and Stanislav Grof, founders, in 1980, of the Spiritual Emergency Network (SEN, subsequently renamed the Spiritual Emergence Network). Pointing to the notion that "some of the dramatic experiences and unusual states of mind that traditional psychiatry diagnoses and treats as mental diseases are actually crises of personal transformation," the Grofs argued that "when these states of mind are properly understood and treated supportively rather than suppressed by standard psychiatric routines, they can be healing and have very beneficial effects on the people who experience them. This positive potential is expressed in the term *spiritual emergency*, which is a play on words, suggesting both a crisis and an opportunity of rising to a new level of awareness, or 'spiritual emergence.' "[32] For the Grofs, this project was personal at least as much as it was professional. Christina Grof first experienced what she subsequently understood to be a Kuṇḍalinī awakening during the birth of her first child. The experience was as traumatic as it was transformational.[33]

The potentially harrowing nature of Kuṇḍalinī awakening is not without its precedents in the historical literature. Here one need only recall the imagery of the thirteenth-century *Jnāneśvarī*, where the newly awakened Kuṇḍalinī sets about devouring the practitioner's body with Her flaming mouth.[34] However, while historical accounts of Kuṇḍalinī may certainly use strong language, cautions against and even more so anxieties about Kuṇḍalinī practice do not tend to be a prominent concern among contemporary Indian communities of practitioners. The modern Western pervasiveness of such fears must therefore be approached as another complex and multilayered cultural and historical phenomenon.

Cautions about the volatile nature of Kuṇḍalinī and the dire dangers of irresponsible or premature awakening appear in Western sources from the earliest outset, starting with the work of the Theosophists. Even in her brief mention of Kuṇḍalinī, Helena Blavatsky is sure to specify that this "electro-spiritual force" is "a creative power which when aroused into action can as easily kill as it can create."[35] Charles Leadbeater advises that it is indeed better to allow this fiery energy to remain dormant until one has reached a sufficient level of moral development, both in strength of will and purity of thought. The "uncontrolled movement" of Kuṇḍalinī, he says, "may readily tear tissues and even destroy physical life."[36] George Arundale similarly says that, unless the individual in question is in full control of himself, body and mind, in awakening

Kuṇḍalinī he risks "the possibility of injury to the heart, to the nervous system through the solar plexus, the individual becoming a chronic invalid with general physical deterioration of the brain, producing a strain also ending in mental unhingement."[37] Such warnings are usually accompanied by lingering Victorian anxieties over sexuality, a danger that both Arundale and Leadbeater treat as even graver than the ordinary physical risks. (We will return to the sexual aspects of Kuṇḍalinī shortly.)

Things get even more complex as these warnings are incorporated into the teachings of popular gurus, where they read as capitalist tactics to corner the market and sew distrust in competitors as much, if not more, than they read as genuine words of caution. Yogi Bhajan, for instance, condemns those who cultivate fear of Kuṇḍalinī, but then arguably proceeds to do exactly this. After exhorting the importance of the "throat lock" (*jālaṅdhara-bandha*), he continues:

> When you do yoga, please, for God's sake, remember you are playing with energy which is the life force of the atom. You can well understand what you are doing. I'm giving you a word of warning. The prana has been described in the shastras (yogic scriptures) as that which makes the atom live. The voltage here in the wall socket is 110? And do you touch it without insulation? No! Then how can you play with the pranic energy? (Proper technique and preparation is the insulation you need.)[38]

Muktananda does the same thing. Despite what "some people" say regarding how Kuṇḍalinī may drive you crazy or afflict your body with terrible diseases, he assures us that there is nothing to fear. There is no disease in Kuṇḍalinī—this is contrary to her divine nature. This is right before he goes on to caution:

> However, some people do attempt to awaken the Kundalini forcibly, through self-effort, either by means of hatha yogic techniques such as mudras and bandhas, or with their own unusual practices, and anything may happen in such a case. If the Kundalini were not to rise in a proper manner, it might prove to be harmful. A person who tries to bring about this kind of awakening on his own with unusual practices does not succeed in raising his Kundalini, he only succeeds in irritating Her. And if the Kundalini is irritated beyond a certain limit, a person might lose his mental balance, or his body might become weak. But if Kundalini awakens through Guru's grace, spontaneously, and in the processes of Kundalini Yoga are set in motion by the Shakti Herself, such adverse reactions would be impossible, because in the kingdom of Kundalini there is no sickness or mental disease.[39]

The notable thing here is that each teacher's approach makes the other's sound, at best, like playing with fire (or a nuclear reactor). According to Yogi Bhajan, training oneself to master proper technique is the only thing that can ensure safety. Why let someone else stick your finger into an electric socket? According to Muktananda, technique alone leaves too much room for error. Why not let the teacher act as your conductor?

Then, of course, there is Osho, whose whole method is based on inducing a state of acute physical and spiritual emergency. This is when Osho would have said to "jump."[40]

Ultimately, the Grofs are perhaps closest to Osho in their approach, despite the fact that Christina Grof came to connect her Kuṇḍalinī journey with receiving *śaktipāt* from Muktananda. In the Grofs' view, as we've seen, crisis opens opportunity. Really, though, it was Sannella's book that finally helped Christina make sense of her experience,[41] and it was in its therapeutic spirit that she and her husband founded SEN in 1980.

SEN did not restrict itself to aiding only those struggling with Kuṇḍalinī awakening. The Grofs understood spiritual emergence quite broadly, but their framework generally resisted the kind of universalizing tendencies we sometimes see around Kuṇḍalinī, including those implicit in Sannella's early work (to say that all mystical experience is Kuṇḍalinī experience). The Grofs' approach is well summarized in their collected volume on the subject, *Spiritual Emergency: When Personal Transformation Becomes a Crisis* (1989). There, the Grofs introduce the following typology of spiritual emergenc(i)es.

1. The shamanic crisis
2. The awakening of Kundalini
3. Episodes of unitive consciousness ("peak experiences")
4. Psychological renewal through return to the center
5. The crisis of psychic opening
6. Past-life experiences
7. Communications with spirit guides and "channeling"
8. Near-death experiences (or NDEs)
9. Experiences of close encounters with UFOs
10. Possession states.[42]

Even without delving into the details, one can easily imagine that there may be substantial areas of overlap between these categories. What differentiates Kuṇḍalinī for the Grofs is that, whatever the contexts in which it may manifest (for instance NDEs or UFO encounters) and whatever "effects" it may have (like feelings of oneness or psychic encounters with superhuman entities), at its core it is an *energetic* phenomenon. That is, Kuṇḍalinī refers to the specific experience of rising energy as it occurs within the body.

The Grofs' description of Kuṇḍalinī is remarkable only in that it perfectly exemplifies what is now indisputably the common standard. An energy—the "serpent power"—is awakened at the base of the spine and rises through the body's subtle channels, clearing out "old traumatic imprints" and opening the "centers of psychic energy" of the *cakras*.[43] The Grofs do not specify the precise trajectory or terminus of Kuṇḍalinī, likely in deference to the divergence found in Sannella's clinical findings—indeed, aside from the Grofs' introduction, a portion of Sannella's book, excerpted under the title "Kundalini: Classical and Clinical," provides the only direct treatment of the subject included in the volume.

The Grofs do, however, provide their own list of the physical and psychological signs of Kuṇḍalinī awakening, which are collected under the blanket term *kriyās* (a rather novel move, given that the term would normally be applied only to formal yogic "exercises," even if these are understood to manifest automatically rather than intentionally), and they run as follows:

> One can experience intense sensations of energy and heat streaming up the spine, associated with violent shaking, spasms, and twisting movements. Powerful waves of seemingly unmotivated emotions, such as anxiety, anger, sadness, or joy and ecstatic rapture, can surface and temporarily dominate the psyche. Visions of brilliant light or various archetypal beings and a variety of internally perceived sounds, as well as experiences of what seem to be memories from past lives, are very common. Involuntary and often uncontrollable behaviors complete the picture: talking in tongues, chanting unknown songs, assuming yogic postures and gestures, and making a variety of animal sounds and movements.[44]

Here, the overlap with other modalities of spiritual emergence becomes clear. But, at this point, it's also useful to take a step back and compare the Grofs' understanding of Kuṇḍalinī awakening, as a state of spiritual emergency, with the kinds of fears and warnings we find in the earlier Western literature. It is important that none of the "symptoms" listed by the Grofs are viewed as abnormal or a sign that something has gone wrong. These are not signs that Kuṇḍalinī has been awakened prematurely, irresponsibly, or improperly, nor that the individual undergoing the experience is somehow physically, mentally, or morally unworthy, immature, or unprepared. In a sense, the Grofs' position is actually closer to the way such potentially alarming phenomena are framed in the historical South Asian sources. This is simply the process. The only "danger" inherent in it, according to the Grofs, is that the experiencer is liable to be misunderstood, misdiagnosed, and mistreated by the medical establishment and the culture at large. What the Grofs were trying to provide in founding SEN was the kind of information and support framework that would have been standard in traditional lineages of practice.

In the end, however, the Grofs and their understanding of spiritual crisis as the opening of an evolutionary-scale transformation cannot be understood apart from their involvement with the Esalen Institute. They lived and taught at Esalen for fourteen years.[45] But before we turn our gaze to the cliff in Big Sur where the Human Potential Movement was born, we need to address an abiding aspect of Kuṇḍalinī that cannot be excluded from any discussion of the countercultural revolution.

THE THING ABOUT SEX

Like the "crisis" aspect of Kuṇḍalinī, its sexual nature can also be found in the historical South Asian literature. In the nondual tantric sources that treat Kuṇḍalinī in Her grandest sense—so, we are not talking about those texts where the concept appears, for instance, simply as an obstruction to be overcome—the Möbius strip of the masculine and feminine is foundational to the nature of reality. That is, reality itself is hermaphroditic and ultimately autoerotic. Without getting into details (some of which we covered in chapter 1), sexual ritual has also had a diverse range of historic roles in such traditions.

However, like all other aspects of Kuṇḍalinī, the modern phenomenon's eroticism can't be understood with reference to these historical South Asian sources alone. After all, Western spirituality has no lack of its own sexual symbolism. In fact, there is something uniquely Western—or, more precisely, biblical—about the anxieties that surround Kuṇḍalinī and sex, and there is something Gnostic in the linkage of sex with Kuṇḍalinī as a way to embrace and redeem it. It was the serpent, after all, who led Adam and Eve to the forbidden fruit with promises of immortality. Layered on top of all this, is an ever-present Orientalist obsession with the inherent eroticism of "Eastern" traditions (and especially tantra), a tendency that arguably has more to do with fantasy and projection than with any genuine engagement with Asian traditions or practices.

A good example here is the work of nineteenth-century American occultist and sexologist Ida C. Craddock, who established a Church of Yoga and used the term in her discussion of sexual intercourse in famous publications such as *Right Marital Living* (1899) and *The Wedding Night* (1900). Craddock herself admits that what she calls "yoga" can just as easily be called "suggestive therapeutics," or else "applied psychology, or mental science, or divine science."[46] As such, her understanding of these matters arguably owes far more to Western metaphysical and harmonial traditions than it does to South Asian ones, but the link she makes surely reinforced the increasingly reflexive identification of Indian traditions with sex, which was already growing into a source of both moral outrage and titillated fascination, depending on whom one asked.

Another prominent data point from this era is Pierre Arnold Bernard (1875–1955), also known as the "Omnipotent Oom," an

American occultist who founded his Tantrik Order as a fashionable secret society in the mold of the Freemasons and Theosophists and attracted a circle of wealthy benefactors-cum-disciples, both male and female. Bernard had a coterie of young female followers, whom he initiated into his order as sacred consorts or "nautch girls."[47] Details of the order's precise practices are lost to history, but it is eminently believable that they included ritualized sex under the banner of "Tantra."

And so, while sexuality certainly had a role to play in certain premodern South Asian tantric, and therefore Kuṇḍalinī-oriented, traditions—and while this history certainly contributed to the colonial denigration of tantra as a perversion—early Western understandings of tantric eroticism were far more firmly based in the concerns (and fanciful imaginings) of Western culture. Insofar as cross-cultural treatments of Kuṇḍalinī from this period had anything to say about sex, these mentions generally amounted to restrictions and words of caution.

This becomes obvious if one examines the early Western (that is, largely Theosophical) literature on Kuṇḍalinī alongside the treatment the topic receives in contemporary works by Indian innovators of yoga. The Indian yogic texts are overwhelmingly concerned with sexual hygiene, up to the point of celibacy. This fits neatly both with the historical importance of sexual fluids as power substances within South Asian tantric traditions, as well as with the more recent historical entanglement of *haṭha* yoga and Vedānta within monastic lineages. Similarly, freedom from sexual impulses is among the most important factors discussed by Arundale to avoid physical and mental damage as a result of Kuṇḍalinī. Unless such impulses have been fully sublimated, Kuṇḍalinī awakening may drain the practitioner of vitality through "sex-obsession."[48] Leadbeater, meanwhile, cautions that, if aroused prematurely, Kuṇḍalinī may flow downward instead of upward and thus it "excites the most undesirable passions—excites them and intensifies their effects to such a degree that it becomes impossible for the man to resist them, because a force has been brought into play in whose presence he is as helpless as a swimmer before the jaws of a shark. Such men become satyrs, monsters of depravity."[49] At first blush, this may evoke South Asian ascetic concerns with seminal retention, but the far more appropriate association here is probably Victorian fears of female nymphomania and especially spermatorrhea, an objectively nonexistent male pathology characterized by "the excessive discharge of sperm caused by illicit or excessive sexual activity, especially masturbation [and] understood to cause anxiety, nervousness, lassitude, impotence, and, in its advanced stages, insanity and death."[50] In short, while this period of cultural melding had its Bernards and Craddocks, the shared sexual conservativism we see among Indian yogis and Western Theosophists, regardless of their respective reasons, was far more typical during the first half of the twentieth century.

Then came the sexual revolution.

As far as second-wave gurus were concerned, the attitudes toward sexuality remained lukewarm at best—the exception being iconoclasts like Osho and Adi Da, and even they generally stopped short of treating sex as the actual engine of transcendence. Muktananda and Desai required celibacy within their communities and encouraged sexual continence more generally among their students. Yogi Bhajan, who billed himself as a householder guru for the masses, also encouraged continence within marriage. The same applied to Sivananda Radha, who likewise did not outright exclude sex, but encouraged reserve and ultimately abstinence. "It is unfortunate that today, when there is a great deal of interest and discussion about kundalini energy," she writes, "it is mainly linked to only one aspect—that of sex. Particularly in the West, it has become a word and a concept that serves as an excuse for many things. Attributing events to kundalini energy and its overwhelming power, men and women throw aside sexual inhibitions and indulge in all sorts of illicit sexual activity. This lack of real understanding of the nature and purpose of kundalini is leading not only to confusion and disaster in human relationships, but also to mental imbalance."[51]

This conservativism, however, was not mirrored within the counterculture at large, where "free love" had become an ecstatic rallying cry. Indeed, Sivananda Radha's comments make it fairly clear that what she is teaching is not what people actually seem to be *doing*, when it comes to Kuṇḍalinī and sex. As we've mentioned, there are important differences between South Asian tantric traditions and the modern global phenomenon that Hugh Urban has called "neo-Tantra,"[52] as well as the slightly more discrete historical movement that Jeffrey J. Kripal has dubbed "American Tantra."[53] As ideologies that seek to deify the sanctity of the individual—as a person, but also as a *principle*—in the form of individual freedom and individual fulfillment, these takes on tantra generally and Kuṇḍalinī specifically are not only modern (Neo-) but, in important ways, Western. This does not render them somehow inferior or inauthentic, but it does render them distinct.

Yet it bears returning to the notion that sexuality *is* (and has been) a feature of South Asian tantric traditions and Kuṇḍalinī awakening. An interesting convergence point of these two takes on tantric sex—the old and the new—is actually one of the first serious in-depth scholarly works on tantric traditions: Lilian Silburn's *Kundalini: The Energy of the Depths* (1983). Silburn (1908–1993) was a French Indologist, with a deep knowledge of medieval tantric literature and a powerful grasp on the Sanskrit language. She was also a practitioner and a student of Swami Laskhman Joo (1907–1991), a Kashmiri guru who instructed her in methods of raising Kuṇḍalinī.[54] The fascinating thing about Silburn's book (especially when one considers that it's a formal academic study) is that it is without doubt the most genuinely erotic treatment of tantra and Kuṇḍalinī to date.

Once again, it's not so much that this eroticism isn't substantiated by the textual tradition (it is), but that there are other features of the textual tradition that could just as easily be emphasized. And so, Silburn's choice to dwell on the erotic, as well as on the symbolism of the serpent, seems to hint not only at her interests as a scholar but at the cultural context that helped her cultivate those interests.

One also wonders how much of Silburn's erotic emphasis is due to her experience as a practitioner. Complex cultural factors aside, from an experiential standpoint, sexuality (if not the more interpretive dimensions of eroticism) seems to be core to Kuṇḍalinī awakening. Gopi Krishna discusses the sexual dimensions of Kuṇḍalinī extensively.[55] Muktananda devotes a significant number of pages in his spiritual autobiography to the experience of being plagued by an erection so fierce that it literally ripped through his loincloth.[56] Experience narratives, both by practitioners and people who experienced apparently spontaneous awakening, frequently remark on the sexual character of their embodied sensations.[57]

For what it's worth, however, according to Michael Murphy, cofounder of Esalen Institute, to which we will now turn, lots of people tried using sex to systematically raise Kuṇḍalinī through the *cakras* during Esalen's countercultural heyday. Reportedly, they didn't get very far.[58] Which is not to say that there were no experiences—they just weren't the systematic kind.

HUMAN POTENTIAL AND A CLIFF

Esalen's cofounders, Michael Murphy (1930–) and Richard Price (1930–1985), met in 1960 at the San Francisco meditation house of Haridas Chaudhuri, a Bengali philosopher who had recently founded the Cultural Integration Fellowship.[59] The Cultural Integration Fellowship, grounded in the Integral Yoga vision of Sri Aurobindo, was a progenitor of the current California Institute of Integral Studies, a private university specializing in comparative and cross-cultural studies in a number of fields ranging from the arts to medicine.[60] Murphy was, at that point, living at Chaudhuri's meditation house, and Price soon joined him.[61]

The two men had much in common. Among other points of convergence, both had studied psychology at Stanford, and both had been influenced by the same professor of Asian philosophy and religion, Fredric Spiegelberg (who the reader might recall wrote the preface to Gopi Krisha's book), during their time there.[62] Murphy had recently spent eighteen months at the Sri Aurobindo Ashram in Pondicherry. Aurobindo was, by then, no longer living; and so, perhaps even more importantly, Murphy had spent this time not only meditating but delving deeply into Aurobindo's magnum opus of evolutionary spirituality *The Life Divine* (1919), which would become a foundational intellectual touchstone to define the rest of Murphy's life.[63] Price, for his part, was more firmly grounded in the ideas of Buddhism and Taoism but, at this point, his most radical defining experience had been the period of spiritual emergency he had undergone in 1955 and the multiyear (coerced and highly damaging) institutionalization he had suffered as a result.[64]

Esalen Institute would come into the world billing itself as "a center to explore those trends in the behavioral sciences, religion and philosophy which emphasize the potentialities and values of human existence."[65] This early version of the institute's credo was inspired by an Aldous Huxley lecture, titled "Human Potentialities," that Price attended in 1960. In this lecture, Huxley argued that the previous twenty thousand years, despite no obvious leaps of anatomical evolution, had "actualized an immense number of things which at that time for many, many centuries thereafter were wholly potential and latent in man," and so—if the neurologists who claimed human beings only used roughly 10 percent of their brain mass were to be believed—many more such potentialities lay on the horizon.[66] During a late-night brainstorming session between Murphy and writer and Integral Transformative Practice cofounder George Leonard (1923–2010), "human potentialities" would become the "Human Potential Movement."[67]

Still, it seems significant that the collaboration that launched Esalen was born of a twin stream of spiritual emergence: evolution and crisis. Murphy does not quite remember when Kuṇḍalinī first appeared on the radar, but it was early enough such that, upon Esalen's founding in 1962, it simply "came with the package." This is borne out by the institute's programming. Kuṇḍalinī makes its first official appearances in Esalen's catalogs as early as 1965 in a workshop titled "Generating and Directing the Kundalini Power," led by psychologist Paul Kurtz. The session promises an exploration of both Indian philosophical and modern psychological understandings of Kuṇḍalinī, "the Sleeping Serpent whose proper awakening is thought to be the goal of existence in various Indian Yoga systems." The catalog description ends by specifying, in faithful Esalen spirit, "Emphasis however will be chiefly on experimentation and experience rather than discussion."[68]

Thus, "experimentation and experience" with regard to human potential signaled by Kuṇḍalinī awakening became one side of the story. Spearheaded by Bentov, as well as "human potential" pioneers like Elmer Green (1917–2017) and Gay Luce (1930–2023), the 1970s and 1980s brought an era of biofeedback and other modes of scientific experimentation geared at inducing, observing, and recording the psycho-physical dynamics of Kuṇḍalinī within the human body. Murphy himself took part in one such session.[69]

The other side, the therapeutic demands of "emergence," is best represented by the Grofs, whose approach to Kuṇḍalinī makes a regular appearance in Esalen catalogs from 1979 to 1985. Featuring large teams of teachers representing a variety of fields, workshops led by the Grofs combined modern medical and psychiatric approaches with practices drawn from a variety of (usually Asian) traditions such as (presumably Hindu) tantra, Zen, Vajrāyana, vipassana meditation, *aikidō*, and nonspecified shamanic practices, as well as from Western schools such as gestalt and Reichian therapy.

However, Kuṇḍalinī's presence at Esalen is certainly not limited to these two streams. In the catalogs, one can also find the term cropping up within explorations of myth and symbolism led by Joseph Campbell. A 1969 workshop by Shyam Bhatnagar offers a Hindu tantric approach. Meanwhile, a 1981 offering by Maureen Lavender evokes Kuṇḍalinī alongside the Holy Spirit.[70] And, beyond this, there is everything that isn't captured in official catalog archives. There are the practices and spontaneous experiences embodied by decades of Esalen residents and visitors.

In addition to Sannella, who, according to Murphy, formed a close relationship with Price, Esalen (and Price, especially) became a magnet for psychiatrists and other professionals interested in exploring crises that would have typically been identified as psychoses through a more holistic lens.[71] These figures included, among others, psychiatrist Thomas Szasz (1920–2012), anthropologist Gregory Bateson (1904–1980), psychotherapists Jay Haley (1923–2007) and Virginia Satir (1916–1988), who both contributed to the development of family therapy, and psychophysiologist Julian Silverman (1933–2001), who went on to serve as Esalen's general manager. At Esalen, psychiatric professionals rubbed shoulders with scholars and practitioners interested in shamanism and psychedelics. Needless to say, there were all sorts of altered states of consciousness on the table.

And this is precisely what makes Kuṇḍalinī at Esalen so slippery, and what makes Esalen such a perfect distillation of the larger patchwork of experience we have been examining. In Murphy's understanding, Esalen has always been a place where the "cafeteria spirituality" approach, which some scholars of religion have decried as a breakdown of tradition driven by shallow pastiche, has been treated as a virtue rather than a sin. Murphy sees Esalen as "recapitulating natural history" within the spiritual domain. Where the scientists of the past may have collected fossils, the researchers (and the practitioners) who come to Esalen "collect experiences."

Needless to say, the counterculture of the 1960s and 1970s yielded a lot of experiences to be collected. "This stuff broke loose doing all sorts of things, in all sorts of ways," says Murphy with regards to Kuṇḍalinī experience—or at least experience that people were inclined to call "Kuṇḍalinī." People meditated. People did drugs. People stopped taking their medications. People got lost in sex. ("Erotomania breaking out," Murphy calls it.) Often people did two or more of these things at once.

For Murphy, though, it comes back to human potential. All sorts of embodied experience, from sex to sports, can descend into a "theater of the occult." When it comes down to it, all sorts of powerful embodied experiences (not just canonically "mystical" ones) can become "a living laboratory of bodily transformation." This is the subject matter of Murphy's masterwork *The Future of the Body* (1992).

"We're a *siddhi* producing race that is pressing to be born in the world," says Murphy. "These are the visionary buds trying to sprout." (One hears the echoes of Aurobindo's evolutionary philosophy here.)

And many of these experiences get mapped as Kuṇḍalinī, Murphy allows, but he is cautious to do so himself. On the one hand, he sees it as a semantic problem. Or perhaps a cartographic one. "You can stylize everything according to the maps you've got to work with," Murphy says, before pointing out, "We're in the hottest of hot zones with old maps." But, for Murphy, this is not simply a matter of interpretation. It's also a matter of how we produce experience through a kind of physical and spiritual mimicry. People—some more than others—are quite good at following maps. Some even manage to incorporate the map into their own bodies. But this has been the advantage of an eclectic and inherently comparative environment like Esalen. At a certain point, one is forced to confront the reality of different maps.

What, then, is Kuṇḍalinī? For Murphy, it might be enough to say that it "points towards something that has a mind of its own . . . an autonomous something within our larger nature, much of which we're unconscious of." There is something that emerges in the human body when we begin "flirting with the edges of homeostasis."

So, what do we do with it? Murphy remains a proponent of the therapeutic reorientation started by Price, and by the Grofs, and others alongside them. But we should not forget that these moves to destigmatize spiritual emergence still imply that the process of transformation should be supported rather than suppressed. It is no coincidence that the birthplace of the Human Potential Movement sits on a cliff. (Though it might be worth mentioning that Price went through an Osho phase and spent two weeks at then Rajneesh's Pune ashram in 1978. He left unimpressed.)[72] And yet, perhaps there is more than one way to jump.

THE TROUBLE WITH NAMING DRAGONS

In philosophy there is something called the fallacy by naming. It means falling into the trap of thinking because we have given something a name we know what it is. We in the West seem to be in danger of falling into this trap over Kundalini. Everyone who is anyone in yoga circles has heard about Kundalini. We not only use the word, we can pronounce it properly, and even spell it. One might almost call it a cult word among meditators and consciousness researchers. But do we really know what the actual phenomenon is to which the sages of ancient India gave this name?[73]

Thus begins Mary Scott's *Kundalini in the Physical World*. Released in 1983, Scott's book would have certainly sat on a shelf alongside the likes of Yogi Bhajan, Muktananda, Sivananda Radha, and Lee Sannella. You can almost see it rubbing covers with the John White volume with which we began this chapter. In fact, though Scott explains that her book was prompted by a volume of the journal *Human Dimensions*, it could have just as easily been an answer to White's collection. "What struck me most about [the journal's] various articles," writes Scott, "was how many Kundalinis there seemed to be. What I had thought a relatively clear-cut and limited phenomenon—the serpent fire of Hinduism, the caduceus power of the hermetic tradition—seemed to have become a mixed bundle of phenomena tied together and labelled 'Kundalini.' "[74]

Scott sets out to offer a corrective to this situation, first by situating Kuṇḍalinī in properly South Asian roots (she draws primarily on Avalon and Aurobindo), and then by seeking to ground the phenomenon in contemporary science, ranging from the biophysical to the planetary. As a work of scholarship, the project is not quite sound, either historically or philosophically. But to critique Scott's work on academic grounds is to miss its point. Perhaps it's easiest to say that she remained a Theosophist at heart. Scott recounts how one of her first exposures to meditative practice came as a result of joining the Esoteric Section of the Theosophical Society.[75] It was also to Theosophical texts that she first went to seek information on Kuṇḍalinī—she betrays these roots when she refers to "the caduceus power of the hermetic tradition"—but she notes that she ultimately found them at odds with the South Asian sources.[76] Of course, Scott's discussion of the correspondences between the individual Kuṇḍalinī that dwells at the base of the spine, Kuṇḍalinī as an "earth force," and "cosmic Kuṇḍalinī" is nevertheless very much in the spirit of Theosophical authors like Charles Leadbeater and George Arundale.[77] Scott's model of physical Kuṇḍalinī, it should be noted, is drawn straight from Bentov and Sannella. And so, in a sense, Scott offers a corrective to the chaos of conflicting models by offering yet another "standard" that is essentially woven together out of strands pulled from that same tangle. Even her "traditional" models (Avalon and Aurobindo) are already works of modern synthesis.

Of course, we might ask whether there was ever a model of Kuṇḍalinī that wasn't a synthesis of something else.

Curiously, Scott would ultimately take a fairly critical approach to Gopi Krishna in the revised edition of her book, reissued under the title *The Kundalini Concept: Its Origin and Value* in 2006. There, Scott would implicitly come to question not only Gopi Krishna's model of Kuṇḍalinī but even the fact that a single force that could be called Kuṇḍalinī was responsible for his experience. "There is no evidence from his books that he ever studied the tantric texts or discussed the nature of Kundalini with tantric scholars or had read *The Serpent Power*," writes Scott. "All Gopi Krishna's theories about Kundalini and the research based upon them rest on what I was to discover in the course of my own research were sadly false assumptions."[78] This, of course, is somewhat ironic, not only because we have every reason to believe that Gopi Krishna consulted Avalon's book and others besides in his initial research, but because the starting point of Gopi Krishna's knowledge about Kuṇḍalinī most likely derived from the very two sources that Scott herself employs: Avalon and Aurobindo. As Gopi Krishna makes quite clear, it wasn't that he didn't know about the historical tantric material, it was that he did not find it very helpful. It is not precisely clear what aspect of Gopi Krishna's model Scott ultimately finds problematic, but she does make it clear that she still prefers to align herself with the Bentov–Sannella physiological framework.

Sannella, meanwhile, appeared to be having a reckoning of his own as early as the 1980s. He reissued an expanded version of his book in 1987. The new edition is a true revision, now more careful with its treatment of both the depth and diversity of Asian traditions, and full to the brim with references to luminaries of the Human Potential Movement. Though, to be fair, Sannella's more intricate treatment of "the classic model" of Kuṇḍalinī appears to be owed chiefly to Arthur Avalon, at least if citations are an accurate gauge. The new edition also contains a great deal more case studies. Most importantly, perhaps, Sannella develops a more circumscribed version of his "physio-kundalini" model. He no longer gestures at the notion that practices not aimed at Kuṇḍalinī, for instance, might be used to guide a practitioner through Kuṇḍalinī awakening in a less forceful fashion. In fact, Sannella had not only grown skeptical of Gopi Krishna's model of Kuṇḍalinī as a universal evolutionary mechanism, but also of the idea that such evolutionary changes in the nervous system had much spiritual import at all—a shift that now seems to stand at odds with the lingering discussion of "spiritual rebirth" at the opening of the book. A new concluding chapter contains a sort of ode to Adi Da and his nondual model of complete transcendence.

(Michael Murphy relates that Fredric Spiegelberg, too, would come to express the opinion that the universalist and evolutionary focus of Gopi Krishna's approach may have done more harm than good. In any case, even before the turn of the millennium, the tensions of so many models rubbing together were mounting, and Gopi Krishna's popularity no doubt made him an easy target.)

Sannella also returns to his claim that Kuṇḍalinī awakening is happening with increased frequency. (He doesn't specify "in the West" this time, but his subsequent reasoning makes this assumption fairly obvious.) On this point, Sannella dismisses the notion that this is all mere appearance, perhaps owed to a shift in the intellectual climate that has allowed people to speak more freely of their experiences. Instead, he says, "people experience kundalini phenomena more frequently because they are actually involved in disciplines and life-styles conducive to psychospiritual transformation."[79] Here he references the common staples of 1970s counterculture: LSD, a slew of Asian meditative traditions, as well as more "domestic" fare such as "dowsing, 'channeling' (mediumism), magic, witchcraft, and psychic healing."[80] It is this particular claim that most clearly shows the hole in Sannella's argument. After all, these are all practices that have been a common staple of European and Euro-American folk religion for centuries, if not longer. But the historical accuracy of the argument is perhaps again not the point.

What is the point, then? There are two angles we could take—and will take, in the final chapter of this book. On the one hand, the perceived "shift" in Western society due to the introduction of Asian spiritual systems is an important development, even if the story is far more complicated (and indeed more bidirectional) than Sannella suggests. On the other hand, as we've seen, a lot of experience happens in the framing. And, just as modern medicine and psychology have pathologized experiences that might have previously been understood differently, so too the evolving framing of Kuṇḍalinī has opened up a space for such experiences to have a new (albeit equally modern) meaning.

8

THE SERPENT IN THE WEB

Contemporary Interweavings

we are all of us
dragons
slouching towards enlightenment

serpents who forgot they could
fly

—AF

We arrive, at last, at the present day. This chapter is a sort of "state of the field," offering snapshots of Kuṇḍalinī across three (at first glance, vastly different) contemporary contexts: current academic research, the digital landscape of the Internet and especially social media, and Indian practitioners of Goddess tantra. Whereas the rest of the book has emphasized the weaving of a web of narrative, here we will focus more on a few of the resulting nodes.

Before we proceed, a content warning is in order. The tail end of this chapter addresses living traditions of Kuṇḍalinī practice in Assam and West Bengal, including explicitly sexual dimensions. Kamala Ma and Sundari Ma's story, in particular, began when the two (now middle-aged) women were trained by their guru, as children, in the bodily disciplines required for sexual ritual. This will no doubt prove disturbing for some readers, especially those unfamiliar with fieldwork involving women in South Asian esoteric traditions and temple culture.

We deliberated whether to include this material, but ultimately decided to do so for several key reasons. First, the women in question were all between forty and sixty years of age at the time of their interviews and shared their stories with the understanding that they would be made public. Second, while social and legal norms may have evolved, these stories remain significant. These things happen. Third, these field notes aim to highlight the challenges inherent in ethnographic research. Ethnographers often meet with complicated data that can be difficult to fit to a single narrative or even interpretation. With this in mind, we have chosen to present the raw data to our readers without imposing value judgments upon our interlocutors' words. And finally, we want to emphasize that this, too, is Kuṇḍalinī. This, too, is modern because it is happening now. This, too, is global because, although it is happening in a small temple town in West Bengal, women like Kamala Ma and Sundari Ma know that the world is much larger than their charnel grounds. They know what people say. Their story matters in part because it is so different from what one finds in scholarly journals, or scattered across social media apps, and yet it is so indelibly entangled with these global threads.

The impact of digital media upon our collective ways of communicating, knowing, and being over the last handful of decades cannot be understated. The world is more connected than ever. Even as we saw the "standard model" of Kuṇḍalinī consolidate itself over the course of the twentieth century, reaching its full-fledged form in the 1960s and 1970s, we were still dealing largely with local networks and communities. With the advent of the Internet, these communities have become global. As we'll see, even seemingly local communities of "traditional" Indian practitioners, some of whom are illiterate and most of whom are not regularly scrolling through TikTok, are not immune to such connections. They, too, are part of the oral back-and-forth that now spans the entire globe. There are lots of buzzwords from the contemporary study of religion we could use here: transnationalism, hybridity, glocalization. But rather than leaning on theory and jargon, we will simply point out that what we see today is in many ways the continuation of a process that has been happening all along. Diverse traditions are consolidated in canonical sources, only to diverge once more in the individual renderings of practitioners. Symbols replicate, blend, and mutate—does it matter if we are referring to literary imagery or Internet memes? Culture is never held entirely in common.

In the end, the seemingly separate spheres of scholarship, pop culture, and tradition turn out to be not so separate after all. Here, we might point to the ways that academic authority, in the form of public scholarship, can even become its own channel of transmission, rendering "tradition" accessible to anyone with an Internet connection. Take, for instance, Christopher D. Wallis, a Sanskritist with advanced degrees from prestigious universities, and a list of academic mentors that includes several luminaries in the field of tantric studies, who runs a popular Internet blog on tantra and leads workshops for spiritual seekers and experiencers.

In short, Kuṇḍalinī today is an object of scholarly and scientific inquiry. Kuṇḍalinī is also the subject of a dizzying flow of imagery and personal experience. And, in some places, to some people, She is still indisputably the Goddess. All of these things are true at once. None of them are simple.

KUṆḌALINĪ ON THE RESEARCHER'S TABLE

Scientific research on Kuṇḍalinī has taken two paths, one centered on Kuṇḍalinī yoga and the other on Kuṇḍalinī experience. When we say "Kuṇḍalinī yoga," what we mostly mean is "Kundalini Yoga as taught by Yogi Bhajan." Explorations of Kuṇḍalinī yoga as therapy and research supporting such goals have primarily been conducted by scholars associated with 3HO and the Kundalini Research Institute.[1] It falls largely along the same lines as other research on the therapeutic effects of yoga practice on mental health and general wellness. This, of course, makes sense in light of the fact that Yogi Bhajan's system ultimately belongs to the same family of practices as other popular forms of modern postural yoga.

Kuṇḍalinī as experience, on the other hand, has mainly thrived in the arena of transpersonal psychology research, where Itzhak Bentov's and Lee Sannella's model of the "physio-kundalini syndrome" has been taken up and elaborated upon by multiple researchers. Though Bentov's theories on the physical mechanisms of Kuṇḍalinī are still referenced, the overall focus has landed not on explanatory models of how and why Kuṇḍalinī works in the body on a physiological level, but on observational maps of how it is experienced. For instance, a 2008 study by Laura Sanches and Michael Daniels introduces a seventy-six-point "Kundalini Awakening Scale."[2] The metrics are grouped into five categories—changes, negative experiences, positive experiences, involuntary positionings, and physical symptoms—and each item is assigned a numerical value based on the subject's experience, which are then tabulated for a total score. Most such studies have focused on individuals experiencing what the pioneers of the field, such as Christina and Stanislav Grof, would have identified as "spiritual emergency." However, other scholars—most notably, perhaps, a recent study of meditators in the Ananda Marga school by Richard Maxwell and Sucharit Katyal—have attempted to track psycho-physical markers of Kuṇḍalinī as they are produced in the context of intentional practice.[3]

Yet, in attempting to systematize Kuṇḍalinī, such studies often run up against a wall of chaotic human experience. For example, a

2015 study by transpersonal psychologist Steve Taylor that attempts to place Kuṇḍalinī experience within a larger typology of spiritual awakening (Taylor associates Kuṇḍalinī specifically with "psycho-sexual" awakening) seems nevertheless unable to pin down precisely what actually "counts" as Kuṇḍalinī. Taylor sums up the issue like this:

> Five participants had kundalini-like experiences, with many of the classic characteristics of the phenomenon; although in four cases they did not specifically locate the "rush of energy" they experienced near the base of the spine, or describe it rising up through the spinal area. This observation suggests either that these four participants were simply unaware of the exact source or trajectory of the energy (perhaps it was the bottom of the spine), or that the upsurge of energy associated with kundalini may sometimes occur in a different form, from a source other than the muladhara-chakra, or through the channel of sushumna.[4]

This, of course, is reminiscent of Sannella's original findings, which he found to disagree on some significant points with his own understanding of the medieval literature as well as with the teachings of contemporary gurus. Though one may find patterns among individual experiencers (and even these are not only self-selecting but ultimately inconsistent), fitting that scatterplot to a single coherent narrative proves to be another matter entirely. In other words, the more one insists on squaring such empirical maps with the "standard model" believed to derive from tradition (that is, the fiery "serpent-like" energy rising up the spine, root to crown), the less the whole thing seems to hold together.

And then there are the bigger questions of meaning. In research contexts, Kuṇḍalinī becomes a technical term for a constellation of symptoms. This, in a way, is the natural outcome of Bentov's and Sannella's "syndrome." A syndrome has no reason and no meaning. However, when couched in the framing of Hindu tantric models as well as the evolutionary frameworks of popularizers like Gopi Krishna (which inevitably show up, in broad strokes, in the introductory sections of such papers), the meanings tend to materialize anyway. The aura of enlightenment lingers.

Here, it may be helpful to look outside of "Kuṇḍalinī research" proper, to get a bit of perspective. The Varieties of Contemplative Experience (VCE) research project led by Drs. Willoughby Britton, Jared Lindahl, and other colleagues at Brown University has been devoted to examining the vast range of experiences—both positive and negative—associated with the practice of meditation.[5] A closer look at the phenomenon they call "energy-like somatic experiences" (ELSEs), led by David Cooper, reveals fascinating patterns in how embodied sensations, including ones that are extreme, prolonged, and even potentially life-disrupting, are interpreted by practitioners in different traditions. All of the practitioners in this study were engaged in a specific type of Buddhist meditation but, by selecting practitioners from Theravada, Tibetan, and Zen traditions, the researchers were able to contrast meditators whose "home traditions" gave them frameworks for interpreting experiences that could be understood as "subtle energy" as well as ones who lacked such models. Interestingly, the team found that practitioners whose traditions included such frameworks were no more likely to report ELSEs than those whose traditions did not. They were, however, more likely to identify their practice as an influencing factor in the ELSE.[6]

Unsurprisingly, when practitioners did not meet with suitable models for such experiences within their own traditions, they sought explanations from other traditions. And, among such practitioners, Kuṇḍalinī was the most common model to be adopted, sometimes based on prior knowledge, but often after the fact. This does not mean, however, that Kuṇḍalinī was their *only* model. It might also be combined with understandings based on traditional systems of medicine (Chinese or Tibetan, for instance) or else of modern psychology and neuroscience. The research team suggested that, for those practitioners who found their ELSEs distressing, simply finding an interpretive framework that helped them make sense of what was happening could prove to be a powerful remedy.[7] However, this could also reveal points of tension with their original tradition of practice. One practitioner of Theravada-style meditation had an energetic experience so dramatic (the energy entered her body as she was sitting in meditation and forcefully banged her back against the wall several times) that she was removed from the retreat in which she was participating when she reported it to her teachers. The teachers removed her without giving any explanations for how and why the experience had come about, and it wasn't until later that she found a therapist who identified her experience with Kuṇḍalinī. The practitioner herself was both relieved and excited; her teachers were less so. "This is what happened to me: I had a *kundalini* release," she reports thinking. "It was like, I know now!' I was like an excited little kid—I know now!' And they said they don't believe in *kundalini* releases."[8]

These findings raise the possibility that it isn't simply the "secular" pathologization of Kuṇḍalinī or Kuṇḍalinī-like experiences that can leave experiencers without proper support. Spiritual traditions where energetic and other subtle body practices do not play a role are not necessarily any better equipped to provide helpful frameworks and satisfying narratives to those who experience such things. And then, of course, the study only examined Western practitioners of Buddhist meditation—meaning that we have to think not only about the secular and the sacred, the modern and the premodern, but also (as the researchers themselves ultimately point out) the "current status of transmission of Buddhism from Asia to the West."[9] And what the VCE researchers say about Buddhism, we could easily extend to Hindu tantra. The key difference would be that, instead of potentially lacking traditional frameworks of explanation for these sorts of embodied experiences, the association between Kuṇḍalinī and the specific historical web of narratives we've traced out in this book has led to the illusion that there is just one model—just one explanation—whereas the reality, even in the "traditional" context, has always been far more complex.

Another important move made by the VCE researchers is to argue that there are distinct interpretive downsides to the "Kuṇḍalinī syndrome" approach, and that these have to do both with the on-the-ground messiness of what embodied energetic experiences actually look like as well as with the accompanying assumption that they must ultimately be a good thing. The research team concludes:

> In light of the heterogeneous phenomenology of ELSEs, their range of impacts, and the various appraisals and responses associated with them, researchers (as well as meditation teachers) should perhaps resist the temptation to assume a spiritual emergency "*kundalini* awakening" framework and the positive spiritual trajectory it typically implies. The archetypal notion popularized by [Stanislav and Christina Grof] and developed through subsequent research in transpersonal psychology in particular, seems to capture neither the full range of ELSEs nor their various trajectories. Rather, as we have argued elsewhere, it may be more appropriate to adopt a person-centered approach that takes the worldviews, values, and proximate and ultimate goals of the practitioner into account when considering which appraisals and remedies to offer. Furthermore, as documented elsewhere in the VCE study, determining the best

> response or intervention for managing ELSEs was, in many cases, more salient than determining the correct appraisal. The interpretations that practitioners gave to ELSEs were often dictated by remedies or responses that worked for managing them. Helpful remedies included normalizing ELSEs, changes in practice type or approach, acupuncture, herbal and pharmacological medicines, and various grounding activities, such as exercise and a change in diet.[10]

In other words, not every spiritual emergency is a rung on the ladder to enlightenment and liberation. Sometimes such experiences are not progressive but simply debilitating. If nothing else, there is no "one size fits all" model, regardless of whether we decide to call it Kuṇḍalinī or not.

The takeaway point, perhaps, is this: Kuṇḍalinī seems to put a word to something that many of us (whether because of "tradition" or "modernity" or both) don't have workable language for. There can be great power in the ability to name a thing. But at what point does the name begin to obscure the thing itself?

LET'S TALK ABOUT SEX (AGAIN)

At this juncture, it's important to remark that, quite often, the thing Kuṇḍalinī names in today's world is sex. As we've seen, the link between Eastern spirituality and sacred sexuality is no novel invention. Refined in the fires of the countercultural revolution and its aftermath, today's incarnations may appear a bit more self-aware—more careful, less naïve. But, on the whole, Neo-Tantra remains alive and well, with all its inherent contradictions. On the one hand, purveyors of Neo-Tantric treatments, workshops, and other resources are meeting a genuine need in a culture where sex is so frequently entangled with repression, anxiety, and profound trauma. On the other hand, there is no denying the utilitarian reality that sex sells.

This is broadly reflected in popular media, especially the documentary format that has experienced a sort of renaissance in the age of streaming platforms. From exposés of infamous gurus, like the Osho-centric *Wild Wild Country* (2018), to more general treatments such as the "Tantric Sex" episode of *(Un)well* (2020), Neo-Tantra is especially well suited to this unique genre of entertainment, which combines the promise of education with titillation and a healthy touch of scandal. The exoticism woven into the sexuality—whether in the trappings of Asia or more homegrown staples of the New Age—is spice added to an already hot commodity. No matter how carefully framed, such portrayals cannot help but reinforce the link between tantra and sex, eliciting both fascination and moral panic.

It's true that we have come a long way from the days of Ida Craddock, the nineteenth-century occultist and activist who married the sacred and the sexual in her "Church of Yoga." Having run afoul of Anthony Comstock—the famously puritanical anti-obscenity crusader whose namesake legislation is still occasionally evoked today—Craddock took her own life rather than endure a five-year prison sentence or confinement to an insane asylum.[11] And yet, it was only in 2016 that Tracy Elise, founder and high priestess of the Phoenix Goddess Temple, was sentenced to just short of five years in prison after being found guilty on twenty-two counts, each variously connected to running a "house of prostitution." Elise refused a plea deal, choosing to serve her time as a testament to her conviction in the sanctity of her practice.[12]

Media accounts aimed at a general audience do not usually contain explicit references to Kuṇḍalinī, but one does not have to dig deep at the intersection of tantra and sex before the term inevitably surfaces. A simple online search quickly produces countless written sources, private sessions, workshops, and retreats hosted anywhere from India to Mexico. Kuṇḍalinī awakening—which can be achieved, among other methods, through massage—is touted as the key to healing, to transformation, to soul-melding relationships and, above all, to cosmically reverberating full-body orgasms.

We are far enough into this book that the reader now knows what to expect: we have no interest in adjudicating whether any of these things represent "genuine" engagements with Kuṇḍalinī. But the tension—between the old and the new, between East and West, between the sacred and the secular, and above all between the promise of healing and the commercial gimmick—seems important to recognize.

KUṆḌALINĪ ONLINE

Beyond the more specialized offerings detailed above, performing a digital search for "kundalini" or "kundalini yoga" yields an easily anticipated slate of results. First come the popular informational sources, both general and more field-specific: there is Wikipedia and Healthline, but also *Yoga Journal* (now a digital platform, but originally a print magazine first published in 1975) and the somewhat newer lifestyle media brand mindbodygreen. Then come the teachers. One finds both the usual suspects stemming from 1960s guru movements—Yogi Bhajan's 3HO and Kundalini Research Institute; Osho; Sivananda's Divine Life Society—as well as newcomers, most notably Sadhguru's Isha Foundation. Sprinkled throughout all of the above content are informational pages from the sites of lower-profile teachers, wellness centers, and lifestyle brands.

In a sense, the migration of Kuṇḍalinī from print to digital media now seems like a minor shift. The content most readily available via online sources does not, in its basic features, differ all that drastically from what the average person could have found in a reasonably stocked bookstore half a century ago. Rather, it is the ready availability in and of itself that presents the greatest change. Yet this appraisal must be revisited if we take into account not simply the most easily discoverable webpages, usually administered by specialists (even if self-styled) and organizations—precisely the type of individuals and entities that would have traditionally had a monopoly on print media—but also the rise of social media, which has had a far more democratizing effect on how we access information as well as each other.

Because social media evolves so quickly, whatever analysis we can provide could be out of date by the time this book actually appears in print. And yet, social media platforms have become so deeply integrated into the fabric of our lives, including in how we obtain and share information, that we cannot simply ignore them in this discussion. With this caveat in mind, then, we'll briefly turn to some of today's most popular social media platforms and offer a few brief reflections on how they might be shaping our common understanding of Kuṇḍalinī.

But where to look? If you perform a traditional search, the first platform (as opposed to simply a website) you are likely to encounter is the video-sharing hub of YouTube. Yet the content shared on YouTube, despite being an important platform when it comes to disseminating information, remains closer in nature to a static webpage rather than a true social media environment. Though commenting is an option on many videos, we rarely find the kind of person-to-person engagement that would be characteristic of a Facebook group, for example. And, at this point in time, YouTube lacks the rapid-fire dynamism of something like Instagram or, even more important as a point of contrast, TikTok. Thus, it is these latter three platforms that we will briefly survey as we try to put our fingers on the pulse of how Kuṇḍalinī is making its way through online spaces. Because they launched roughly half a decade apart (which may as well be eons in "Internet time"), considering the three in succession also gives us a sense of how content sharing and social interaction have evolved since the initial introduction of such spaces.

Facebook technically launched in 2004, but it did not achieve anything like its present form until 2007. Having opened to the general public only a year prior, the company introduced a "Pages" function, available to companies but also allowing pages focused on a specific theme, which in turn paved the way for the introduction of "Groups" in 2010. For our intents and purposes, it is this group function that stands out as perhaps most important, since it allows users to easily make connections beyond their personal "Friends" networks. By joining a group, a user can share content and interact with hundreds and even thousands of others who share their specific interests. In 2017, Facebook shifted its business model to foreground this feature, because it was seen as unique among the growing slate of competing platforms.

Today, Facebook's various Kuṇḍalinī groups are a place for people to share experiences, resources, and occasionally rants. One popular group boasts more than three-quarters of a million members. Posts there regularly receive dozens, even hundreds of comments. Some of these are superficial one-liners, but many others show sustained engagement and discussion among participants. Impressionistically speaking, a large percentage of the participants in such groups report having experienced their Kuṇḍalinī awakening spontaneously. Some groups are specifically targeted at those seeking guidance and support in the midst of a Kuṇḍalinī awakening. To some extent, this may add further fuel to the anxieties and fear surrounding Kuṇḍalinī experiences, especially the notion that Kuṇḍalinī should not be raised until one is physically, mentally, and spiritually "ready."

Social media-based groups also generally lack any formal sense of structure to support their members. While groups may be administered by a specific individual (such as a teacher) or an organization (for instance, an ashram), many are not moderated closely, which is especially true of the largest and liveliest groups. This means that there is no expert vetting of the information that is shared, even when it comes to basic accuracy. Indeed, a sizeable portion of the posts in larger groups are not about Kuṇḍalinī at all, and they veer into a variety of other esoteric and spiritual topics such as manifestation, Jungian "shadow work," and even Christian evangelism. While, as proposed by the researchers of the VCE project, even a basic acknowledgement and affirmation of an otherwise destabilizing psycho-physical "energetic" experience can have a great deal of positive value, this value ultimately depends on gaining a functional interpretive framework. Whether or not Facebook groups provide such a framework is debatable.

While Facebook groups can certainly be eclectic in their content, this is even more true of platforms that are not focused on thematic subunits. Searching for "kundalini" on Instagram (launched in 2010, now a subsidiary of Meta, along with Facebook, by which it was acquired in 2012) yields a flood of images, drawn from every possible source. Chinese meridians blend with Indian *cakras*. Depth psychology meets New Age prosperity gospel. Everywhere, serpents slither and rainbows radiate. If Facebook is still primarily modeled on interpersonal engagement, including through the groups feature, which can expand one's social circle to an unprecedented size, Instagram is based more firmly in creator-to-consumer content delivery. While some posts (especially those made by popular accounts) may elicit a large number of comments, there is little dialogue in the manner of Facebook groups. Engagements are short, transient, and rarely involve more than two users. More than anything else, then, Instagram allows us to gauge what Kuṇḍalinī literally *looks* like at this specific moment in time. To give an executive summary: things have certainly become more chaotic (to be expected). And yet, the fundamental imagery we have been tracking throughout this book still occupies a plurality of posts. *Cakras* are common, but they are largely rainbow-colored and decidedly seven in number. There are lots of serpents, most often appearing in a caduceus-like double helix, which now additionally evokes the spiraling structure of DNA. And there is fire, electricity, light.

TikTok (launched in 2016), being newer than the other two platforms and skewing younger in its demographics, combines their basic features and turns the result up to eleven. Here, narrative explodes with frenetic imagery and sound. You can find anything from personal testimonies to instructions and demonstrations of practices, to warnings about demonic possession, to explanations of how the sun can "upgrade your DNA." Unlike other "creator-focused" platforms (like YouTube or Instagram), however, the comments are a lively space where users connect with one another by agreeing and disagreeing, offering their own experiences, reassuring one another, and occasionally calling out what they perceive to be inauthentic or otherwise dubious content. Because of the relative brevity of most TikTok videos—currently in-app recordings have a maximum limit of three minutes, though uploaded videos are permitted up to ten—it seems unlikely that most users are looking to gain in-depth information. In other words, someone is more likely to "discover" Kuṇḍalinī for the first time via TikTok rather than turn to it for research. But this discovery effect should not be treated as superficial. Because TikTok is known for its highly personalized algorithm, it may be uniquely adapted to introducing Kuṇḍalinī to exactly the demographic with whom such concepts are most likely to resonate.

In short, across the different types of social media, we see the collective evolution of Kuṇḍalinī narratives acquire an unprecedented degree of interconnectivity, exposure, reach, and above all immediacy. A book can only give impressionistic descriptions. On video, you can see a body jerk and spasm as a teacher performs energy work. On social media, you can view dozens of such videos in the space of a few minutes. Such access undoubtedly comes with both benefits and shortfalls. Even platforms that make space for longer-form narrative content (Facebook or YouTube) encourage mass, rapid consumption of individual contributions. Each source is always vying for attention with thousands of others. In this environment, familiar images thrive. A baseline level of familiarity, after all, is the essence of a meme. The ability to present a familiar image allows a content creator to communicate content more rapidly when working within allotted timespans (due as much to formal platform restrictions as to restricted attention spans). This is not a phenomenon that is novel or unique to online content, much less to social media. But, like so many other human traits, individual and social alike, technology has augmented and intensified the way it functions.

So what does this mean for Kuṇḍalinī? On the one hand, we can expect to see a strengthening of what cultural commentators have long referred to as "monoculture," drawing on an agricultural metaphor that refers to populating a given area with only a single variety of crop. As the same images and the same narratives are shared and reshared, they become an ever more universal standard. This is true not only of algorithmically driven social media platforms, but also of seemingly more static online content which is nevertheless accessed primarily via the invisible algorithms of search engines. One simple yet stark example: typing "Who is the father of Kundalini yoga?" into Google immediately returns a seemingly unambiguous answer. The engine sprawls "Harbhajan Singh Khalsa" (that is, Yogi Bhajan) across the top of the results page in large, bolded letters. This isn't technically false, of course. But it is missing at least one fairly important qualifier.

Such flattening of nuance through a focus on the ever more efficient delivery of information is unlikely to reverse its course. As we wrap up our work on this book in the fall of 2023, we can safely say that the past year alone has been transformational when it comes to the role of Large Language Model (LLM) artificial intelligence in the way that we generate, transmit, and receive information. LLMs operate by distilling patterns and connections between words and phrases. And so, if we are interested in problematizing the idea of "standard models" and "common narratives," then we might have good reason to be concerned about tools that are built to produce precisely these things on an unprecedented scale. The LLM speaks the language of the least common denominator.

On the other hand, however, online resources and platforms have undoubtedly allowed for an unprecedented proliferation of individual narratives. To say that these must inherently act as a counterbalance to the monoculture born of algorithmic reductionism and increasing interconnectedness would be as simplistic as it would be naïve. After all, what does it matter how many people are telling a story if they're all telling the exact same one? And yet, stories, much less experiences, never are quite the same from telling to telling.

THE SERPENT IN THE FIELD: SRAVANA'S RESEARCH DIARY

But what of the people engaging in Kuṇḍalinī practice just as they have always done, on the ground? Indeed, what of those engaging in it on the very same ground where the term first appeared, over a millennium ago now? How has Kuṇḍalinī changed for them, if it has changed at all? The stories that follow were gathered as part of Sravana Borkataky-Varma's doctoral dissertation research in Assam and

Western Bengal over a period of four years (2011–2015). Though the analysis below contains reflections by both authors, for the sake of clarity, the "I" telling these stories remains Sravana. All names are fictitious to protect the privacy of these practitioners. The names of temples have been changed only if they threatened to divulge the identity of the presiding guru.

When I first embarked on studying the modern practices of Kuṇḍalinī yoga, it was part of a larger (and somewhat different) project than the one presented in this book. This project was specifically focused on shedding light upon the role of women in living Goddess tantra traditions—the ways they are revered, but also the ways that they are marginalized and perhaps even stymied in the pursuit of their own enlightenment (rather than that of their partners). For this reason, the stories below come primarily from women. This is not a representative sample of Indian tantric practitioners as a whole. Instead, it offers what I believe to be an important and often ignored angle. Even a corrective. In some ways, we can view these accounts as a counterbalance to the historical accounts of Kuṇḍalinī we examined in chapter 1, which inevitably assume that the practitioner is male.

I also share these women's stories here because—though they are many other things—they are a perfect encapsulation of how even the local and the seemingly "traditional" is nevertheless yet another tangled thread in the global and the inescapably modern. The women I interviewed are part of this world, and they are part of these conversations. They don't only talk, they listen. As a researcher, I became deeply aware of the role that I myself was playing in this transmission of Kuṇḍalinī—how the questions I asked and the language I used were taken in, absorbed, and adapted by those I spoke to.

In the years after I completed my doctoral work, I conducted a few more informal interviews, largely because I felt that I was not done with the topic—or rather, that it was not done with me. My interlocutors were people I met at workshops in various Indian cities, and some were simply introduced to me by mutual friends. The conversations, needless to say, were fascinating. In the interest of both research ethics and personal privacy, I will not address their stories directly here. Nevertheless, I offer a few general observations.

First, though I generally encountered them in India, all of these individuals were of Euro-American descent—that is, while many were clearly serious practitioners, they were not embedded in the same culture as the people whose stories follow below. To be blunt, they were white, largely affluent people. Many of them can be found dressed in fine shawls from inner Mongolia, or wearing "quiet luxury" Indian brands, and for some reason they love wearing flower garlands and carry water bottles everywhere they go. This is the very group of people—some of whom are more or less professional seekers if not outright spiritual influencers—who play a crucial role in the export-import transmission history of Kuṇḍalinī that now thrives on social media. Their high-resolution photos are captivating. Their captions frequently sound like excerpts from *Eat, Pray, Love*. Having said all the above, I do not want to imply that they are not true seekers. They are. They simply belong to a specific culture.

What was striking about these people's answers to my questions was how easily they seemed to derive from the histories and especially from the "web" of sources we have treated in this book. Their understanding of Kuṇḍalinī was often rather abstract, occasionally even vague. And yet, Kuṇḍalinī—especially the experience of it—seemed to have a palpable presence in their spiritual lives. Often, though not always, this presence was also fundamentally sexual, sometimes even bordering perhaps on sexual fantasy. ("When orgasm is experienced along with a raised Kuṇḍalinī, you experience oneness," one woman told me. "This oneness is then seen in every being, be it an ant, a tree, or a human being. It is intoxicating. Once you have experienced this, you cannot ever go back to bedroom sex.") The power of the feminine loomed large, with women being believed to have easier access to Kuṇḍalinī. One of my conversation partners told me this was because "women have less ego." Another attributed it to the power of female sexual fluids. They had slightly different ideas on where Kuṇḍalinī resided, or how it should be raised, but most seemed to agree with the idea of oneness, of bliss. In a sense, their answers were often contracted versions of the sort of accounts one finds in books like *Kundalini Rising*, by Gurmukh Kaur Khalsa and others, or in similar sources by Western teachers and experiencers.

The Indian practitioners to whom I spoke by and large did not have access to such sources. Many were illiterate. And yet, woven into their language I found some of the same terms ("buzzwords"), often rendered in English, that we see in the Western literature and in global online communities.

Mai of Devi Mandir at Guwahati

Mai was born in a small village called Naddi in Nalbari, Assam. Her father was a devoted Brahmin and tantric practitioner (*sādhaka*). He initiated his daughter into his practice and taught her how to do *sādhana*. One day when Mai was around twelve or thirteen years old, as she sat meditating, she was bestowed with special powers (*siddhi*) that made her clairvoyant. In the few years after, Mai's reputation spread far and wide, and she gained a large following of devotees. This was also how she met her partner. One night she dreamt of her wedding, and, in this dream, she was introduced to a man who would soon become her husband. At this stage, it's important to note that a skeptic may interpret Mai's precognition of her future marriage as a desire to marry a particular man, perhaps based on other sources of knowledge acquired by ordinary means. That is not how Mai understands the dream, however, nor do her followers question it. Indeed, what many would call "clairvoyance" is taken for granted by the followers of tantric adepts and gurus. It is simply a reality. This, and other *siddhis*, are a product of Kuṇḍalinī rising. In any case, Mai told her father of the dream and gave a general description of her future husband's family and the location of his village. Her family then set forth to find the man. The two were married soon after. A few years later, Mai's husband also joined her practice and is now the head priest of her temple.

Mai's cherished goddess (*iṣṭa-devī*)—the form of the divine to whom she devotes her *sādhana* as well as her love—is Caṇḍī or Caṇḍīkā (the "Fierce One"). Mai had no plans to move out of her village, but one night Caṇḍī came to her and said, "There is an old devotee who takes care of me. He lives in Guwahati, but he will die soon. I direct you to go there; live and make a temple there."

The next few months were very confusing, Mai tells me. At first, she was nervous about moving her young family out of their home. Mai intuited that she was looking for a particular shed in Guwahati, where she would find the devotee the Goddess spoke of—but how to find the shed? She prayed for many days, and soon she decided to move to Guwahati. She and her husband walked for days together, scouting around and asking the locals about this mysterious shed. She found it at last, but by this time the old priest had passed away, and the shed was in shambles. Mai tells me, tenderly now, how she cried for the devout priest, and of the dilapidated state in which she found the sacred icon (*mūrti*) of Caṇḍī. Mai cleaned the place up and, from that day until the present, she has continued to live there. In that time (about thirty-five years), the shed has grown into a sprawling temple complex. The present temple has been constructed so that its inner sanctum stands on the exact spot of the old shed, where it houses the sacred icon of Caṇḍī that the old priest used to pray to. This is Mai's "seat." Today, she is the presiding guru of her temple, a position of high honor.

In speaking with me, Mai admits to practicing Śākta tantra since she believes that Caṇḍī is only pleased by this kind of *sādhana.* Kuṇḍalinī, Mai tells me, is a "kind of light" (*jyoti*), which gets activated when one seeks to genuinely know the mysteries of the divine. Who is the divine? Where is the divine? Mai explains that when Kuṇḍalinī is at play and activated, an individual gets restless and feels a deep urge to find the answers to such questions.

I ask her to describe this "kind of light," and Mai explains a visualization of the light as akin to a white dot. She uses many English words to explain the "light." The white dot is present in every human being, she says, but it only starts to rise when one continues to meditate with single-pointed concentration (*ekodhyano*). According to her, the white dot is Kuṇḍalinī, the cosmic power that has created the entire universe and is planted as a seed in all human beings. It is the agent in the nervous system that remains dormant for most people. But, with determination and single-pointed concentration, Kuṇḍalinī can be raised. Once it rises, it is systematically absorbed in the body and blends in with the "entire nervous system" which in turn activates each cell in the body. (Here, Mai uses the terms "nervous system" and "cell" in English.) This eventually leads to the formation of a "new body." Mai describes this new body as a second body that is inside us. "We have two bodies. What you see," she says as she points at her hands and feet, "is the physical body. It is a shell, a cover, a shield of some sort." Then she continues:

> After Kuṇḍalinī has risen, it creates a new inner body. The new body is formed; each cell in the body, each nerve gets charged; there is a distinct sensation, almost like a vibration, similar to goose bumps, but the goose bumps surface internally and not externally. Each and every cell in the body will have bumps.

Not a single cell is left untouched. One will have no desire or energy left to move away from this state. Once individuals—male or female—get Kuṇḍalinī to rise, they are never the same again. Something alters within the individual permanently. People come to me with problems. For example, they want to know if their child will get better, if their husband will survive cancer, if their daughter will get married, if the financial hardships will end, and so forth. When they come into the temple and I make eye contact, I instantly know the reason for their visit; I do not need to hear the question from their mouth. At the moment I make eye contact, I am *jñāt*, that is, I am in a "conscious mind state."[13] It is with this mind I ask, "What problem does this person have? Why is this person looking so troubled? What is bothering this family? What is the solution to their problem?" But it is here the conscious mind state ends. Since I search for answers, the answers, the solutions come from the state of being *cetanāhen*, the unconscious mind state.[14] I cannot find that answer in the conscious mind state. If I come up with an answer in the conscious mind state, my solution will be ineffective, wrong, and may be even damaging. I must draw the solution or the answer from the unconscious mind state. So in some ways it is a dual existence. I keep entering the conscious mind state and the unconscious mind state constantly. It is physically exhausting. The unconscious mind state is where you find pure reality. What I find there is absolutely and totally pure. There are no illusions. It is not diluted; it is a clear vision, a vision in which I see the solution and that is what I communicate to the people. But once your nerves get activated by Kuṇḍalinī, you remain altered. Since Kuṇḍalinī rose in me as a child, I have never gone back to the state I was in or experienced before it arose. I live somewhere in between the conscious mind state and the unconscious mind state at all points in time. Also,

> Kuṇḍalinī never goes back to sleep. It is always active: as I sleep, while I am up, when I sit, when I walk, when I talk, when I bathe, all the time.

Mai makes some significant claims about this "new body," and about living constantly in a "twilight zone" in between consciousness and unconsciousness—claims that make most scholars nervous.

The use of terms like "conscious," "unconscious," and "pure reality" is deservedly problematic and fraught with all sorts of cross-cultural complexities. When Mai refers to terms like *jñāt* and *cetanāhen* and relates that she constantly operates out of these mind states, she has in some ways constructed a third category of existence, a "twilight mind existence," as it were. This is a state that exists in most people but of which they are generally unaware. In the case of Mai herself, she is mindful of these states and over the years has cultivated them to reach a level of perfection. Such constructions do force a scholar to probe further into the ontological claims. I certainly did. I questioned her further about the "new body," which I understood to be the "subtle body." But soon I arrived at the conclusion that, unlike Western scholars, Mai does not worry about or ponder over such matters of ontology. For her, it is given. It is the truth. There is nothing to ask or explain. In her view, it is a state that simply happens.

Later, I ask Mai about the role of men and women in each other's practice of Kuṇḍalinī yoga. This is not an easy conversation to initiate. Mai skirts the line of questioning several times. Finally, Mai tells me there are four kinds of practitioners: unmarried men, married men, unmarried women, and married women. In her view, for a man, "a female partner is essential for the practice of Kuṇḍalinī yoga." A man cannot proceed on this path unless he is married and has a devoted wife who will practice with him. Therefore, success comes to married men only. But women, Mai says, do not require the support of anyone because they already have all the energies that are required. They do not need a male partner or a husband for the energy to rise or for the practice to bear fruit. If a woman has self-will, determination, and blessings from the Goddess, she will succeed. This is a powerful statement, if considered in light of the social and cultural norms that surround Mai, where women are not whole if not defined by their relationships to men—as daughters, sisters, wives, and finally as mothers of the sons they may bear. Mai's words turn patriarchy on its head.[15]

Mai's power is attributed, by herself and by her followers, to Kuṇḍalinī. The scholar in me is skeptical of her *siddhis* and finds it difficult to believe in her claimed efficacy. Yet, what I can vouch for is that she has some sort of spiritual power or *presence*, even if I am not sure what it is or how to define it.

Over the months of my fieldwork, I chat with many devotees who come to the temple to seek advice. Many of them are repeat visitors, while some are there for the first time. It is fascinating to observe their interactions with Mai. According to most, the reason she gives them for their visit is accurate. This, in turn, makes them committed to following everything she asks them to do: to offer prayers, fast, make a donation, feed the poor, and so forth. Interestingly enough, those whose reasons for coming contradict the reason stated by Mai do not blame her. Instead, they either blame themselves or justify the discrepancy by stating that they were caught up in the present and that Mai identified the cause of their perils as something in the past, sometimes even many generations ago. Over the many years I have continued to visit, I have yet to find an individual who would call Mai a sham. There are a few skeptics who step into the temple, but I have noticed that, by the time they leave, Mai has managed to convince them that their skepticism is the result of a lack of faith, which itself is the result of a mistake that either they or someone in their family has made in the past.

Ranjan, an Ardent Follower of Mai

I hear it said over and over among practitioners of Kuṇḍalinī yoga: Women embody the maternal principle, and they are supremely powerful. The energies reside in them naturally. But in the case of a man, he lacks purity. A man will need to be purified by women ritually. This is the case with Ranjan, an ardent follower of Mai, and an adherent of her *sādhana*. Kuṇḍalinī is a type of power, Ranjan tells me, before adding:

> Now, do not ask me what power is. Power is power. If now you were to close your eyes, and with your eyes closed, using your inner eye, you were to focus, you would find a white dot coming toward you. While that white dot would originate, it would not come and hit you in the forehead because you do not do *sādhana*. Only if you keep doing *sādhana* on the *jyoti*, slowly and slowly the *jyoti* will come toward you. The day it hits your forehead, that will be the day you will realize that Kuṇḍalinī has risen within you. This does not mean you have gained all knowledge and have become super intelligent. No, when Kuṇḍalinī has risen, your body has become pure, and you have clarity in your vision, which will help you look at things differently. You will be able to look into a person's past like Mai can. You will be blessed with special powers; you will have *siddhi*.

Over the many years he has spent with Mai, Ranjan has found (just as I have) that Mai gives simple solutions—like watering a plant, obtaining a sacred icon, seeking forgiveness, and so forth—to people's grave life problems. I come to understand that Mai's suggested solutions provide people with a type of strength. In other words, it seems like giving them something to do encourages them to take some agency and some responsibility for their situation, even as it also encourages them to rely on an external source of power and help.

People and families come to Mai broken, but Mai helps them go home convinced that the bad days will be over soon. This is the norm among Indian healers and psychics, and many scholars have discussed this form of healing.

Ranjan often wonders how Mai is able to state people's thoughts accurately, time and time again. What quality does she have that others do not have? In his understanding, this is the power of *siddhi.* People with *siddhis* can identify the causes of mysterious situations and problems, whereas a common person cannot. Many people in modern times tend to believe that if something cannot be explained, it cannot be understood. If it cannot be understood, it cannot be taught. If it cannot be taught, it cannot be learned. If it cannot be learned, then it contains no truth. If it contains no truth, it cannot exist. But according to Ranjan, that is not how faith works. People who come to Devi Mandir believe that Mai has special powers, or they have been told so by someone close to them. They do not operate within the matrix of logical explanation and do not seek proof for the existence of what they cannot see.

Nirupama of a Small Town Outside of Guwahati

Nirupama, whom I found in a small town just outside the sprawling city of Guwahati, is another female guru, holding the seat of honor at her own temple. Indeed, she has many similarities with Mai. They even look similar, though perhaps this is largely a result of similar dress preferences and mannerisms. Like Mai, Nirupama is soft-spoken, and both are careful in their choice of words and descriptions of rituals pertaining to the practice of Kuṇḍalinī yoga. While Nirupama's ashram is smaller than Mai's large temple structure, the layout is more or less identical. In both compounds, the inner sanctum is the sacred space, inaccessible to all outsiders, while in the main temple everyone is welcome. And, in both cases, the temple is managed by the female guru's husband. Both Mai's and Nirupama's husbands hold the designation of chief priest. They offer prayers and are primarily responsible for the everyday running of the temple and keeping its accounts.

Nirupama tells me that Kuṇḍalinī is a type of energy (*śakti*). It is the energy of the chosen and cherished goddess (*iṣṭa-devī*) that rises within the practitioner. For Nirupama, Kuṇḍalinī is "the true presence of the goddess Durgā within her." Nirupama meditates on Durgā. For her, Durgā is the supreme energy, and it is only when Durgā comes into her that she is able to provide answers to people. She follows a meticulous process every day. First, she cleans her body in order to communicate with the divine energy. Then, she must clean her mind, reciting mantras and offering *pūjā* (worship) by performing *bhūtaśuddhi* (purification of the body's essences). Once her mind and body are cleansed, she meditates for seven to eight hours, keeping her focus only on Durgā. While Nirupama maintains her focus, she gradually slows down her breathing.

"It is only when my breathing is at a bare minimum and my mind is clear of all thoughts that Ma Durgā slowly enters my body," Nirupama says. I ask her to explain how she feels when Durgā enters her body. Nirupama tells me, "First I get small tremors, and then as Durgā melts into me, my body is on fire. I feel very hot, and I am no longer the same person you are seeing now. My body is transformed." It is only from this "Durgā-melted body" that Nirupama seeks answers, and the solutions she gives to people come from "that mind" and the speech from "that body."

Ashok of the Kāmākhyā Temple at Guwahati

Ashok is only twenty-six years old when I speak with him for the first time. I was introduced to him through a family of priests who are permitted to give initiation (*dīkṣā*) in the Kāmākhyā tradition. Despite his young age, he is believed to have progressed very well in the path of Kuṇḍalinī yoga. Ashok views tantra as a *guru mukhi vidyā*, that is, "face-to-face wisdom from the spiritual teacher." *Guru mukhi vidyā* is understood to be a method of teaching and learning whereby the lessons are taught in a private setting or a smaller setting. The knowledge is communicated directly by the teacher to the disciple with the understanding that the disciple will either keep the teachings secret or seek prior permission from the guru if they intend to share it in a public forum. This lineage of training is historically situated in a well-defined ancient tradition. The disciple must have a strong desire to learn and follow the path of Śākta tantra, and only then can they seek a teacher and be initiated. It is the guru who teaches the disciple to follow a progressive path in which the body (*tanu*) is the medium to access the "self" (*ātman*), with the final goal of achieving *ātman darśan*: a vision of and communion with the true self.

This self cannot be created, Ashok tells me, nor can it ever die. When someone dies, this energy is transferred or converted. In other words, tantra is a type of energy practice. The *ātman* resides in the body like a dot (*bindu*). The objective of tantric practice is to become one with this *bindu*, like a drop of water disappearing into the ocean. Once this happens, there is no dual existence. One cannot differentiate between the *ātman* and the cosmos (*brahmāṇḍa*); the world inside us replicates the world outside us. The *bindu* is you, and you are the *bindu*. For practitioners to arrive at the point of "becoming one," they must have active Kuṇḍalinī.

The color of Kuṇḍalinī is red, says Ashok, as it is of feminine gender. He describes Kuṇḍalinī to me like this:

> Kuṇḍalinī is a coiled snake in the *mūlādhāra chakra*, which is present in everyone's body. This energy must be raised from the

> *mūlādhāra chakra* to the *sahasrāra chakra*. But one must not get confused or fixated on the snake imagery. The imagery evolves as one proceeds along this path. The human body is made of *tattvas*, which are present in the universe. The objective of Kuṇḍalinī yoga is to successfully identify the presence of *tattvas* in one's body and be able to channel the elements. At the initial stages of the practice, the practitioner needs to get some of the *tattvas* from outside into their body. A successful absorption of elements leads to a heightened realization of the presence of elements within their own physical body. However, once the practitioner masters the experience and is able to identify and channel the *tattvas*, the need for outside substances is eliminated.

Ashok elaborates on his description by first explaining *tattva*, which he defines along traditional lines in accordance with Hindu esoteric traditions and Śākta tantra. There are five *tattvas* that create global energy cycles of *tattvic* tides. The list begins with *ākāśa* (space or "ether") and continues with *vāyu* (air), *tejas* (fire), *āpas* (water), and *pṛthivī* (earth). Most people live their entire lives without coming to any realization of how the *tattvas* affect the constitution of the human body and nature, whereas for a tantric adept the functioning of the *tattvas* is of utmost importance. As the practitioner gets better at identifying and taking command over the *tattvas*, they get to experience the presence of Kuṇḍalinī. To do so, the practitioner, regardless of gender, must have a guru, a deep desire, commitment, and a partner (who is usually their spouse). This is a significant shift in understanding between Mai and Ashok. In Mai's understanding, it is only men who need a (female) partner.

Identifying the guru is the first step. One must examine the guru carefully before becoming completely subservient to them. Experience, personality, and ability are key to identifying one's proper guru. Once a guru is identified, one takes *dīkṣā*; that is, one is initiated. Then one simply follows the guidance and teachings of the guru.

The second step is to identify a cherished goddess or god (*iṣṭa-devatā*) to complement the unique personality (*prakṛti*) of the practitioner. As part of the initiation ceremony, the guru looks at the practitioner's nature and then assigns an appropriate deity. The divine personality should be such that it melts into the seeker, similar to the way butter melts into a baking cake. You can taste the butter, even though you cannot see it, and you know instantly when it's missing. The practitioner must not be afraid of the deity's presence, their physical attributes, their looks, or their nature. Yet, at the same time, the practitioner must not become so enamored that they fall in love and forget the end goal of the practice. Once the initiation has been completed, the guru whispers to the disciple the sacred seed words (*bīja mantra*), which must never be divulged to others. The mere recitation of the seed words activates the disciple's bodily functions for the practice (*sādhana*), so that when Kuṇḍalinī rises, She takes the form of the cherished goddess or god.

And, finally, a partner is needed for this practice. The role of the partner is largely to physically draw the "outside bodily elements" into the practice. Typically, the wives of male tantric adepts take *dīkṣā* and get instructed by the same guru as their husbands. According to Ashok, for Kuṇḍalinī to rise, one must experience ultimate pleasure—climax—and, for that, one needs three people: the guru, oneself, and the partner. It is essential to differentiate sexual activities done for pleasure or procreation from those done as ritual sexual acts. A male practitioner accepts help from his female partner (wife) until such a time as he is able to identify and channel the feminine energy latent within himself. Once the practitioner masters the art of channeling the feminine, he is barred from using a woman as part of Kuṇḍalinī yoga.

The process is the same for women. That is, they use a male partner (typically the husband) for the ritual. But women in the tradition are believed to have the ability to more quickly master the art of getting Kuṇḍalinī to rise than men. This understanding is derived largely from the normative assumption that women naturally carry the germplasm of God, called the clan fluid (*kula dravya* or *kula amṛta*), that is, the vital energies required for the practice. Sometimes, Ashok tells me, it takes many human births to get to the stage of successful identification of all the energies and getting Kuṇḍalinī to rise. There are no guarantees that a guru can provide access to such experiences or assure success in truly raising Kuṇḍalinī.

If and when Kuṇḍalinī rises through each *cakra*, the practitioner's internal energy generated from the elements is transmitted back to the cosmos (*brahmāṇḍa*). As this happens, the dross material in the body is shed, and the physical body is transformed into a pure body. As Ashok explains to me, if you have not started a car for a long time, it gets rusty. After the initial preparations, when you start the engine, some rusted dust particles and dried oil residue will fall off the engine. In the same way, when Kuṇḍalinī rises, the dross elements from the body are flushed out. A strange kind of *śakti* called "creator power" (*sṛṣṭi śakti*) starts to appear, and a kind of heat gets generated. When this happens, it is very important to have a guru. It can be a very scary stage, since people will not necessarily know how to handle this intense experience.

When Kuṇḍalinī rises, hitting each *cakra* in turn, a *siddhi* or magical power is said in the texts (Ashok refuses to mention the specific texts to which he is referring) to result from each center's "awakening." As one succeeds in awakening a particular *cakra*, one gains its particular powers, explained in the ancient texts as *siddhis*. A *siddhi* in this context can be understood as a type of power that provides the person with certain special abilities, such as the ability to see into a person's past, to communicate with a departed soul, and so on, much as we see with mediums and psychics in the West. But these are small *siddhis*. The ultimate *siddhi* is when Kuṇḍalinī hits the *sahasrāra cakra* at the top of the skull and the adept gains *mokṣa*, that is, becomes one with the *ātman*. Once one attains *mokṣa*, there is no point in returning to *saṃsāra*, the worldly existence, because there is nothing to return to. But for the former to happen, one must master Kuṇḍalinī, including making it rise and withdraw at one's command.

Ashok also tells me that it is believed that for male adepts' female partners play a very important role in this practice. "Without women, the result of the *sādhanā* will be adulterated or false," he says. "Since the [male] practitioner starts identifying and channeling the *tattvas*, he must also be able to identify the feminine energies present in them. He can only do so with the help of a woman practitioner."

This comment raises a multitude of questions in my mind. After I ask several questions on the status of the women, such as whether all of them are the adepts' wives, Ashok states that "most male practitioners are married, and the wife almost always takes *dīkṣā* with the husband and performs her duties every day as prescribed. However, there are unmarried practitioners who need the presence of women consorts. In some tantric traditions, unmarried women are frowned upon. But in Kāmākhyā, unmarried women who aid adepts in their *sādhanā* are not looked down upon. They are fewer in number and are well accepted. It is much easier if the practitioner is married, as no one asks questions."

Later, it occurs to me to ask whether male consorts are provided to unmarried female practitioners. I finally pose this question more than a year later, when I go back for more interviews. It's an uphill task to broach the topic and almost impossible to get an answer. At last, I am informed that it is rare for women to take *dīkṣā* in Kāmākhyā for the purpose of their own practice. Most women take *dīkṣā* to aid their husbands. In recent times, there have been some married women, mostly from the West, who have taken *dīkṣā* for themselves, with their husbands. However, very rarely an unmarried woman walks through the gates of Kāmākhyā seeking to take *dīkṣā*. If she is sincere and truly dedicated, the guru will arrange for a male consort.

I try hard, and for a very long time, to seek interviews with married women pursuing their own practice, as well as with consorts. After what feels like an age of hard toil, I am able to get a joint interview with two wives married to two separate tantric adepts, but I am unable to get any exclusive interviews with unmarried men who practice with consorts, nor with any female consorts. While I hang around in the temple at different times of the day, my contacts point out the consorts, but I am not allowed to approach them. When I persist in being introduced, I am subtly told to correct my requests, or I will get into a lot of trouble.

My interactions with Ashok over the years help me gain insights into the multifarious lives and experiences in Kāmākhyā. Kāmākhyā continues to mesmerize me. The energies in the temple call and compel me to visit it every so often. With each new visit over the years, I start to question more and more of Ashok's statements, which are representative of how most adepts think in Kāmākhyā: "As a man, I will have to practice a thousand times to get to each stage, and that too if I am lucky, but for you as a woman, you will be successful in less than fifty times."

Since I heard this statement and similar thoughts repeated over the years, I have often wondered whether women get left out of experiencing the mystical power of Kuṇḍalinī rising only because they are constantly reminded of the ease of the path for women. If a woman persists and is diligent in her *sādhanā*, she is either reminded of her easy access and quick success on this path, or she is told that, in this lifetime, she can be 99 percent ready, but she needs to be born as a man in the next to be completely successful. Neither provides her with the necessary support on the hard path to liberation. In my observations, and during many subsequent conversations, I see most women get relegated to being mere accessories to the success of male practitioners.

Ashok's interpretation and explanation of Kuṇḍalinī can be traced to a combination of Sanskrit texts, specifically the *Yoginī Tantra* and *Kālikā Purāṇa*. Ashok read them in Sanskrit with both Assamese and Bengali translations under his guru's guidance. When I first met Ashok, he was considered to be a young, promising tantric adept. Over the years, through my repeated meetings, I saw him become more and more popular. He became more difficult to access; the wait times increased. But the most interesting shift I found was in his attitude toward women. He continued to believe that Kuṇḍalinī could successfully be raised in women, but only in a select few. He now believed most female practitioners were expected to perform their duties as taught by the guru to aid the male adept. Ashok was less and less sympathetic toward women and their needs in the path of Śākta tantra, and indeed he was comfortable accepting that women should be a mere means to an end goal for the male adept. I often wondered what prompted the change in Ashok's attitude.

One speculative theory led me to attribute Ashok's change in attitude to his wedding. Ashok was a bachelor when I first met him, and two years later he was a married man. My guess is that post-wedding he chose the traditional narrative path of defining his wife in relation to himself and projected that identity onto women generally. Another reason could possibly be something simpler, such as being exposed to different, more conservative teachers or readings. It is in Mai's personal interest to subvert the reigning patriarchal status quo. Less so, for Ashok. Kuṇḍalinī may be the path to transcendence, but that path still runs through the mire of society.

Kamala Ma and Sundari Ma of the Charnel Grounds at Tārāpīṭh

Kamala Ma and Sundari Ma are sisters, both trained by their guru from a young age in Kuṇḍalinī yoga. They are middle-aged by the time that I meet them, somewhere around fifty perhaps, with a decade or so between them. Before proceeding, it is worth highlighting that their stories may prove challenging for some readers, in light of the sexual nature of their practice and especially given the age at which their training first began. Still, I present Kamala Ma's and Sundari Ma's experience without passing explicit judgment because to do so would be to erase not only its complexity but ultimately the agency of these two (now adult) women. More so than any of my other interlocutors, they challenge me to think about the role of sex in Kuṇḍalinī practice—and, for them, this looks quite different than for my Western subjects, for whom Neo-Tantra is often cloaked in an air of orgasmic mysticism.

Kamala Ma and Sundari Ma tell me Kuṇḍalinī is the energy that resides in the vagina (*jōni* or *yoni*) of women, and in men it is stored in the penis. Here, they do not use specific words like *bara* or *liṅg*. Instead, they point to the groin of a man passing by and say, "It is in that part the Kuṇḍalinī resides in men." When all the elements in the body become pure, Kuṇḍalinī will rise upward. It takes many years for the body to get trained. There may be an accidental rise of Kuṇḍalinī in an untrained body, but the practitioner will not be able to command a strong hold upon it. It is only a trained practitioner, guided by their guru for many years, who can successfully let it rise and settle it back again. A guru is also important for understanding the reactions and sensations one feels when Kuṇḍalinī is active. Without the guru, the practitioner is sure to lose all mental composure. "We began this training when we were little girls," they tell me. "The first step is to train one's *jōni* (vagina). The vagina has to be very strong for women to be successful. You have to be able to hold/grab the *liṅg* (penis) tight for a long time, in such a way that not even a single drop of semen is leaked."

I keep asking both sisters to give me more information on "training the vagina." They refuse multiple times. But after a few months, I accidentally meet them in Kāmākhyā. They are attending the famous Ambubachi Mela. Kamala Ma and Sundari Ma interpret this unexpected meeting as a sign from goddess Kālī. They remember that I wanted to know more about training the vagina, and they ask me if I was successful in getting more information. I tell them I was not, and so, at last, they explain. After a few hours, we find a small shed where Kamala Ma exposes herself and shows me the strength of her vagina.

Kamala Ma explains that their daily set of rituals entails the bodily disciplines prescribed by *haṭha* yoga: cleansing practices (*dhauti*), postures (*āsana*), and locks (*bandha*), integrated with breath control (*prāṇāyāma*). Kamala Ma adds that, along with these disciplines, sexual intercourse (real or imagined) is essential to the process of Kuṇḍalinī rising. She, too, emphasizes that it is crucial to separate sexual activities undertaken for pleasure or procreation from those performed as ritual acts. The ritualized sexual acts are real and essential at the early stages of the training. They are an orientation exercise to lead the physical body to experience the bodily reactions felt while Kuṇḍalinī rises. In order for that to happen, both men and women must not release their bodily fluids immediately after climax. Instead, both must mindfully use the *mūla-bandha* (root lock) to lock in the fluids at the peak of the act. If one successfully manages to perform the *bandha*, one must then swiftly move the fluids and the breath by applying the *uḍḍiyāna-bandha* (stomach lock) and then the *jālandhara-bandha* (throat lock). Kamala Ma clarifies that, over the years, once the practitioner had mastered these *bandhas*, he or she would no longer need to actually perform the sexual act.

In the confines of the little shed, Sundari Ma provides the commentary while Kamala Ma performs the exercise. There are no male partners present and, instead of holding on to a penis, Kamala Ma uses a small plastic bottle. She begins by praying to Kālī and seeking forgiveness in advance for any errors she might make while demonstrating this secret (*gupt*) training. Then she prays to her guru. Finally, she blesses me. Once we complete the ritual blessings, Kamala Ma uses her vagina to grab onto the small plastic bottle, takes an enormous deep breath, and carefully, swiftly, performs the *mūla-bandha*, moves to the *uḍḍiyāna-bandha*, and finishes with the *jālaṅdhara-bandha*. With all three bandhas engaged, Kamala Ma remains in this position, eyes open, not blinking, nor breathing for a long time. (My guess is that it lasts about two to three minutes.)

Sundari Ma, meanwhile, explains that for Kuṇḍalinī to rise in a woman, she must be on top of the man. This is how the practice works:

> The bottle that *dīdī* [sister, i.e. Kamala Ma] is using would be the penis in real practice, and when she takes a deep breath in and holds the breath in that fashion, the semen is released in her body. Since the vagina is holding tightly to the penis and because she is not breathing, a vacuum is created, due to which the semen rises upwards, mixed with her own fluids, and starts hitting the *cakras*. While the fluids rise, it causes pain and discomfort. It takes many years of practice for someone to get comfortable with the pain and to train their body.

Kamala Ma comes out of her trance-like demonstration all flushed and sweating. She starts to breathe again and gently releases the plastic bottle from the grasp of her vagina. It takes her almost thirty minutes to cool her body down. When I probe further into how long it took Kamala Ma to learn to hold her breath effectively and be comfortable with all the three *bandhas*, she says, "Many, many years. Our Guru taught us. This training over the years is done by using different types of objects, and the duration of time for which we have to hold onto the object is increased." As for men, Kamala Ma says, they too have to go through many years of training. "They have to train their penis to be a suction cup and be able to absorb things. But it is very difficult for men. You know, they do not have a hole like women. It is a lot more painful. Women learn to control and channel Kuṇḍalinī faster than men. The path is the same. The only difference is men have to be on top if they want their Kuṇḍalinī to rise."

This notion of a man or woman needing to be on top if they want to raise their Kuṇḍalinī brings to mind interesting memories of iconographic representations. One thinks, for instance, of the goddess Kālī, so often pictured naked, straddling or standing on top of Śiva. Most imagery of this type uses the Hindu cremation ground as the larger scene of the ritual, which is, after all, precisely where I find the sisters. The medieval texts may assume a male body when they describe their practices, but perhaps the images tell a different side of the story.

Unlike Mai and Nirupama, enthroned in their temples, Kamala Ma and Sundari Ma, though teachers in their own right, live in "the liminal." This includes physically residing between the living and the dead: their little thatched residence shares a border with the Tārāpīṭh cremation grounds. The information they have shared on the training men and women undergo in order to effectively raise Kuṇḍalinī is unlike anything else I have heard during my field research. I probe them on this, and they tell me that everyone goes through this training, but people are scared to talk about it. Most people take the pledge to never disclose it and simply state that it is a secret (*gupt*). What's more, it is believed that if the initiated ever spoke of it, they and their entire kin would go to hell.

At this point, a modern reader might be tempted to point to such dynamics as hallmarks of abuse. Perhaps. Certainly, such an analysis would not be out of line with contemporary understandings—both popular and academic—of sexual exploitation, especially given (as we have already noted) that Kamala Ma and Sundari Ma's training as tantric consorts began when they were both still children. However, it is equally important to point out that this is not how *they* see their practice. And they do have a practice, which is their own, and not solely in service to the practice of their male partners. Like Mai, Kamala Ma and Sundari Ma also have a way of turning patriarchy on its head. Or perhaps of straddling it in the charnel grounds. On-the-ground reality is messy, and an ethnographer must learn to navigate the gray areas of her subjects' lived experience. In this case, my subjects do not see themselves as victims of oppression—or, at least, this is not how they see their practice. Instead, oppression is something that imposes itself as an external force, through hypocritical judgments and through failures of understanding. The only reason Kamala Ma and Sundari Ma give for their decision to share their knowledge with me is that they are tired of being misunderstood and misrepresented. Our unexpected meeting in the Kāmākhyā temple was the final sign. They have been on the Śākta tantric path for most of their lives, and it is a heritage in which they take pride.

Here we are then, having gone there and back again (indeed, more than once), to wind up on a charnel ground in northern India. It might seem like these practitioners live in a different world from the ones explaining how to use Kuṇḍalinī and the power of the sun to reprogram your DNA on TikTok. Perhaps that is so. What would Mai or Kamala Ma make of Sanchez and Daniels's seventy-six-point Kundalini Awakening Scale? Would they laugh? Or would the experiential breakdown make sense to them?

We will not speculate.

We can only conclude by pointing out that all of these things coexist. All of them are called, by someone, Kuṇḍalinī. And, if one follows the threads carefully enough, one eventually sees that they *are* all related.

It is impossible to say what Kuṇḍalinī will look like in another decade, or two, or three. All we feel confident saying is that the web will undoubtedly grow larger. Its nodes will continue to multiply. Perhaps from some angles it will look more uniform. Perhaps messier. Probably both. How many heads can a serpent grow before it ceases to be a serpent?

It does not feel fitting to write a conclusion to this book. The subject matter spurns conclusiveness.

Is there one Kuṇḍalinī of which there are many experiences? Or are there in fact many Kuṇḍalinīs? The only possible answer is: both. We are reminded of the old parable of the blind men and the elephant. One feels the elephant's trunk and concludes it's a serpent. Another grasps the tail and decides the elephant is a brush. A third, touching the ear, finds a banana leaf. Kuṇḍalinī is a bit like this. Except in this case, it's highly possible that the elephant is also a shape shifter.

But then, the alchemists have long told us this. Original matter has no shape. And, when the shape emerges, sometimes it is simply our own.

NOTES

PROLOGUE

1. Gopi Krishna, *Kundalini: The Evolutionary Energy in Man* (New Delhi: Ramadhar and Hopman, 1967), 14.
2. See Hugh B. Urban, *Tantra: Sex, Secrecy, Politics, and Power in the Study of Religion* (Berkeley: University of California Press, 2003); see Jeffrey J. Kripal, *Esalen: America and the Religion of No Religion* (Chicago: University of Chicago Press, 2007).
3. See Ana Laura Funes Maderey, "Kuṇḍalinī Rising and Liberation in the Yogavāsiṣṭha: The Story of Cūḍālā and Śikhidhvaja," *Religions* 8, no. 11 (November 2017): 248.
4. We thank Jason Schwartz for this insight.
5. The image of the serpent is, of course, not absolute. In fact, some eminent scholars have asserted that "according to Vedic mythology, descending Kuṇḍalinī has the form of a horse. . . . The oldest manifestation of ascending Kuṇḍalinī is the trunk of Ganesh." (Karl Baier, Private Occult Tour of Vienna, April 30, 2022.) This, dear reader, is a joke. Probably. Our point is: don't let the serpent lead you astray—that's not what it's here for.
6. Jeffrey J. Kripal, *The Serpent's Gift: Gnostic Reflections on the Study of Religion* (Chicago: University of Chicago Press, 2007), 123.
7. See Wouter J. Hanegraaff, *Esotericism and the Academy: Rejected Knowledge in Western Culture* (Cambridge, UK: Cambridge University Press, 2012), 191–207, for an explication of "alchemical" thought. See Simon

Paul Cox, *The Subtle Body: A Genealogy* (New York: Oxford University Press, 2022), 174–75, and Christopher Jain Miller, *Embodying Transnational Yoga: Eating, Singing, and Breathing in Context* (London: Routledge, forthcoming), for examples of how this might be applied.

8. See Ann Taves and Egil Asprem, "Experience as Event: Event Cognition and the Study of (Religious) Experiences," *Religion, Brain & Behavior* 7, no. 1 (2017): 43–62.
9. Kripal, *Esalen*, 23.
10. Walter H. Capps, *Religious Studies: The Making of a Discipline* (Minneapolis: Fortress Press, 1995), 156.
11. I have primarily drawn on definitions offered by the following works: Douglas Renfrew Brooks, *The Secret of the Three Cities: An Introduction to Hindu Sakta Tantrism* (Chicago: University of Chicago Press, 1990); David Kinsley, *Tantric Visions of the Divine Feminine: The Ten Mahavidyas* (Berkeley: University of California Press, 1997); David Gordon White, ed., *Tantra in Practice* (Princeton, NJ: Princeton University Press, 2000); André Padoux, *The Hindu Tantric World: An Overview* (Chicago: University of Chicago Press, 2017); André Padoux, *Vāc: The Concept of the Word in Selected Hindu Tantras*, trans. Jacques Gontier (Albany: State University of New York Press, 1990); Hillary Peter Rodrigues, *Ritual Worship of the Great Goddess: The Liturgy of the Durgā Pūjā with Interpretations* (Albany: State University of New York Press, 2003); Prem Saran, *Yoga, Bhoga, and Ardhanariswara: Individuality, Wellbeing, and Gender in Tantra* (London: Routledge, 2008); and Hugh B. Urban, *The Power of Tantra: Religion, Sexuality and the Politics of South Asian Studies* (London: I. B. Tauris, 2009).
12. I acknowledge that some of the resulting practices may be used for certain practical outcomes and not necessarily liberation. For example, the *ṣaṭkarman* rituals. The "six results" (*ṣaṭkarman*) in Hindu magic rituals are *śānti* (tranquilizing), *vaśīkaraṇa* (subjugating), *stambhana* (immobilizing), *mohana* (bewildering), *vidveṣana* (dissent), *uccāṭana* (eradicating), *ākarṣaṇa* (attracting), and *mārana* (murder). These too fall under the larger umbrella of tantra.
13. Anya Foxen, *Inhaling Spirit: Harmonialism, Orientalism, and the Western Roots of Modern Yoga* (New York: Oxford University Press, 2020), 3.
14. See Nika Kuchuk, "Genealogies of Transnational Religion: Translation, Revelation, and Discursive Technologies in Two Female Gurus of

Esoteric Vedanta" (PhD diss., University of Toronto, 2021), for an excellent discussion of the dynamics of translation in this context.

15. Jonathan Z. Smith, "In Comparison a Magic Dwells," in *Imagining Religion: From Babylon to Jonestown*, ed. Jonathan Z. Smith (Chicago: University of Chicago Press, 1982), 19–35.
16. See Hanegraaff, *Esotericism and the Academy*.
17. Hanegraaff, 2.

1. SOUTH ASIAN ROOTS

1. Following the thought of Henry Corbin (1903–1978).
2. James Mallinson and Mark Singleton, *Roots of Yoga: A Sourcebook from the Indic Traditions* (London: Penguin Classics, 2017), 179.
3. This is why it's worth expanding our lens somewhat. Relatedly, see Robert Czyżykowski, "The Problem of Kuṇḍalinī in the Context of Yogic Aspects of the Bengali Tantric Vaiṣṇava (Sahajiyā) Tradition," *Religions of South Asia* 12, no. 2 (2018): 185–206, for a discussion of Kuṇḍalinī-like concepts in the Vaiṣṇava Sahajiyā traditions of Bengal. In these sources, the most analogous concept to Kuṇḍalinī may actually be a fish, which begins to make a lot of sense once you consider the fact that these traditions imagine the *cakras* not just as lotuses (as is typical) but as ponds.
4. Mallinson and Singleton, *Roots of Yoga*, 179.
5. Gerrit Lange, "Cobra Deities and Divine Cobras: The Ambiguous Animality of Nāgas," *Religions* 10, no. 8 (August 2019): 2. It's worth noting that when Nāginīs (female Nāgas) appear in modern pop cultural contexts such as film, they are frequently portrayed as morally ambiguous "vamp" figures.
6. Lange, "Cobra Deities," 7. Vṛtra persists as the most important Vedic serpent, but there is also Ahirbundhya, "the serpent of the depths," who holds the universe. See Lilian Silburn, *Kuṇḍalinī: The Energy of the Depths; A Comprehensive Study Based on the Scriptures of Nondualistic Kashmir Shaivism*, trans. Jacques Gontier (Albany: State University of New York Press, 1988), 16.
7. Lange, "Cobra Deities," 6–7.
8. David Gordon White, *The Alchemical Body: Siddha Traditions in Medieval India* (Chicago: University of Chicago Press, 1996), 215.

9. White, *The Alchemical Body*, 221.
10. David Gordon White, *Sinister Yogis* (Chicago: University of Chicago Press, 2009), 135–37.
11. Patrick Olivelle, *The Early Upaniṣads: Annotated Text and Translation* (New York: Oxford University Press, 1998), 21.
12. Johannes Bronkhorst, *Greater Magadha: Studies in the Culture of Early India* (Leiden, the Netherlands: Brill, 2007), 52; Johannes Bronkhorst, *The Two Traditions of Meditation in Ancient India* (Delhi: Motilal Banarsidass Publishers, 2000), 43–50.
13. Walter O. Kaelber, *Tapta Mārga: Ascetism and Initiation in Vedic India* (Albany: State University of New York Press, 1989), 15–20.
14. James Mallinson, "Yoga and Yogis," *Nāmarūpa* 3, no. 15 (March 2012): 10–12.
15. White, *Sinister Yogis*, 33, 60.
16. See Paul Eduardo Muller-Ortega, *The Triadic Heart of Śiva: Kaula Tantricism of Abhinavagupta in the Non-Dual Shaivism of Kashmir* (Albany: State University of New York Press, 1997).
17. Translation adapted from Olivelle, *The Early Upaniṣads*, 279.
18. David Gordon White, ed., *Tantra in Practice* (Princeton, NJ: Princeton University Press, 2000), 25–28.
19. Quoted in Mallinson and Singleton, *Roots of Yoga*, 175.
20. David Gordon White, *The Kiss of the Yoginī: "Tantric Sex" in Its South Asian Contexts* (Chicago: University of Chicago Press, 2002), 224.
21. White, *The Kiss of the Yoginī*, 225.
22. White, 195.
23. White, 106–12; Anya Foxen previously called this latter term "sexually transmitted enlightenment"—see Anya Foxen and Christa Kuberry, *Is This Yoga? Concepts, Histories, and the Complexities of Modern Practice* (New York: Routledge, 2021)—but she would like to thank Travis Chilcott for the invaluable moment of casual peer review that yielded this new and improved turn of phrase and the acronym it allows for.
24. White, *The Kiss of the Yoginī*, 219–57.
25. White, *Sinister Yogis*, 140.
26. Mallinson, "Yoga and Yogis," 11–12.
27. Jason Birch, "The Meaning of Haṭha in Early Haṭhayoga," *Journal of the American Oriental Society* 131, no. 4 (October–December 2011): 527–54.

28. Mallinson and Singleton, *Roots of Yoga*, 197, 214.
29. White, *The Alchemical Body*, 243.
30. Mallinson and Singleton, *Roots of Yoga*, 202.
31. Mallinson and Singleton, 179.
32. All brackets in the source material. Translated in André Padoux, *Vāc: The Concept of the Word in Selected Hindu Tantras*, trans. Jacques Gontier (Albany: State University of New York Press, 1990), 128–30; also quoted in White, *The Kiss of the Yoginī*, 229–30.
33. White, *The Kiss of the Yoginī*, 230; Mallinson and Singleton, *Roots of Yoga*, 179.
34. Mallinson and Singleton, 213.
35. Mallinson and Singleton, 194.
36. Gavin D. Flood, *The Tantric Body: The Secret Tradition of Hindu Religion* (London: I. B. Tauris, 2006), 140–41.
37. Mallinson and Singleton, *Roots of Yoga*, 206–7.
38. Mallinson and Singleton, 208.
39. Mallinson and Singleton, 176–77.
40. Mallinson and Singleton, 179.
41. Mallinson and Singleton, 216–17.
42. Mallinson and Singleton, 211.
43. Somadeva Vasudeva, *The Yoga of the Mālinīvijayottaratantra: Chapters 1-4, 7, 11-17* (Pondicherry, India: Institut français de Pondichéry, Ecole française d'Extrême-Orient, 2004), 434–36.
44. Mallinson, "Yoga and Yogis," 7.
45. Mallinson and Singleton, *Roots of Yoga*, 74–86.
46. Mallinson and Singleton, 206.
47. Mallinson, "Yoga and Yogis," 6.
48. Catharina Kiehnle, "The Secret of the Nāths: The Ascent of *Kuṇḍalinī* according to *Jñāneśvarī* 6.151–328," *Bulletin des Études Indiennes* 22–23 (2004–2005): 447.
49. Catharina Kiehnle, *Songs on Yoga: Texts and Teachings of the Mahārāṣṭrian Nāths* (Stuttgart, Germany: Franz Steiner Verlag Stuttgart, 1997), 10. The account that follows is drawn primarily from Kiehle's work.
50. Kiehnle, "The Secret of the Nāths," 467.
51. Kiehnle, 469.
52. Kiehnle, 470.

53. Kiehnle, 471.
54. Kiehnle, 472.
55. Kiehnle, 473.
56. Kiehnle, 476.
57. Kiehnle, 481.
58. Kiehnle, 481.
59. Kiehnle, 485.

2. WESTERN ROOTS

1. For a dynamic, modern instance of such a tradition, see the artistic work of Dr. Marques Redd, as well as his organization: Rainbow Serpent, https://www.therainbowserpent.org.
2. See for instance Carl W. Ernst, "The Islamization of Yoga in the 'Amrtakunda' Translations," *Journal of the Royal Asiatic Society* 13, no. 2 (July 2003): 199–226, and Shaman Hatley, "Mapping the Esoteric Body in the Islamic Yoga of Bengal," *History of Religions* 46, no. 4 (May 2007): 351–68.
3. See for example David Gordon White, *Daemons Are Forever: Contacts and Exchanges in the Eurasian Pandemonium* (Chicago: University of Chicago Press, 2021).
4. The preceding account is largely adapted from Tuomas Rasimus, "Ophite Gnosticism, Sethianism and the Nag Hammadi Library," *Vigiliae Christianae* 59, no. 3 (August 2005): 237–38. It is derived from Irenaeus's *Adversus Haereses* 1.30, which Rasimus describes as likely summarizing a written source similar to a number of other Gnostic tracts of an Ophite bend.
5. Rasimus, "Ophite Gnosticism," 238; Tuomas Rasimus, *Paradise Reconsidered in Gnostic Mythmaking: Rethinking Sethianism in Light of the Ophite Myth and Ritual* (Leiden, the Netherlands: Brill, 2009), 100. This is mirrored by the famous biblical line in Matthew 10:16: "Behold, I send you forth as sheep in the midst of wolves: be ye therefore wise as serpents, and harmless as doves."
6. Rasimus, "Ophite Gnosticism," 241.

7. Roelof Van den Broek, "Gnosticism and Hermetism in Antiquity: Two Roads to Salvation," in *Gnosis and Hermeticism from Antiquity to Modern Times*, ed. Roelof Van den Broek and Wouter J. Hanegraaff (Albany: State University of New York Press, 1998), 10. This is not an absolute evaluation as there are likewise a number of passages in the philosophical Hermetica that express the more standard negative view of the cosmos. See Roelof Van den Broek, "Hermetism," in *Dictionary of Gnosis & Western Esotericism*, ed. Wouter J. Hanegraaff et al. (Leiden, the Netherlands: Brill, 2006), 562. Similarly, for a different formulation of Gnosticism that includes the Hermetists, see April D. DeConick, *The Gnostic New Age: How a Countercultural Spirituality Revolutionized Religion from Antiquity to Today* (New York: Columbia University Press, 2016).
8. Lucas Siorvanes, *Proclus: Neo-Platonic Philosophy and Science* (Edinburgh: Edinburgh University Press, 1996), 304–5.
9. Siorvanes, *Proclus*, 306.
10. Charles G. Gross, "Aristotle on the Brain," *The Neuroscientist* 1, no. 4 (July 1995): 245–50; Christopher Gill, "Galen and the Stoics: Mortal Enemies or Blood Brothers?," *Phronesis: A Journal for Ancient Philosophy* 52, no. 1 (January 2007): 88–120.
11. E. R. Dodds, *Stoicheiosis Theologike: The Elements of Theology* (Oxford: Clarendon Press, 1963), 313n4.
12. See A. P. Bos, *The Soul and Its Instrumental Body: A Reinterpretation of Aristotle's Philosophy of Living Nature* (Leiden, the Netherlands: Brill, 2003), on *pneuma* as the soul's "instrumental body" in Aristotle. Bos states that the chief difference between Plato's and Aristotle's doctrines of the soul is that for Plato the soul is a "self-mover" whereas for Aristotle it is an "unmoved mover." Aristotle is then forced to explain how something that is not itself in motion is capable of producing it (53–54).
13. John M. Rist, "On Greek Biology, Greek Cosmology and Some Sources of Theological Pneuma," in *Man, Soul, and Body: Essays in Ancient Thought from Plato to Dionysius*, ed. D. W. Dockrill and R. G. Tanner (Auckland, New Zealand: University of Auckland, 1985), 32.
14. John F. Finamore, *Iamblichus and the Theory of the Vehicle of the Soul* (Chico, CA: Scholars Press, 1985), 1.

15. For an outline of the usage of theurgy in late antiquity and medieval sources, as well as general historiographic trends, see Claire Fanger, "Introduction," in *Invoking Angels: Theurgic Ideas and Practices; Thirteenth to Sixteenth Centuries*, ed. Claire Fanger (University Park: Pennsylvania State University Press, 2015), 15–27.
16. Gregory Shaw, *Theurgy and the Soul: The Neoplatonism of Iamblichus* (University Park: Pennsylvania State University Press, 1995), 222–23. The below synthesis likewise appears in Shaw's work on these same pages. Lacking any concrete evidence of influence one way or the other, I would have to concur with Shaw in simply calling such similarities "suggestive."
17. Ruth Majercik, ed., *The Chaldean Oracles: Text, Translation, and Commentary*, trans. Ruth Majercik (Leiden, the Netherlands: Brill, 1989), 38–39. See also Radcliffe G. Edmonds, "Did the Mithraists Inhale?," *Ancient World* 32, no. 1 (2001): 10–24. Edmonds compares textual evidence from the Mithras Liturgy, technically an unnamed section within a set of fourth-century Greco-Egyptian magical papyri, with that from the Chaldean Oracles and material evidence including Mithraic monuments and frescoes to conclude that the practice of theurgic ascent along the rays of the sun was likely an authentic feature of Mithraism, at least as an esoteric practice employed by the initiated individual.
18. Hans Dieter Betz, ed., *The Greek Magical Papyri in Translation, Including the Demotic Spells* (Chicago: University of Chicago Press, 1986), 48. Also quoted in Shaw, *Theurgy and the Soul*, 223.
19. Sarah Iles Johnson, "Rising to the Occasion: Theurgic Ascent in Its Cultural Milieu," in *Envisioning Magic: A Princeton Seminar and Symposium*, ed. Peter Schäfer and Hans Kippenberg (Leiden, the Netherlands: Brill, 1997), 183.
20. Shaw, *Theurgy and the Soul*, 47–50.
21. April D. DeConick, "The Road for the Souls Is Through the Planets: The Mysteries of the Ophians Mapped," in *Practicing Gnosis: Ritual, Magic, Theurgy, and Liturgy in Nag Hammadi, Manichaean and Other Ancient Literature: Essays in Honor of Birger A. Pearson*, ed. April D. DeConick, Gregory Shaw, and John D. Turner (Leiden, the Netherlands: Brill, 2013), 37–74.
22. DeConick, "Road for the Souls," 57.

23. Christoph Riedweg, *Pythagoras: His Life, Teaching, and Influence*, trans. Steven Rendall and Andreas Schatzmann (Ithaca, NY: Cornell University Press, 2005), 29–30, 84–89. See also Anya Foxen, *Inhaling Spirit: Harmonialism, Orientalism, and the Western Roots of Modern Yoga* (New York: Oxford University Press, 2020), 43–89.
24. James H. Charlesworth, *The Good and Evil Serpent: How a Universal Symbol Became Christianized* (New Haven, CT: Yale University Press, 2010); Daniel Ogden, *Drakon: Dragon Myth and Serpent Cult in the Greek and Roman Worlds* (Oxford: Oxford University Press, 2013), 247–49.
25. Arlene Allan, *Hermes* (London: Routledge, 2018), 5.
26. Roelof Van den Broek, "Hermes Trismegistus I: Antiquity," in *Dictionary of Gnosis & Western Esotericism*, ed. Wouter J. Hanegraaff et al. (Leiden, the Netherlands: Brill, 2006), 475.
27. Allan, *Hermes*, 115.
28. Homer, *The Odyssey*, trans. Emily R. Wilson (New York: Norton, 2020), 181.
29. Van den Broek, "Hermes Trismegistus I: Antiquity," 475.
30. Ogden, *Drakon*, 311.
31. Charlesworth, *The Good and Evil Serpent*, 160.
32. Roelof Van den Broek, "Hermetic Literature I: Antiquity," in *Dictionary of Gnosis & Western Esotericism*, ed. Wouter J. Hanegraaff et al. (Leiden, the Netherlands: Brill, 2006), 493.
33. Van den Broek, "Hermetic Literature I," 494.
34. Rebecca Lesses, "Image and Word: Performative Ritual and Material Culture in the Aramaic Incantation Bowls," in *Practicing Gnosis: Ritual, Magic, Theurgy, and Liturgy in Nag Hammadi, Manichaean and Other Ancient Literature; Essays in Honor of Birger A. Pearson*, ed. April D. DeConick, Gregory Shaw, and John D. Turner (Leiden, the Netherlands: Brill, 2013), 387–88.
35. Lawrence Principe, *The Secrets of Alchemy* (Chicago: University of Chicago Press, 2013), 25–26.
36. Tuomas Rasimus, *Paradise Reconsidered in Gnostic Mythmaking: Rethinking Sethianism in Light of the Ophite Myth and Ritual* (Leiden, the Netherlands: Brill, 2009), 70.
37. Ogden, *Drakon*, 297–309; Bernard D. Haage, "Alchemy II: Antiquity–12th Century," in *Dictionary of Gnosis & Western Esotericism*, ed. Wouter J. Hanegraaff et al. (Leiden, the Netherlands: Brill, 2006), 24.

38. Van den Broek, "Hermes Trismegistus I: Antiquity," 478.
39. Arthur Versluis, *Wisdom's Children: A Christian Esoteric Tradition* (Albany: State University of New York Press, 1999), 183.
40. Quoted in Versluis, *Wisdom's Children*, 31. Square brackets are from the source.
41. See Foxen, *Inhaling Spirit*, 86.
42. See also Versluis, *Wisdom's Children*, 180–2 for a description of this series.
43. Versluis, 162.
44. See Foxen, *Inhaling Spirit*, 93–94.
45. Emanuel Swedenborg, *Arcana Caelestia*, trans. J. C. Ager, vol. 1, 8 vols. (New York: American Swedenborg Printing and Publishing Society, 1882), 359.
46. Swedenborg, *Arcana Caelestia*, 360–62.
47. Heinrich August Wrisberg, *Observationum anatomicarum de nervis viscerum abdominalium* (Göttingen, Germany: Ioann Christian Dietrich, 1780), 38.
48. Wouter J. Hanegraaff, *Esotericism and the Academy: Rejected Knowledge in Western Culture* (Cambridge, UK: Cambridge University Press, 2012), 260.
49. Foxen, *Inhaling Spirit*, 91–93.
50. Robert Darnton, *Mesmerism and the End of the Enlightenment in France* (Cambridge, MA: Harvard University Press, 1968), 8.
51. Bertrand Meheust, "Animal Magnetism/Mesmerism," in *Dictionary of Gnosis & Western Esotericism*, ed. Wouter J. Hanegraaff et al. (Leiden, the Netherlands: Brill, 2006), 82.
52. Karl Baier, "Theosophical Orientalism and the Structures of Intercultural Transfer: Annotations on the Appropriation of the Cakras in Early Theosophy," in *Theosophical Appropriations: Esotericism, Kabbalah, and the Transformation of Traditions*, ed. Julie Chajes and Boaz Huss (Beer Sheva, Israel: Ben-Gurion University of the Negev Press, 2016), 339.
53. Baier, "Theosophical Orientalism," 339.

3. WEST MEETS EAST

1. Rudolf Steiner, *Kundalini: Spiritual Perception and the Higher Element of Life*, ed. Andreas Meyer (Forest Row, UK: Rudolf Steiner Press, 2019), 3.

2. Arthur Avalon, *The Serpent Power* (Madras, India: Ganesh & Co., 1950), 14. See also Julian Strube, *Global Tantra: Religion, Science, and Nationalism in Colonial Modernity* (New York: Oxford University Press, 2022), 228–29.
3. Karl Baier, "Theosophical Orientalism and the Structures of Intercultural Transfer: Annotations on the Appropriation of the Cakras in Early Theosophy," in *Theosophical Appropriations: Esotericism, Kabbalah, and the Transformation of Traditions*, ed. Julie Chajes and Boaz Huss (Beer Sheva, Israel: Ben-Gurion University of the Negev Press, 2016), 322.
4. This is a text more formally known as the *Yogayājñavalkya*, whose teachings on Kuṇḍalinī are based on those of the earlier *Pādma Saṃhitā* (see James Mallinson and Mark Singleton, *Roots of Yoga: A Sourcebook from the Indic Traditions* [London: Penguin Classics, 2017], 5n21).
5. Strube, *Global Tantra*, 43–8.
6. T. Subba Row, "The Twelve Signs of the Zodiac," in *Five Years of Theosophy* (London: Reever and Turner, 1885), 111n. Originally printed in the November 1881 issue of *The Theosophist*. It is conceivable that Row himself based his comments on an even earlier article by Baradakanta Majumdar, published in *The Theosophist* in April 1880, which refers to Kuṇḍalinī, stating that "modern science also teaches us that heat, light, electricity, magnetism, &c., are but the modifications of one great force" (see Strube, *Global Tantra*, 46). Row returns to the topic of Kuṇḍalinī in "Notes on Hata Yoga," *The Theosophist* 8, no. 87 (December 1886), 138–39. There, he offers a brief account of the raising of Kuṇḍalinī through the seven *cakras* as a means of attaining *rāja* yoga. Importantly, he associates the *cakras* with the seven planetary spheres and finishes the piece by enumerating a number of other traditional methods of attaining *rāja* yoga (*mahāvākyam*; contemplation of *parabrahman*; contemplation of the guru; repetition of the *praṇava* [*oṃ*]; cultivation of the will). With regards to which of these methods is the true one, Row advises his reader that all are necessary, and more besides—on this topic, he refers the reader to *Light on the Path*, a visionary text authored by the British Theosophist Mabel Collins: Mabel Collins, *Light on the Path* (Boston: Cupples, Upham and Company, 1886). Row's recommendation of Collins's text suggests an already deep

entanglement between South Asian and Western thought, not only with regards to concepts, but also spiritual practice.

7. H. P. Blavatsky, *The Secret Doctrine: The Synthesis of Science, Religion and Philosophy*, vol. 1 (London: Theosophical Publishing Company, 1888), 293.
8. The other two, according to Leadbeater, are Mabel Collins's *Light on the Path* (1885) and *At the Feet of the Master* (1910), published under the name Alcyone and attributed to the young Jiddu Krishnamurti, who was then in the early days of being positioned by the Theosophical Society as the new World Teacher.
9. H. P. Blavatsky, *The Voice of the Silence* (London: Theosophical Publishing Company, 1889), vi.
10. Blavatsky, *The Voice of the Silence*, 12.
11. Blavatsky, 9.
12. Blavatsky, 76n24.
13. Baier, "Theosophical Orientalism," 327.
14. *The Dream of Ravan: A Mystery* (London: The Theosophical Publishing Society, 1895), 190. Also quoted in Baier, "Theosophical Orientalism," 327. It is in fact this former source, referenced by an anonymous author known only as "Truth seeker" in the January 1880 edition of *The Theosophist*, that puts Kuṇḍalinī on the radar of Western Theosophists (Baier, "Theosophical Orientalism," 327; Strube, *Global Tantra*, 43).
15. Nicholas Goodrick-Clarke, "The Esoteric Uses of Electricity: Theologies of Electricity from Swabian Pietism to Ariosophy," *Aries* 4, no. 1 (January 2004): 70–72.
16. Kurt Leland, *Rainbow Body: A History of the Western Chakra System from Blavatsky to Brennan* (Lake Worth, FL: Ibis Press, 2016), 102–27. In this context, Blavatsky taught a very distinctive system of *cakras* and related practices, probably influenced by the teachings of Sabhapati Swami (Baier, "Theosophical Orientalism," 329; Strube, *Global Tantra*, 106–107; see also Keith Edward Cantú, *Like a Tree Universally Spread: Sri Sabhapati Swami and Śivarājayoga* [New York: Oxford University Press, 2023]).
17. Leland, *Rainbow Body*, 122–24.
18. See Anya Foxen, *Inhaling Spirit: Harmonialism, Orientalism, and the Western Roots of Modern Yoga* (New York: Oxford University Press, 2020), 89–90.

19. James Morgan Pryse, "Memorabilia of H. P. B.," *The Canadian Theosophist* 16, no. 1 (March 1935): 1–5. Actually, Pryse traced his and Blavatsky's acquaintance considerably further into the past. In this same account, he revealed his belief that she was a reincarnation of the sixteenth-century Swiss physician and alchemist Paracelsus, whom he had known in one of his own former lives and was destined to meet again.
20. James Morgan Pryse, "An Important Statement by Mr. J. M. Pryse," *The Canadian Theosophist* 7, no. 6 (September 1926): 140, 141.
21. James Morgan Pryse, *The Apocalypse Unsealed: Being an Esoteric Interpretation of the Initiation of Iôannês Commonly Called the Revelation of St. John, with a New Translation* (Los Angeles: J. M. Pryse, 1910), unpaginated preface.
22. Pryse, *The Apocalypse Unsealed*, 1.
23. Pryse, 11–12.
24. Pryse, 16.
25. See again Baier, "Theosophical Orientalism," 329; Strube, *Global Tantra*, 106–107; and Cantú, *A Tree Universally Spread*. Generally, Sabhapati Swami's work appears to have been widely enough circulated to be available to the careful researcher. For instance, William J. Flagg casually cites Swami on the matter of the soul's ascent in his wide-ranging *Yoga or Transformation* (New York: J. W. Bouton, 1898), 303.
26. April D. DeConick, "The Road for the Souls Is Through the Planets: The Mysteries of the Ophians Mapped," in *Practicing Gnosis: Ritual, Magic, Theurgy and Liturgy in Nag Hammadi, Manichaean and Other Ancient Literature; Essays in Honor of Birger A. Pearson*, ed. April D. DeConick, Gregory Shaw, and John D. Turner (Leiden, the Netherlands: Brill, 2013), 65.
27. Pryse, *The Apocalypse Unsealed*, 22–23.
28. Pryse, 44.
29. Pryse, 23–24.
30. We thank Nathan Fredrickson for this insight.
31. Indra Devi, *Yoga for Americans* (Englewood Cliffs, NJ: Prentice-Hall, 1959), 135.
32. Gopi Krishna, *Yoga: A Vision of Its Future* (New Delhi: Kundalini Research and Publication Trust, 1978), 76.
33. C. W. Leadbeater, *The Inner Life* (Adyar, India: Theosophical Publishing House, 1917), 298–99.

34. Simon Paul Cox, *The Subtle Body: A Genealogy* (New York: Oxford University Press, 2022), 126.
35. C. W. Leadbeater, *The Chakras* (Wheaton, IL: Theosophical Publishing House, 1927), 187.
36. C. W. Leadbeater, *Clairvoyance* (London: The Theosophical Publishing Society, 1899), 17; partially quoted also in Leland, *Rainbow Body*, 186.
37. Leadbeater, *The Chakras*, 24–30.
38. Leadbeater, 27.
39. Leadbeater, 27–28.
40. Leadbeater, 28–30. Note that Leadbeater seems to conflate his forces here. Elsewhere he indicates that the "primary" life force comes from the Second Outpouring while the vital force comes from the sun.
41. Peter Kingsley, *Ancient Philosophy, Mystery, and Magic: Empedocles and Pythagorean Tradition* (Oxford: Clarendon Press, 1995), 54–56. We see something like this image in Johann Georg Gichtel's images of spiritual awakening. In *The Secret Doctrine*, Blavatsky likewise repeatedly refers to a "Central Spiritual Sun," but for her this entity seems more akin to the Pythagorean model of a central fire that exists beyond the earth rather than inside it. See also Nicholas Goodrick-Clarke, *Black Sun: Aryan Cults, Esoteric Nazism, and the Politics of Identity* (New York: New York University Press, 2002) for an analysis of this image in modern fascism.
42. Leadbeater, *The Chakras*, 32.
43. George Sydney Arundale, *A Fragment of Autobiography* (Adyar, India: Kalakshetra, 1940), 5.
44. George Sydney Arundale, *Kundalini: An Occult Experience* (Adyar, India: Theosophical Publishing House, 1938), 11.
45. Arundale, *Kundalini*, 50–51.
46. Arundale, 13.
47. Arundale, 59.
48. Arundale, xiv.
49. Arundale, 41.
50. Arundale, 41–43.
51. Arundale, 80–81.
52. Arundale, 71.

53. C. G. Jung, "Lecture IX, 11 December 1935," in *Nietzsche's* Zarathustra*: Notes of the Seminar Given in 1934–1939*, ed. James L. Jarrett (Princeton, NJ: Princeton University Press, 1988), 748.
54. Cox, *The Subtle Body*, 181.
55. Tuomas Rasimus, *Paradise Reconsidered in Gnostic Mythmaking: Rethinking Sethianism in Light of the Ophite Myth and Ritual* (Leiden, the Netherlands: Brill, 2009), 87–89; Jung, "Lecture IX," 748.
56. Cox, *The Subtle Body*, 165.
57. Sonu Shamdasani, "Introduction: Jung's Journey to the East," in *The Psychology of Kundalini Yoga: Notes of the Seminar Given in 1932*, ed. Sonu Shamdasani (Princeton, NJ: Princeton University Press, 1996), xlv.
58. C. G. Jung, "Yoga and the West," in *Psychology and the East*, trans. R. F. C. Hull (Princeton, NJ: Princeton University Press, 1978), 77–86.
59. C. G. Jung, *The Red Book: Liber Novus*, ed. Sonu Shamdasani, trans. Mark Kyburz, John Peck, and Sonu Shamdasani (New York: Norton and Company, 2009), 237, 239, 244, 270.
60. Jung, *The Red Book*, 251–53.
61. Jung, 352.
62. Jung, 325–27.
63. Jung, 318, 322–29.
64. Jung, 247.
65. Shamdasani, "Introduction," xxvi.
66. See C. G. Jung, *The Psychology of Kundalini Yoga: Notes of the Seminar Given in 1932*, ed. Sonu Shamdasani (Princeton, NJ: Princeton University Press, 1996), 22n41 for Shamdasani's opinion that this may have been influenced by Avalon's *The Serpent Power*. The original reference in Avalon (see Avalon, *The Serpent Power*, 295) refers to the internalization of the feminine principle in tantric ritual, specifically as represented by the *haṭhayogic* texts of the medieval Nāths, where ascetic concerns led to a rejection of external sexual ritual. See James Mallinson, "Yoga and Yogis," *Nāmarūpa* 3, no. 15 (March 2012): 8.
67. Jung, *The Psychology of Kundalini Yoga*, 22.
68. Jung, 68–69. It's important not to mistake Jung's exaltation of the feminine for an actual elevation of women: "And that is the secret of the anima, human on the one side and that most paradoxical and incomprehensible thing on the other. On the one side she is an inferior

woman with all the bad qualities of a merely biological woman, an intriguing and plotting devil who always tries to entangle a man and make a perfect fool of him; yet she winds up with that snake's tail, with that peculiar insight and awareness. She is a psychopompos, and leads you into the understanding of the collective unconscious just by the way of the fool." Jung, "Lecture IX," 751.

69. Gopi Krishna, *Kundalini for the New Age: Selected Writings*, ed. Gene Kieffer (Toronto: Bantam Books, 1988), 43. With these words, Gopi Krishna is technically addressing Jung's commentary on *The Secret of the Golden Flower*, but he goes on to state that this is precisely the case with Jung's approach to Kuṇḍalinī.
70. For instance, Harold Coward summarized the matter as follows: "What Jung's 'Commentary' accomplished then, and still does today, is to provide added insight into *his* understanding of the *process of Individuation*, not an accurate description of Kundalini." See Harold Coward, *Jung and Eastern Thought* (Albany: State University of New York Press, 1985), 123. Quoted in Shamdasani, "Introduction," xliii.
71. Shamdasani, "Introduction," xliv.
72. Shamdasani, xlv.
73. Kathleen Taylor, *Sir John Woodroffe, Tantra and Bengal: "An Indian Soul in a European Body?"* (London: Routledge, 2001), 11–13.
74. Taylor, *Sir John Woodroffe*, 37.
75. Taylor, 97; Strube, *Global Tantra*, 220.
76. Strube, *Global Tantra*, 220.
77. Strube, 8. Strube specifies that the latter two men were also disciples of Shivachandra.
78. Strube, 221.
79. See Taylor, *Sir John Woodroffe*, 147–48.
80. Strube, *Global Tantra*, 226–27.
81. Avalon, *The Serpent Power*, 299–301.
82. Baier, "Theosophical Orientalism," 313.
83. Mallinson and Singleton, *Roots of Yoga*, 176–77. Mallinson and Singleton suggest that the six(-plus-one)-*cakra* systems endured better than competing models by virtue of their association with India's most prominent and still-active orders of ascetic yogis. Strube importantly points out that the elevation of the "six-plus-one" *cakra*

system found in the *Ṣaṭcakra Nirūpaṇa* has a longer history among Bengali thinkers (Strube, *Global Tantra*, 52). Thus, Avalon's privileging of it was not a novel phenomenon, but it was instrumental in carrying this focus over to a global audience. For an account of the modern evolution of this Southern Transmission, known today as Śrīvidyā, see Meera Jo Kachroo, "Śrīvidyā's Rahasya: Public Esotericism in a Contemporary Tantric Tradition" (PhD diss., McGill University, 2022).

84. Avalon, *The Serpent Power*, 5.
85. Avalon, 7.
86. Avalon, 21.
87. Avalon, 22.
88. Avalon, 159.
89. Avalon, 161–62.

4. EAST MEETS WEST

1. Mark Singleton, *Yoga Body: The Origins of Modern Posture Practice* (New York: Oxford University Press, 2010), 51.
2. Singleton, *Yoga Body*, 50–53. See also Kurt Leland, *Rainbow Body: A History of the Western Chakra System from Blavatsky to Brennan* (Lake Worth, FL: Ibis Press, 2016), 99–101, 250–52; Julian Strube, *Global Tantra: Religion, Science, and Nationalism in Colonial Modernity* (New York: Oxford University Press, 2022), 121–22.
3. James Mallinson, "Yoga and Yogis," *Nāmarūpa* 3, no. 15 (March 2012): 11–12.
4. Alexis Sanderson, "The Śaiva Age: The Rise and Dominance of Śaivism During the Early Medieval Period," in *Genesis and Development of Tantrism*, ed. Shingo Einoo (Tokyo: Institute of Oriental Culture, University of Tokyo, 2009), 41–350.
5. James Mallinson, "*Hathayoga*'s Philosophy: A Fortuitous Union of Non-Dualities," *Journal of Indian Philosophy* 42, no. 1 (March 2014): 225–47.
6. Christian Bouy, *Les Nātha-yogin et les Upaniṣads: Étude d'histoire de la littérature hindoue* (Paris: Diffusion De Boccard, 1994) and Jeffrey Clark Ruff, "Yoga in the Yoga Upaniṣads: Disciplines of the Mystical OṂ Sound," in *Yoga in Practice*, ed. David Gordon White

(Princeton, NJ: Princeton University Press, 2012), 97–116. See also Jason Schwartz, "Parabrahman Among the Yogins," *International Journal of Hindu Studies* 21, no. 3 (December 2017): 345–89.

7. Swami Vivekananda, *The Complete Works of Swami Vivekananda*, vol. 1 (Calcutta: Advaita Ashrama, 1915), 185.
8. Quoted in Anya Foxen, *Biography of a Yogi: Paramahansa Yogananda and the Origins of Modern Yoga* (New York: Oxford University Press, 2017), 51.
9. Foxen, *Biography of a Yogi*, 51.
10. Elizabeth De Michelis, *A History of Modern Yoga: Patañjali and Western Esotericism* (London: Continuum, 2004), 104.
11. Vivekananda, *The Complete Works*, 187.
12. Vivekananda, 264–65.
13. See also Strube, *Global Tantra*, 120–21, for a treatment of Basu. Strube identifies Basu as perhaps the first published attempt to identify the *cakras* with nerve plexuses.
14. Vivekananda, *The Complete Works*, 182.
15. Vivekananda, 185.
16. Vivekananda, 185.
17. Vasant G. Rele, *The Mysterious Kundalini* (Bombay, India: D. B. Taraporevala Sons & Co., 1931), xxi–xxii.
18. Rele, *The Mysterious Kundalini*, x.
19. Rele, xi.
20. Rele, 22.
21. Rele, 25–26.
22. Rele, 65.
23. Rele, x.
24. Rele, 77.
25. Rele, 79.
26. Edwin F. Bryant, *The Yoga Sutras of Patañjali: A New Edition, Translation, and Commentary; With Insights from the Traditional Commentators* (New York: North Point Press, 2009), 358.
27. David Gordon White, *The Yoga Sutra of Patanjali: A Biography* (Princeton, NJ: Princeton University Press, 2014), 127.
28. Jason Birch, "Rājayoga: The Reincarnations of the King of All Yogas," *International Journal of Hindu Studies* 17, no. 3 (December 2013): 408.

29. Jason Birch, "The Proliferation of Āsana-s in Late-Mediaeval Yoga Texts," in *Yoga in Transformation: Historical and Contemporary Perspectives on a Global Phenomenon*, ed. Karl Baier, Philip A. Maas, and Karin Preisendanz (Göttingen, Germany: Vandenhoeck & Ruprecht Unipress, 2018), 101–80.
30. Joseph S. Alter, *Yoga in Modern India: The Body Between Science and Philosophy* (Princeton, NJ: Princeton University Press, 2004), 73–108; and Elliott Goldberg, *The Path of Modern Yoga: The History of an Embodied Spiritual Practice* (Rochester, VT: Inner Traditions, 2016), 75–88.
31. Quoted in Goldberg, *The Path of Modern Yoga*, 84.
32. Srimat Kuvalayananda, "Prāṇāyāma," *Yoga-Mīmānsa* 3, no. 1 (1928): 267n4.
33. Kuvalayananda, "Prāṇāyāma," 267n4.
34. Kuvalayananda, 268n4.
35. Srimat Kuvalayananda, "Kapālabhāti," *Yoga-Mīmānsa* 4, no. 2 (1930): 174n1.
36. Srimat Kuvalayananda, "Preparing Oneself for Āsanas," *Yoga-Mīmānsa* 4, no. 3 (1933): 223.
37. Srimat Kuvalayananda, "Scientific Survey of Cultural Poses," *Yoga-Mīmānsa* 4, no. 3 (1933): 245.
38. Srimat Kuvalayananda, "Pressure Experiments in Prāṇāyāma," *Yoga-Mīmānsa* 4, no. 1 (1930): 12.
39. Kuvalayananda, "Pressure Experiments in Prāṇāyāma," 13.
40. Kuvalayananda, "Scientific Survey," 232.
41. Srimat Kuvalayananda, *Popular Yoga: Prâṇâyâma* (Bombay, India: Kaivalyadhama, 1931), 128.
42. Swami Sivananda, *Yogic Home Exercises: Easy Course of Physical Culture for Modern Men and Women* (Bombay, India: D. B. Taraporevala Son and Co., 1939), 51.
43. Swami Sivananda, *Kundalini Yoga* (Shivanandanagar, India: The Divine Life Society, 1994), 37.
44. Sivananda, *Kundalini Yoga*, 35.
45. Singleton, *Yoga Body*, 178–84.
46. Mark Singleton and Tara Fraser, "T. Krishnamacharya, Father of Modern Yoga," in *Gurus of Modern Yoga*, ed. Mark Singleton and Ellen Goldberg (New York: Oxford University Press, 2014), 93.

47. Simon Atkinson, *Krishnamacharya on Kuṇḍalinī: The Origins and Coherence of His Position* (Sheffield, UK: Equinox, 2022).
48. Atkinson, *Krishnamacharya on Kuṇḍalinī.*
49. Atkinson, 131.
50. Frederick M. Smith and Joan White, "Becoming an Icon: B. K. S. Iyengar as a Yoga Teacher and a Yoga Guru," in *Gurus of Modern Yoga*, ed. Mark Singleton and Ellen Goldberg (New York: Oxford University Press, 2014), 134–35.
51. De Michelis, *A History of Modern Yoga*, 244.
52. B. K. S. Iyengar, *Light on Yoga: Yoga Dipika* (New York: Schocken Books, 1979), 130.
53. Iyengar, *Light on Yoga*, 273.
54. Iyengar, 440.
55. B. K. S. Iyengar, *Light on Prāṇāyāma: Prāṇāyāma Dīpikā* (London: Unwin Paperbacks, 1983), 179–80.
56. B. K. S. Iyengar, *Light on the Yoga Sūtras of Patañjali* (London: Thorsons, 2002), 184; also partially quoted in De Michelis, *A History of Modern Yoga*, 243.
57. Bryant, *The Yoga Sutras of Patañjali*, 408; Vivekananda, *The Complete Works*, 309.
58. Bryant, *The Yoga Sutras of Patañjali*, 409–10.
59. Vivekananda, *The Complete Works*, 310.
60. Foxen, *Biography of a Yogi*, 99.
61. Swami Satyeswarananda Giri, *Kriya: Finding the True Path* (San Diego, CA: Sanskrit Classics, 1991), 150.
62. Foxen, *Biography of a Yogi*, 134.
63. See Foxen, 133–36, for a general outline of Kriya Yoga practice.
64. Paramahansa Yogananda, "Awakening of Kundalini, or Serpent Force," *Yogoda Sat-Sanga Fortnightly Instructions*, n.d.; Paramahansa Yogananda, *The Second Coming of Christ: The Resurrection of the Christ Within You; A Revelatory Commentary on the Original Teachings of Jesus* (Los Angeles: Self-Realization Fellowship, 2008), 47.
65. Yogananda, "Awakening of Kundalini"; Yogananda, *The Second Coming of Christ*, 263.
66. Yogananda, 790. There is some ambiguity around the authorship of texts published by the SRF after Yogananda's passing. Because they contain substantial additions and edits that depart from

Yogananda's work as published during his lifetime, literal authorship can only be assigned by way of attribution. However, a similar issue arises with regards to Yogananda's autobiography, which was created through a process of intensive editorial collaboration. For our intents and purposes, the ideas articulated here fall close enough to fragments found in Yogananda's earlier work and to the overall character of his thought.

67. Paramahansa Yogananda, *Autobiography of a Yogi* (Nevada City, CA: Crystal Clarity Publishers, 1995), 239.
68. Yogananda, *Autobiography of a Yogi*, 397.
69. See for instance Sri Sailendra Bejoy Dasgupta, *Kriya Yoga*, trans. Yoga Niketan (Lincoln, NE: iUniverse, 2009).
70. Yogananda, *Autobiography of a Yogi*, 49, 426.
71. Sri Aurobindo, *The Complete Works of Aurobindo: Autobiographical Notes and Other Writings of Historical Interest*, vol. 36 (Pondicherry, India: Sri Aurobindo Ashram Press, 2006), 98–99.
72. Sri Aurobindo, *The Complete Works of Aurobindo: Letters on Yoga II*, vol. 29 (Pondicherry, India: Sri Aurobindo Ashram Press, 2013), 459.
73. Ann Gleig and Charles I. Flores, "Remembering Sri Aurobindo and the Mother: The Forgotten Lineage of Integral Yoga," in *Gurus of Modern Yoga*, ed. Mark Singleton and Ellen Goldberg (New York: Oxford University Press, 2014), 55.
74. Peter Heehs, *The Lives of Sri Aurobindo* (New York: Columbia University Press, 2008), 239.
75. Aurobindo, *The Complete* Works, vol. 29, 460.
76. Aurobindo, 462.
77. Aurobindo, 460.
78. Aurobindo, 377.
79. Heehs, *The Lives of Sri Aurobindo*, 274.
80. Heehs, 273.
81. Sri Aurobindo, *The Complete Works of Aurobindo: Essays Divine and Human*, vol. 12 (Pondicherry, India: Sri Aurobindo Ashram Press, 1997), 166.
82. Aurobindo, *The Complete Works of Aurobindo*, vol. 12, 157.
83. See Heehs, *The Lives of Sri Aurobindo*, 274.
84. Sri Aurobindo, *The Complete Works of Aurobindo: Letters on Yoga III*, vol. 30 (Pondicherry, India: Sri Aurobindo Ashram Press, 2014), 216.
85. Aurobindo, *The Complete Works*, vol. 29, 462–64.

5. WHEN THE SERPENT RISES

1. Dick Russell, *The Life and Ideas of James Hillman: Volume I; The Making of a Psychologist* (New York: Helios Press, 2013), 335.
2. Russell, *Ideas of James Hillman*, 305.
3. Russell, 335.
4. Teri Degler, *Gopi Krishna: A Biography; Kundalini, Consciousness, and Our Evolution to Enlightenment* (Markdale, Canada: Institute for Consciousness Research, 2023), 94.
5. For a more specific analysis of Gopi Krishna's situatedness in scientific understandings of Kuṇḍalinī, see also Marleen Thaler, "Approaching a Universal Pattern? Gopi Krishna's Transformational Kuṇḍalinī Experience Within the Frame of Universalism and Religious Scientism," in *Intentional Transformative Experiences*, eds. Sarah Perez, Jens Schlieter, and Bastiaan Vanrijn (Berlin: De Gruyter, forthcoming).
6. Gopi Krishna, *Kundalini: The Evolutionary Energy in Man* (New Delhi: Ramadhar and Hopman, 1967), 17.
7. Krishna, *Kundalini*, 14.
8. Letter from Gopi Krishna to Sri Aurobindo, 1938 (Pondicherry, India: Sri Aurobindo Ashram Archives). All quotations from Gopi Krishna's correspondences with Aurobindo, unless otherwise specified, derive from this source.
9. Krishna, *Kundalini*, 24–25.
10. Krishna, 3.
11. Krishna, 107–8.
12. Krishna, 100.
13. Krishna, 106.
14. Krishna, 108–9.
15. Krishna, 167.
16. Krishna, 176.
17. Krishna, 179.
18. Krishna, 189–90, 201.
19. Krishna, 219–30.
20. Krishna, 236.
21. Krishna, 238–42, 249–57.
22. Krishna, 249.

23. Krishna, 281.
24. Krishna, 56.
25. Krishna, 54.
26. Krishna, 54.
27. Krishna, 54.
28. Krishna, 71.
29. Krishna, 75.
30. Krishna, 68.
31. Krishna, 69.
32. Krishna, 66.
33. Krishna, 136–37.
34. Joseph S. Alter, "Shri Yogendra: Magic, Modernity, and the Burden of the Middle-Class Yogi," in *Gurus of Modern Yoga*, ed. Mark Singleton and Ellen Goldberg (New York: Oxford University Press, 2013), 71.
35. Krishna, *Kundalini*, 206.
36. Krishna, 206.
37. Krishna, 102.
38. Krishna, 273.
39. Krishna, 193–94.
40. Krishna, 209.
41. Krishna, 42–44.
42. Krishna, 83.
43. Gopi Krishna, *Kundalini for the New Age: Selected Writings*, ed. Gene Kieffer (Toronto: Bantam Books, 1988), 43.
44. Gopi Krishna, *The Biological Basis of Religion and Genius* (New York: Harper & Row, 1972), 28–29.
45. Krishna, *Biological Basis of Religion*, 4.
46. Krishna, 42–43.
47. Krishna, *Kundalini for the New Age*, 189.
48. Krishna, 190.
49. Russell, *Ideas of James Hillman*, 337.
50. Krishna, *Kundalini*, 69.
51. Russell, *Ideas of James Hillman*, 342.
52. Krishna, *Kundalini*, 289. Contrast with Gopi Krishna's own gendered statement on the dynamics of these energies: "Nothing can convey my condition more graphically than the representation of

Shiva and Sakti, pictured by an ancient master, in which the former is shown lying helpless and supine while the latter in an absolutely reckless mood dances gleefully on his prostrate frame." Krishna, *Kundalini*, 179–80. Hillman remarks but does not follow through on this dominant feminine principle. His framework does not allow for it.

53. Russell, *Ideas of James Hillman*, 351.
54. Russell, 351–52.
55. Russell, 359.
56. Russell, 459.
57. Sonu Shamdasani, "Introduction: Jung's Journey to the East," in *The Psychology of Kundalini Yoga: Notes of the Seminar Given in 1932*, ed. Sonu Shamdasani (Princeton, NJ: Princeton University Press, 1996), xxxvii; Dimitry Okropiridze, " 'East' and 'West' in the Kaleidoscope of Transculturality—The Discursive Production of the Kuṇḍalinī as a New Ontological Object Within and Beyond Orientalist Dichotomies," in *Eastspirit: Transnational Spirituality and Religious Circulation in East and West*, ed. Jørn Borup and Marianne Qvortrup Fibiger (Leiden, the Netherlands: Brill, 2017), 136.

6. THE SERPENT IN THE MARKETPLACE

1. Andrea R. Jain, "Muktananda: Entrepreneurial Godman, Tantric Hero," in *Gurus of Modern Yoga*, ed. Mark Singleton and Ellen Goldberg (New York: Oxford University Press, 2014), 196.
2. Ronald M. Davidson, *Indian Esoteric Buddhism: Social History of the Tantric Movement* (Delhi: Motilal Banarsidass, 2004), 25–30.
3. Daniel Gold, *The Lord as Guru: Hindi Sants in North Indian Tradition* (New York: Oxford: Oxford University Press, 1987), 4.
4. Gavin D. Flood, *The Tantric Body: The Secret Tradition of Hindu Religion* (London: I. B. Tauris, 2006), 11.
5. David Gordon White, *Sinister Yogis* (Chicago: University of Chicago Press, 2009), 140.
6. Jain, "Muktananda," 200.
7. Lola Williamson, "The Perfectibility of Perfection: Siddha Yoga as a Global Movement," in *Gurus in America*, ed. Thomas A. Forsthoefel and

Cynthia Ann Humes (Albany: State University of New York Press, 2005), 151–52; Jain, "Muktananda," 195, 199–201.

8. Jain, "Muktananda," 209n8.
9. See, for instance, the now-classic Jeremy R. Carrette and Richard King, *Capitalist Spirituality: The Silent Takeover of Religion* (London: Routledge, 2004).
10. Swami Satyeswarananda Giri, *Kriya: Finding the True Path* (San Diego, CA: Sanskrit Classics, 1991), 150.
11. Swami Muktananda, *Kundalini: The Secret of Life* (Fallsburg, NY: SYDA Foundation, 1994), 36.
12. Amanda Lucia, "Guru Sex: Charisma, Proxemic Desire, and the Haptic Logics of the Guru-Disciple Relationship," *Journal of the American Academy of Religion* 86, no. 4 (December 2018): 953–88.
13. Jeffrey J. Kripal, *The Superhumanities: Historical Precedents, Moral Objections, New Realities* (Chicago: University of Chicago Press, 2022), 127.
14. Kripal, *The Superhumanities*, 127–28.
15. Philip Deslippe, "From Maharaj to Mahan Tantric: The Construction of Yogi Bhajan's Kundalini Yoga," *Sikh Formations* 8, no. 3 (December 2012): 370.
16. Deslippe, "Maharaj to Mahan Tantric," 370.
17. Deslippe, 371–72.
18. Deslippe, 372.
19. Joseph S. Alter, *The Wrestler's Body: Identity and Ideology in North India* (Berkeley: University of California Press, 1992), 82–83; Jason Birch and Mark Singleton, "The Yoga of the Haṭhābhyāsapaddhati: Haṭhayoga on the Cusp of Modernity," *Journal of Yoga Studies* 2 (December 2019): 47–48; Jerome Armstrong, "Uncovering Vyāyāma in Yoga," *Journal of Yoga Studies* 4 (April 2023): 271–302.
20. See Anya Foxen, *Biography of a Yogi: Paramahansa Yogananda and the Origins of Modern Yoga* (New York: Oxford University Press, 2017), 135–44 and Anya Foxen, *Inhaling Spirit: Harmonialism, Orientalism, and the Western Roots of Modern Yoga* (New York: Oxford University Press, 2020), 244–47.
21. Martin Douglas, "Yogi Bhajan, 75, 'Boss' of Worlds Spiritual and Capitalistic, Dies," *The New York Times*, October 9, 2004, https://www.nytimes.com/2004/10/09/us/yogi-bhajan-75-boss-of-worlds-spiritual-and-capitalistic-dies.html.

22. Deslippe, "Maharaj to Mahan Tantric," 373.
23. Harbhajan Singh Khalsa, *The Teachings of Yogi Bhajan* (New York: Hawthorn Books, Inc., 1977), 182.
24. Gurucharan Singh Khalsa and Yogi Bhajan, "Exploring the Myths and Misconceptions of Kundalini," in *Kundalini: Evolution and Enlightenment*, ed. John White (New York: Paragon House, 1979), 133.
25. Khalsa and Bhajan, "Exploring the Myths," 147.
26. Khalsa and Bhajan, 147.
27. Khalsa and Bhajan, 144.
28. Khalsa and Bhajan, 144.
29. Khalsa and Bhajan, 146–47.
30. Khalsa and Bhajan, 145.
31. See Foxen, *Inhaling Spirit.*
32. Doris Jakobsh, "3HO/Sikh Dharma of the Western Hemisphere: The 'Forgotten' New Religious Movement?," *Religion Compass* 2, no. 3 (May 2008): 385–408; Constance Waeber Elsberg, *Graceful Women: Gender and Identity in an American Sikh Community* (Knoxville: The University of Tennessee Press, 2003).
33. Elsberg, *Graceful Women*, 73–80.
34. Khalsa, *The Teachings of Yogi Bhajan,* 184.
35. Khalsa, 177.
36. Khalsa and Bhajan, "Exploring the Myths," 144.
37. Khalsa and Bhajan, 147.
38. Williamson, "The Perfectibility of Perfection," 87.
39. Ellen Goldberg, "Swami Kṛpālvānanda: The Man behind Kripalu Yoga," in *Gurus of Modern Yoga*, ed. Mark Singleton and Ellen Goldberg (New York: Oxford University Press, 2014), 176. See also Christopher D. Wallis, "The Descent of Power: Possession, Mysticism, and Initiation in the Śaiva Theology of Abhinavagupta," *Journal of Indian Philosophy* 36, no. 2 (April 2008): 247–95.
40. See Jain, "Muktananda," 191–92.
41. Muktananda, *Kundalini*, 11.
42. Swami Muktananda, *Play of Consciousness* (San Francisco: Harper & Row, 1974), 64.
43. Muktananda, *Play of Consciousness*, 64–65.
44. Quoted in Jain, "Muktananda," 201.

45. Paul Zweig, "Shaktipat," in *Kundalini: Evolution and Enlightenment*, ed. John White (New York: Paragon House, 1979), 176–77.
46. Muktananda, *Play of Consciousness*, xxi.
47. Muktananda, *Kundalini*, 15–16.
48. Muktananda, xvii.
49. Muktananda, *Play of Consciousness*, 24.
50. "Just as a seed contains a whole tree in potential form, Kundalini contains all the different forms of yoga, and when She is awakened through the grace of the Guru, She makes all yogas take place within you spontaneously. The process which begins when you receive Shaktipat is called Siddha Yoga, the 'perfect yoga,' or Maha Yoga, the 'great yoga.' . . . Siddha Yoga is called Maha Yoga because it encompasses all other yogas. There are many kinds of yogas: hatha yoga, the practice of physical exercises; bhakti yoga, the path of love; raja yoga, which is attained through meditation; mantra yoga; laya yoga; jnana yoga and many others. When Kundalini is awakened, all these other yogas take place automatically. You don't have to make any effort to practice them; they come to you on their own." Muktananda, *Kundalini*, 18.
51. Muktananda, *Play of Consciousness*, 19.
52. Ellen Goldberg, "Amrit Desai and the Kripalu Center for Yoga and Health," in *Homegrown Gurus: From Hinduism in America to American Hinduism*, ed. Ann Gleig and Lola Williamson (Albany: State University of New York Press, 2014), 63.
53. Gene R. Thursby, "Hindu Movements Since Mid-Century: Yogis in the States," in *America's Alternative Religions*, ed. Timothy Miller (Albany: State University of New York Press, 1995), 201.
54. Thursby, "Hindu Movements Since Mid-Century," 202.
55. Yogi Amrit Desai, *Kripalu Yoga: Meditation-in-Motion* (Lenox, MA: Kripalu Publications, 1985), 23–25.
56. Desai, *Kripalu Yoga*, 27–29.
57. Desai, 30.
58. Desai, 36.
59. Desai, 10–11.
60. James Mallinson and Mark Singleton, *Roots of Yoga: A Sourcebook from the Indic Traditions* (London: Penguin Classics, 2017), 179.
61. Goldberg, "Swami Kṛpālvānanda," 181.

62. Desai, *Kripalu Yoga*, 77.
63. Desai, 79.
64. Stephen Cope, *Yoga and the Quest for the True Self* (New York: Bantam Books, 1999), 69. Also quoted in Ellen Goldberg, "Amrit Desai and the Kripalu Center for Yoga and Health," in *Homegrown Gurus: From Hinduism in America to American Hinduism*, ed. Ann Gleig and Lola Williamson (Albany: State University of New York Press, 2014), 75–76.
65. Despite the fact that Osho generally went by "Rajneesh" during the period of his career that we are addressing here, we refer to him as Osho throughout to avoid confusion for non-specialist readers. "Osho" is the name that the techniques in question are associated with when one looks them up today.
66. Hugh B. Urban, "Osho, from Sex Guru to Guru of the Rich: The Spiritual Logic of Late Capitalism," in *Gurus in America*, ed. Thomas A. Forsthoefel and Cynthia Ann Humes (Albany: State University of New York Press, 2005), 172–73.
67. Urban, "Osho, from Sex Guru," 181–82.
68. Urban, 174–76.
69. Urban, 173–74.
70. Hugh B. Urban, *Zorba the Buddha: Sex, Spirituality, and Capitalism in the Global Osho Movement* (Oakland: University of California Press, 2016), 60.
71. Urban, *Zorba the Buddha*, 60.
72. Bhagwan Shree Rajneesh, *Meditation: The Art of Ecstasy* (New York: Harper & Row, 1978), 65.
73. Rajneesh, *Meditation*, 65.
74. Rajneesh, 65–66.
75. Rajneesh, 82.
76. Rajneesh, 86.
77. Rajneesh, 233.
78. "OSHO Dynamic Meditation," OSHO, OSHO International Foundation, accessed July 21, 2023, https://www.osho.com/meditation/osho-active-meditations/osho-dynamic-meditation.
79. Bhagwan Shree Rajneesh, *The Orange Book* (Rajneeshpuram, OR: Rajneesh Foundation International, 1983), 135–36.
80. Rajneesh, *Meditation*, 72.

81. Rajneesh, 73.
82. Rajneesh, 73.
83. Rajneesh, 185.
84. Rajneesh, 76.
85. Rajneesh, 67.
86. Rajneesh, 69.
87. Rajneesh, 74–75.
88. Rajneesh, 75–76.
89. See, for instance, Osho, *The Sword and the Lotus: Talks in the Himalayas* (Cologne, Germany: Rebel Publishing House, 1986) and Osho, *In Search of the Miraculous: Kundalini Yoga*, vol. 2 (New Delhi: Sterling, 1998).
90. Urban, *Zorba the Buddha*, 62.
91. Thursby, "Hindu Movements Since Mid-Century," 205.

7. THE SERPENT IN THE MELTING POT

1. John White, ed., *Kundalini: Evolution and Enlightenment* (New York: Paragon House, 1979), 16.
2. White, *Kundalini*, 17.
3. White, 17.
4. Swami Rama (1925–1996) was the founder of the Himalayan Institute of Yoga, which persists into today.
5. See Thomas A. Forsthoefel and Cynthia Ann Humes, eds., *Gurus in America* (Albany: State University of New York Press, 2005) and Ann Gleig and Lola Williamson, eds., *Homegrown Gurus: From Hinduism in America to American Hinduism* (Albany: State University of New York Press, 2014).
6. Swami Sivananda Radha, *Kundalini Yoga* (Delhi: Motilal Banarsidass, 2011), 13.
7. Sivananda Radha, *Kundalini Yoga*, 4.
8. Swami Sivananda Radha, *Hatha Yoga: The Hidden Language; Symbols, Secrets, and Metaphor* (Boston: Shambhala, 1987), 279.
9. Jeffrey J. Kripal, "Riding the Dawn Horse: Adi Da and the Eros of Non-duality," in *Gurus in America*, ed. Thomas A. Forsthoefel and Cynthia Ann Humes (Albany: State University of New York Press, 2005), 214n1.
10. Kripal, "Riding the Dawn Horse," 202–203.
11. Kripal, 199.

12. Quoted in Lee Sannella, *The Kundalini Experience: Psychosis or Transcendence?* (Lower Lake, CA: Integral Publishing, 1987), 122.
13. See Anya Foxen, *Inhaling Spirit: Harmonialism, Orientalism, and the Western Roots of Modern Yoga* (New York: Oxford University Press, 2020), 189–222, 255–56.
14. Da Avabhasa, *The Knee of Listening* (Clearlake, CA: The Dawn Horse Press, 1992), 68–69, 99.
15. Da Avabhasa, *The Knee of Listening*, 41.
16. Itzhak Bentov, *Stalking the Wild Pendulum: On the Mechanics of Consciousness* (New York: Bantam Books, 1977), 178.
17. Bentov, *Stalking the Wild Pendulum*, 181.
18. Lee Sannella, *Kundalini: Psychosis or Transcendence?* (San Francisco: H. S. Dakin Company, 1976), 87–88.
19. Bentov, *Stalking the Wild Pendulum*, 183.
20. Bentov, 182.
21. Randi Rossman, "Lee Sherman Sannella," *The Press Democrat*, March 22, 2010, https://www.pressdemocrat.com/article/news/lee-sherman-sannella/.
22. Sannella, *Kundalini*, 13.
23. Sannella, 44–51.
24. Sannella, 11.
25. Sannella, 55.
26. Stanislav Grof and Christina Grof, eds., *Spiritual Emergency: When Personal Transformation Becomes a Crisis* (Los Angeles: Jeremy P. Tarcher, 1989), 15.
27. Sannella, *Kundalini*, 12–13.
28. Sannella, 11.
29. Sannella, 63.
30. Sannella, 24.
31. Sannella, 64.
32. Sannella, x.
33. Jeffrey J. Kripal, *Esalen: America and the Religion of No Religion* (Chicago: University of Chicago Press, 2007), 264.
34. Catharina Kiehnle, "The Secret of the Nāths: The Ascent of Kuṇḍalinī According to Jñāneśvarī 6.151–328," *Bulletin Des Études Indiennes* 22–23 (2005–2004), 476.

35. H. P. Blavatsky, *The Voice of the Silence* (London: Theosophical Publishing Company, 1889), 76n24.
36. C. W. Leadbeater, *The Chakras* (Wheaton, IL: Theosophical Publishing House, 1927), 81.
37. George Sydney Arundale, *Kundalini: An Occult Experience* (Adyar, India: Theosophical Publishing House, 1938), 22.
38. Gurucharan Singh Khalsa and Yogi Bhajan, "Exploring the Myths and Misconceptions of Kundalini," in *Kundalini: Evolution and Enlightenment*, ed. John White (New York: Paragon House, 1979), 143.
39. Swami Muktananda, *Kundalini: The Secret of Life* (Fallsburg, NY: SYDA Foundation, 1994), 24.
40. Bhagwan Shree Rajneesh, *Meditation: The Art of Ecstasy* (New York: Harper & Row, 1978), 72.
41. Kripal, *Esalen*, 264.
42. Grof and Grof, *Spiritual Emergency*, 13–14.
43. Grof and Grof, 15.
44. Grof and Grof, 15.
45. Kripal, *Esalen*, 269.
46. Ida Craddock, *Sexual Outlaw, Erotic Mystic: The Essential Ida Craddock*, ed. Vere Chappell (San Francisco: Weiser Books, 2010), 212. See also Andrea R. Jain, *Selling Yoga: From Counterculture to Pop Culture* (New York: Oxford University Press, 2014), 24–25.
47. See Robert Love, *The Great Oom: The Improbable Birth of Yoga in America* (New York: Viking, 2010).
48. Arundale, *Kundalini*, 21.
49. Leadbeater, *The Chakras*, 82.
50. Ellen Bayuk Rosenman, *Unauthorized Pleasures: Accounts of Victorian Erotic Experience* (Ithaca, NY: Cornell University Press, 2003), 16.
51. Swami Sivananda Radha, "Kundalini: An Overview," in *Kundalini: Evolution and Enlightenment*, ed. John White (New York: Paragon House, 1979), 51.
52. See Hugh B. Urban, *Tantra: Sex, Secrecy, Politics, and Power in the Study of Religion* (Berkeley: University of California Press, 2003).
53. See Kripal, *Esalen*.
54. Jacqueline Chambron, *Lilian Silburn: Une vie mystique* (Paris: Almora, 2015), 31–34.

55. See for instance Gopi Krishna, *Kundalini: The Evolutionary Energy in Man* (New Delhi: Ramadhar and Hopman, 1967), 102, 150, 175.
56. Swami Muktananda, *Play of Consciousness* (San Francisco: Harper & Row, 1974), 95.
57. See for instance Sannella, *Kundalini*, 53, 67–68, 90.
58. Unless noted otherwise, all subsequent information, ideas, and quotes attributed to Michael Murphy derive from a personal interview with the authors, conducted on June 20 and June 21, 2023. Further, one of the co-authors (Borkataky-Varma) leads several public workshops at Esalen Institute and is also one of the Board of Trustees, as of 2023.
59. Kripal, *Esalen*, 82.
60. Robert McDermott, "A Brief History of California Institute of Integral Studies," California Institute of Integral Studies, November 17, 2017, https://www.ciis.edu/discover-ciis/our-history.
61. Kripal, *Esalen*, 82.
62. Kripal, 82.
63. Kripal, 60–61.
64. Kripal, 79–81.
65. Mission statement quoted in Kripal, *Esalen*, 28.
66. Kripal, 85–86.
67. Kripal, 87.
68. Esalen Institute, "Seminars at Big Sur Hot Springs and Redwood Lodge," (Winter/Spring 1965), n.p.
69. Marleen Thaler, "The Rising Serpent at Esalen," Esalen, Esalen Institute and Esalen Theory & Research, May 24, 2023, https://www.esalen.org/post/the-rising-serpent-at-esalen-052323.
70. We would like to offer our deep gratitude to Marleen Thaler for her tireless work in the Esalen catalog archives and for sharing the fruits of that research with us.
71. See Linda Sargent Wood, *A More Perfect Union: Holistic Worldviews and the Transformation of American Culture After World War II* (New York: Oxford University Press, 2010), 190.
72. Kripal, *Esalen*, 365–66.
73. Mary Scott, *Kundalini in the Physical World* (London: Routledge & Kegan Paul, 1983), 1.
74. Scott, *Kundalini in the Physical World*, 1.
75. Scott, 3.

76. Scott, 24–25.
77. For an examination of Kuṇḍalinī in the context of terrestrial spiritual models, see also Marleen Thaler, "Gaia's Energy Flows: The Interplay of Eco-Spirituality and Terrestrial Energy Healing," in *Subtle Energies in Therapy, Spirituality, Arts, and Politics, 1800–Present*, ed. Julian Strube, Marleen Thaler, and Dominic Zoehrer (Leiden, the Netherlands: Brill, forthcoming).
78. Mary Scott, *The Kundalini Concept: Its Origin and Value* (Fremont, CA: Jain Publishing, 2006), xv. Scott also somewhat misrepresents the nature of Gopi Krishna's model based on just one of his early collaborations: "In writing his *Kundalini: The Evolutionary Energy in Man* he collaborated with James Hillman, then Director of the C.G. Jung Institute in Zurich, who produced a commentary analyzing Gopi Krishna's experiences along Jungian lines. As there was no reference to *The Serpent Power* and the Tantric source of the concept, this meant that the research orientation of Gopi Krishna's Research Foundation was Jungian rather than Tantric." Scott, *The Kundalini Concept*, xvi. Arguably, the research orientation of Gopi Krishna's various research initiatives was neither Jungian nor tantric (see the later portion of Teri Degler's biography on this point), but we might also question whether this is, at every level, a meaningful distinction—after all, both the Jungian and tantric angles are essentially alchemical in their logic.
79. Sannella, *The Kundalini Experience*, 18.
80. Sannella, 18–19.

8. THE SERPENT IN THE WEB

1. See, for instance, the work of Sat Bir Singh Khalsa, such as Sat Bir Singh Khalsa, "Treatment of Chronic Primary Sleep Onset Insomnia with Kundalini Yoga: A Randomized Controlled Trial with Active Sleep Hygiene Comparison," *Journal of Clinical Sleep Medicine* 17, no. 9 (September 2021): 1841–52, as well as Gurucharan Singh Khalsa.
2. Laura Sanches and Michael Daniels, "Kundalini and Transpersonal Development: Development of a Kundalini Awakening Scale and a Comparison Between Groups," *Transpersonal Psychology Review* 12, no. 1 (January 2008): 73–83.

3. Richard W. Maxwell and Sucharit Katyal, "Characteristics of Kundalini-Related Sensory, Motor, and Affective Experiences During Tantric Yoga Meditation," *Frontiers in Psychology* 13 (June 2022), https://www.frontiersin.org/articles/10.3389/fpsyg.2022.863091. Also see Maxwell and Katyal's article for a useful overview of previous such research.
4. Steve Taylor, "Energy and Awakening: A Psycho-Sexual Interpretation of Kundalini Awakening," *The Journal of Transpersonal Psychology* 47, no. 2 (2015): 229.
5. Jared R. Lindahl, "Somatic Energies and Emotional Traumas: A Qualitative Study of Practice-Related Challenges Reported by Vajrayāna Buddhists," *Religions* 8, no. 8 (August 2017), https://doi.org/10.3390/rel8080153.
6. David J. Cooper et al., " 'Like a Vibration Cascading through the Body': Energy-Like Somatic Experiences Reported by Western Buddhist Meditators," *Religions* 12, no. 12 (December 2021), https://doi.org/10.3390/rel12121042, 13.
7. Cooper, "Like a Vibration," 19.
8. Cooper, 15.
9. Cooper, 24.
10. Cooper, 22–23.
11. See Leigh Eric Schmidt, *Heaven's Bride: The Unprintable Life of Ida C. Craddock; American Mystic, Scholar, Sexologist, Martyr, and Madwoman* (New York: Basic Books, 2010).
12. Danielle Quijada, "Ariz. Temple Leader Sentenced on Prostitution Charges," *USA Today*, May 19, 2016, https://www.usatoday.com/story/news/nation-now/2016/05/19/ariz-temple-leader-sentenced-prostitution-charges/84623744/.
13. I was not sure of what Mai meant by "I am *jñāt*." My confusion must have been apparent, since before I could ask any further questions, Mai translated *jñāt* as "conscious mind state." She said "conscious mind state" in English. But further discussions led me to understand that what Mai meant by *jñāt* was more strictly "someone to whom knowledge has come."
14. Mai translated *cetanāhen* as "unconscious mind state," without any verbal prompting. We can also understand *cetanāhen* as a state where her mind exists as conscious awareness only, without an object of consciousness—an altered state.

15. In the margins of the diary I maintained during my interviews with Mai, over a few occasions, I wrote: "The dynamic between Mai and her husband seems reversed. He is much younger, or at least so it appears. I am not sure if it is the age difference that leads me to believe that the dynamic is skewed or something else, or maybe it is a combination of many factors: he is younger; she is socially powerful; his social standing is directly proportionate to her power; Mai's ardent followers believe that her husband does not have any *siddhis*, must remain as the priest of the temple, and finally should be there to serve her."

BIBLIOGRAPHY

Allan, Arlene. *Hermes*. London: Routledge, 2018.

Alter, Joseph S. "Shri Yogendra: Magic, Modernity, and the Burden of the Middle-Class Yogi." In *Gurus of Modern Yoga*, ed. Mark Singleton and Ellen Goldberg, 60–82. New York: Oxford University Press, 2013.

——. *The Wrestler's Body: Identity and Ideology in North India*. Berkeley: University of California Press, 1992.

——. *Yoga in Modern India: The Body Between Science and Philosophy*. Princeton, NJ: Princeton University Press, 2004.

Armstrong, Jerome. "Uncovering Vyāyāma in Yoga." *Journal of Yoga Studies* 4 (April 2023): 271–302.

Arundale, George Sydney. *A Fragment of Autobiography*. Adyar, India: Kalakshetra, 1940.

——. *Kundalini: An Occult Experience*. Adyar, India: Theosophical Publishing House, 1938.

Atkinson, Simon. *Krishnamacharya on Kuṇḍalinī: The Origins and Coherence of His Position*. Sheffield, UK: Equinox, 2022.

Aurobindo, Sri. *The Complete Works of Aurobindo: Autobiographical Notes and Other Writings of Historical Interest*. Vol. 36. Pondicherry, India: Sri Aurobindo Ashram Press, 2006.

——. *The Complete Works of Aurobindo: Essays Divine and Human*. Vol. 12. Pondicherry, India: Sri Aurobindo Ashram Press, 1997.

——. *The Complete Works of Aurobindo: Letters on Yoga II*. Vol. 29. Pondicherry, India: Sri Aurobindo Ashram Press, 2013.

——. *The Complete Works of Aurobindo: Letters on Yoga III*. Vol. 30. Pondicherry, India: Sri Aurobindo Ashram Press, 2014.

Avalon, Arthur. *The Serpent Power*. Madras, India: Ganesh & Co., 1950.

Baier, Karl. "Theosophical Orientalism and the Structures of Intercultural Transfer: Annotations on the Appropriation of the Cakras in Early Theosophy." In *Theosophical Appropriations: Esotericism, Kabbalah, and the Transformation of Traditions*, ed. Julie Chajes and Boaz Huss, 309–54. Beer Sheva, Israel: Ben-Gurion University of the Negev Press, 2016.

Bentov, Itzhak. "Micromotion of the Body as a Factor in the Development of the Nervous System." In *Kundalini: Psychosis or Transcendence?*, by Lee Sannella, 71–93. San Francisco: H. S. Dakin Company, 1976.

——. *Stalking the Wild Pendulum: On the Mechanics of Consciousness*. New York: Bantam Books, 1977.

Betz, Hans Dieter, ed. *The Greek Magical Papyri in Translation, Including the Demotic Spells*. Chicago: University of Chicago Press, 1986.

Birch, Jason. "The Meaning of Haṭha in Early Haṭhayoga." *Journal of the American Oriental Society* 131, no. 4 (October–December 2011): 527–54.

——. "The Proliferation of Āsana-s in Late-Mediaeval Yoga Texts." In *Yoga in Transformation: Historical and Contemporary Perspectives on a Global Phenomenon*, ed. Karl Baier, Philip A. Maas, and Karin Preisendanz, 101–80. Göttingen, Germany: Vandenhoeck & Ruprecht Unipress, 2018.

——. "Rājayoga: The Reincarnations of the King of All Yogas." *International Journal of Hindu Studies* 17, no. 3 (December 2013): 399–442.

Birch, Jason, and Mark Singleton. "The Yoga of the Haṭhābhyāsapaddhati: Haṭhayoga on the Cusp of Modernity." *Journal of Yoga Studies* 2 (December 2019): 3–70.

Blavatsky, H. P. *The Secret Doctrine: The Synthesis of Science, Religion and Philosophy*. Vol. 1. London: Theosophical Publishing Company, 1888.

——. *The Voice of the Silence*. London: Theosophical Publishing Company, 1889.

Bos, A. P. *The Soul and Its Instrumental Body: A Reinterpretation of Aristotle's Philosophy of Living Nature*. Leiden, the Netherlands: Brill, 2003.

Bouy, Christian. *Les Nātha-yogin et les Upaniṣads: Étude d'histoire de la littérature hindoue*. Paris: Diffusion De Boccard, 1994.

Bronkhorst, Johannes. *Greater Magadha: Studies in the Culture of Early India*. Leiden, the Netherlands: Brill, 2007.

——. *The Two Traditions of Meditation in Ancient India*. Delhi: Motilal Banarsidass Publishers, 2000.

Bryant, Edwin F. *The Yoga Sutras of Patañjali: A New Edition, Translation, and Commentary; With Insights from the Traditional Commentators*. New York: North Point Press, 2009.

Cantú, Keith Edward. *Like a Tree Universally Spread: Sri Sabhapati Swami and Śivarājayoga*. New York: Oxford University Press, 2023.

Capps, Walter H. *Religious Studies: The Making of a Discipline*. Minneapolis: Fortress Press, 1995.

Carrette, Jeremy R., and Richard King. *Capitalist Spirituality: The Silent Takeover of Religion*. London: Routledge, 2004.

Chambron, Jacqueline. *Lilian Silburn: Une vie mystique*. Paris: Almora, 2015.

Charlesworth, James H. *The Good and Evil Serpent: How a Universal Symbol Became Christianized*. New Haven, CT: Yale University Press, 2010.

Cooper, David J., Jared R. Lindahl, Roman Palitsky, and Willoughby B. Britton. "'Like a Vibration Cascading Through the Body': Energy-Like Somatic Experiences Reported by Western Buddhist Meditators." *Religions* 12, no. 12 (December 2021). https://doi.org/10.3390/rel12121042.

Coward, Harold. *Jung and Eastern Thought*. Albany: State University of New York Press, 1985.

Cox, Harvey. *Turning East: The Promise and Peril of the New Orientalism*. New York: Simon and Schuster, 1977.

Cox, Simon Paul. *The Subtle Body: A Genealogy*. New York: Oxford University Press, 2022.

Craddock, Ida. *Sexual Outlaw, Erotic Mystic: The Essential Ida Craddock*. Ed. Vere Chappell. San Francisco: Weiser Books, 2010.

Czyżykowski, Robert. "The Problem of Kuṇḍalinī in the Context of Yogic Aspects of the Bengali Tantric Vaiṣṇava (Sahajiyā) Tradition." *Religions of South Asia* 12, no. 2 (2018): 185–206.

Da Avabhasa. *The Knee of Listening*. Clearlake, CA: The Dawn Horse Press, 1992.

Darnton, Robert. *Mesmerism and the End of the Enlightenment in France*. Cambridge, MA: Harvard University Press, 1968.

Davidson, Ronald M. *Indian Esoteric Buddhism: Social History of the Tantric Movement*. Delhi: Motilal Banarsidass, 2004.

De Michelis, Elizabeth. *A History of Modern Yoga: Patañjali and Western Esotericism*. London: Continuum, 2004.

DeConick, April D. *The Gnostic New Age: How a Countercultural Spirituality Revolutionized Religion from Antiquity to Today*. New York: Columbia University Press, 2016.

——. "The Road for the Souls Is Through the Planets: The Mysteries of the Ophians Mapped." In *Practicing Gnosis: Ritual, Magic, Theurgy and Liturgy in Nag Hammadi, Manichaean and Other Ancient Literature; Essays in Honor of*

Birger A. Pearson, ed. April D. DeConick, Gregory Shaw, and John D. Turner, 37–74. Leiden, the Netherlands: Brill, 2013.

Degler, Teri. *Gopi Krishna: A Biography; Kundalini, Consciousness, and Our Evolution to Enlightenment*. Markdale, Canada: Institute for Consciousness Research, 2023.

Desai, Yogi Amrit. *Kripalu Yoga: Meditation-in-Motion*. Lenox, MA: Kripalu Publications, 1985.

Deslippe, Philip. "From Maharaj to Mahan Tantric: The Construction of Yogi Bhajan's Kundalini Yoga." *Sikh Formations* 8, no. 3 (December 2012): 369–87.

Dodds, E. R. *Stoicheiosis Theologike: The Elements of Theology*. Oxford: Clarendon Press, 1963.

Douglas, Martin. "Yogi Bhajan, 75, 'Boss' of Worlds Spiritual and Capitalistic, Dies." *The New York Times*, October 9, 2004. https://www.nytimes.com/2004/10/09/us/yogi-bhajan-75-boss-of-worlds-spiritual-and-capitalistic-dies.html.

The Dream of Ravan: A Mystery. London: The Theosophical Publishing Society, 1895.

Edmonds, Radcliffe G. "Did the Mithraists Inhale?" *Ancient World* 32, no. 1 (2001): 10–24.

Elsberg, Constance Waeber. *Graceful Women: Gender and Identity in an American Sikh Community*. Knoxville: The University of Tennessee Press, 2003.

Esalen Institute. "Seminars at Big Sur Hot Springs and Redwood Lodge." Winter/Spring 1965.

Fanger, Claire. "Introduction." In *Invoking Angels: Theurgic Ideas and Practices, Thirteenth to Sixteenth Centuries*, ed. Claire Fanger, 1–36. University Park: Pennsylvania State University Press, 2015.

Finamore, John F. *Iamblichus and the Theory of the Vehicle of the Soul*. Chico, CA: Scholars Press, 1985.

Flood, Gavin D. *The Tantric Body: The Secret Tradition of Hindu Religion*. London: I. B. Tauris, 2006.

Forsthoefel, Thomas A., and Cynthia Ann Humes, eds. *Gurus in America*. Albany: State University of New York Press, 2005.

Foxen, Anya. *Biography of a Yogi: Paramahansa Yogananda and the Origins of Modern Yoga*. New York: Oxford University Press, 2017.

——. *Inhaling Spirit: Harmonialism, Orientalism, and the Western Roots of Modern Yoga*. New York: Oxford University Press, 2020.

Foxen, Anya, and Christa Kuberry. *Is This Yoga? Concepts, Histories, and the Complexities of Modern Practice*. New York: Routledge, 2021.

French, Brendan. "The Mercurian Master: Hermes' Gift to the Theosophical Society." *Aries* 1, no. 2 (January 2001): 168–205.

Funes Maderey, Ana Laura. "Kuṇḍalinī Rising and Liberation in the Yogavāsiṣṭha: The Story of Cūḍālā and Śikhidhvaja." *Religions* 8, no. 11 (November 2017): 248.

Gill, Christopher. "Galen and the Stoics: Mortal Enemies or Blood Brothers?" *Phronesis: A Journal for Ancient Philosophy* 52, no. 1 (January 2007): 88–120.

Gleig, Ann, and Charles I. Flores. "Remembering Sri Aurobindo and the Mother: The Forgotten Lineage of Integral Yoga." In *Gurus of Modern Yoga*, ed. Mark Singleton and Ellen Goldberg, 38–59. New York: Oxford University Press, 2014.

Gleig, Ann, and Lola Williamson, eds. *Homegrown Gurus: From Hinduism in America to American Hinduism*. Albany: State University of New York Press, 2014.

Gold, Daniel. *The Lord as Guru: Hindi Sants in North Indian Tradition*. New York: Oxford University Press, 1987.

Goldberg, Ellen. "Amrit Desai and the Kripalu Center for Yoga and Health." In *Homegrown Gurus: From Hinduism in America to American Hinduism*, ed. Ann Gleig and Lola Williamson, 63–86. Albany: State University of New York Press, 2014.

——. "Swami Kṛpālvānanda: The Man behind Kripalu Yoga." In *Gurus of Modern Yoga*, ed. Mark Singleton and Ellen Goldberg, 171–89. New York: Oxford University Press, 2014.

Goodrick-Clarke, Nicholas. "The Esoteric Uses of Electricity: Theologies of Electricity from Swabian Pietism to Ariosophy." *Aries* 4, no. 1 (January 2004): 69–90.

Grof, Stanislav, and Christina Grof, eds. *Spiritual Emergency: When Personal Transformation Becomes a Crisis*. Los Angeles: Jeremy P. Tarcher, 1989.

Gross, Charles G. "Aristotle on the Brain." *The Neuroscientist* 1, no. 4 (July 1995): 245–50.

Haage, Bernard D. "Alchemy II: Antiquity–12th Century." In *Dictionary of Gnosis & Western Esotericism*, ed. Wouter J. Hanegraaff, Antoine Faivre, Roelof Van den Broek, and Jean-Pierre Brach, 16–34. Leiden, the Netherlands: Brill, 2006.

Hanegraaff, Wouter J. *Esotericism and the Academy: Rejected Knowledge in Western Culture*. Cambridge, UK: Cambridge University Press, 2012.

Heehs, Peter. *The Lives of Sri Aurobindo*. New York: Columbia University Press, 2008.

Homer. *The Odyssey*. Trans. Emily R. Wilson. New York: Norton, 2020.

Iyengar, B. K. S. *Light on Prāṇāyāma: Prāṇāyāma Dīpikā*. London: Unwin Paperbacks, 1983.

——. *Light on the Yoga Sūtras of Patañjali*. London: Thorsons, 2002.

——. *Light on Yoga: Yoga Dipika*. New York: Schocken Books, 1979.

Jain, Andrea R. "Muktananda: Entrepreneurial Godman, Tantric Hero." In *Gurus of Modern Yoga*, ed. Mark Singleton and Ellen Goldberg, 190–209. New York: Oxford University Press, 2014.

——. *Selling Yoga: From Counterculture to Pop Culture*. New York: Oxford University Press, 2014.

Jakobsh, Doris. "3HO/Sikh Dharma of the Western Hemisphere: The 'Forgotten' New Religious Movement?" *Religion Compass* 2, no. 3 (May 2008): 385–408.

Johnson, Sarah Iles. "Rising to the Occasion: Theurgic Ascent in Its Cultural Milieu." In *Envisioning Magic: A Princeton Seminar and Symposium*, ed. Peter Schäfer and Hans Kippenberg, 165–94. Leiden, the Netherlands: Brill, 1997.

Jung, C. G. "Lecture IX, 11 December 1935." In *Nietzsche's* Zarathustra*: Notes of the Seminar Given in 1934–1939*, ed. James L. Jarrett, 748–64. Princeton, NJ: Princeton University Press, 1988.

——. *The Psychology of Kundalini Yoga: Notes of the Seminar Given in 1932*. Ed. Sonu Shamdasani. Princeton, NJ: Princeton University Press, 1996.

——. *The Red Book: Liber Novus*. Ed. Sonu Shamdasani. Trans. Mark Kyburz, John Peck, and Sonu Shamdasani. New York: Norton and Company, 2009.

——. "Yoga and the West." In *Psychology and the East*, trans. R. F. C. Hull, 77–86. Princeton, NJ: Princeton University Press, 1978.

Kachroo, Meera Jo. "Śrīvidyā's Rahasya: Public Esotericism in a Contemporary Tantric Tradition." PhD diss., McGill University, 2022.

Kaelber, Walter O. *Tapta Mārga: Asceticism and Initiation in Vedic India*. Albany: State University of New York Press, 1989.

Khalsa, Gurucharan Singh, and Yogi Bhajan. "Exploring the Myths and Misconceptions of Kundalini." In *Kundalini: Evolution and Enlightenment*, ed. John White, 132–48. New York: Paragon House, 1979.

Khalsa, Harbhajan Singh. *The Teachings of Yogi Bhajan*. New York: Hawthorn Books, Inc., 1977.

Khalsa, Sat Bir Singh. "Treatment of Chronic Primary Sleep Onset Insomnia with Kundalini Yoga: A Randomized Controlled Trial with Active Sleep Hygiene Comparison." *Journal of Clinical Sleep Medicine* 17, no. 9 (September 2021): 1841–52.

Kiehnle, Catharina. "The Secret of the Nāths: The Ascent of Kuṇḍalinī According to Jñāneśvari 6.151–328." *Bulletin Des Études Indiennes* 22–23 (2004–2005).

——. *Songs on Yoga Texts and Teachings of the Mahārāṣṭrian Nāths*. Stuttgart, Germany: Franz Steiner Verlag Stuttgart, 1997.

Kripal, Jeffrey J. *Esalen: America and the Religion of No Religion*. Chicago: The University of Chicago Press, 2007.

——. "Riding the Dawn Horse: Adi Da and the Eros of Nonduality." In *Gurus in America*, ed. Thomas A. Forsthoefel and Cynthia Ann Humes, 193–218. Albany: State University of New York Press, 2005.

——. *The Serpent's Gift: Gnostic Reflections on the Study of Religion*. Chicago: The University of Chicago Press, 2007.

——. *The Superhumanities: Historical Precedents, Moral Objections, New Realities*. Chicago: The University of Chicago Press, 2022.

Krishna, Gopi. *The Biological Basis of Religion and Genius*. New York: Harper & Row, 1972.

——. *Kundalini for the New Age: Selected Writings*. Ed. Gene Kieffer. Toronto: Bantam Books, 1988.

——. *Kundalini: The Evolutionary Energy in Man*. New Delhi: Ramadhar and Hopman, 1967.

——. *Yoga: A Vision of Its Future*. New Delhi: Kundalini Research and Publication Trust, 1978.

Kuchuk, Nika. "Genealogies of Transnational Religion: Translation, Revelation, and Discursive Technologies in Two Female Gurus of Esoteric Vedanta." PhD diss., University of Toronto, 2021.

Kuvalayananda, Srimat. "Kapālabhāti." *Yoga-Mīmānsa* 4, no. 2 (1930): 161–78.

——. *Popular Yoga: Prâṇâyâma*. Bombay, India: Kaivalyadhama, 1931.

——. "Prāṇāyāma." *Yoga-Mīmānsa* 3, no. 1 (1928): 258–74.

——. "Preparing Oneself for Āsanas." *Yoga-Mīmānsa* 4, no. 3 (1933): 221–31.

——. "Pressure Experiments in Prāṇāyāma." *Yoga-Mīmānsa* 4, no. 1 (1930): 9–46.

——. "Scientific Survey of Cultural Poses." *Yoga-Mīmānsa* 4, no. 3 (1933): 232–46.

Lange, Gerrit. "Cobra Deities and Divine Cobras: The Ambiguous Animality of Nāgas." *Religions* 10, no. 8 (August 2019).

Leadbeater, C. W. *The Chakras*. Wheaton, IL: Theosophical Publishing House, 1927.

——. *Clairvoyance*. London: The Theosophical Publishing Society, 1899.

——. *The Inner Life*. Adyar, India: Theosophical Publishing House, 1917.

Leland, Kurt. *Rainbow Body: A History of the Western Chakra System from Blavatsky to Brennan*. Lake Worth, FL: Ibis Press, 2016.

Lesses, Rebecca. "Image and Word: Performative Ritual and Material Culture in the Aramaic Incantation Bowls." In *Practicing Gnosis: Ritual, Magic, Theurgy and Liturgy in Nag Hammadi, Manichaean and Other Ancient Literature; Essays in Honor of Birger A. Pearson*, ed. April D. DeConick, Gregory Shaw, and John D. Turner, 377–408. Leiden, the Netherlands: Brill, 2013.

Lindahl, Jared R. "Somatic Energies and Emotional Traumas: A Qualitative Study of Practice-Related Challenges Reported by Vajrayāna Buddhists." *Religions* 8, no. 8 (August 2017). https://doi.org/10.3390/rel8080153.

Love, Robert. *The Great Oom: The Improbable Birth of Yoga in America*. New York: Viking, 2010.

Lucia, Amanda. "Guru Sex: Charisma, Proxemic Desire, and the Haptic Logics of the Guru-Disciple Relationship." *Journal of the American Academy of Religion* 86, no. 4 (December 2018): 953–88.

Majercik, Ruth, ed. *The Chaldean Oracles: Text, Translation, and Commentary*. Trans. Ruth Majercik. Leiden, the Netherlands: Brill, 1989.

Mallinson, James. "Hathayoga's Philosophy: A Fortuitous Union of Non-Dualities." *Journal of Indian Philosophy* 42, no. 1 (March 2014): 225–47.

——. "Yoga and Yogis." *Nāmarūpa* 3, no. 15 (March 2012): 1–27.

Mallinson, James, and Mark Singleton. *Roots of Yoga: A Sourcebook from the Indic Traditions*. London: Penguin Classics, 2017.

Maxwell, Richard W., and Sucharit Katyal. "Characteristics of Kundalini-Related Sensory, Motor, and Affective Experiences During Tantric Yoga Meditation." *Frontiers in Psychology* 13 (June 2022). https://www.frontiersin.org/articles/10.3389/fpsyg.2022.863091.

McDermott, Robert. "A Brief History of California Institute of Integral Studies." California Institute of Integral Studies, November 17, 2017. https://www.ciis.edu/discover-ciis/our-history.

Miller, Christopher Jain. *Embodying Transnational Yoga: Eating, Singing, and Breathing in Context*. London: Routledge, forthcoming.

Muktananda, Swami. *Kundalini: The Secret of Life*. Fallsburg, NY: SYDA Foundation, 1994.

——. *Play of Consciousness*. San Francisco: Harper & Row, 1974.

Muller-Ortega, Paul Eduardo. *The Triadic Heart of Śiva: Kaula Tantricism of Abhinavagupta in the Non-Dual Shaivism of Kashmir*. Albany: State University of New York Press, 1997.

Ogden, Daniel. *Drakon: Dragon Myth and Serpent Cult in the Greek and Roman Worlds*. Oxford: Oxford University Press, 2013.

Okropiridze, Dimitry. "'East' and 'West' in the Kaleidoscope of Transculturality—The Discursive Production of the Kuṇḍalinī as a New Ontological Object Within and Beyond Orientalist Dichotomies." In *Eastspirit: Transnational Spirituality and Religious Circulation in East and West*, ed. Jørn Borup and Marianne Qvortrup Fibiger, 120–45. Leiden, the Netherlands: Brill, 2017.

Olivelle, Patrick. *The Early Upaniṣads: Annotated Text and Translation*. New York: Oxford University Press, 1998.

OSHO. "OSHO Dynamic Meditation." OSHO International Foundation. Accessed July 21, 2023. https://www.osho.com/meditation/osho-active-meditations/osho-dynamic-meditation.

Padoux, André. *Vāc: The Concept of the Word in Selected Hindu Tantras*. Trans. Jacques Gontier. Albany: State University of New York Press, 1989.

Principe, Lawrence. *The Secrets of Alchemy*. Chicago: University of Chicago Press, 2013.

Pryse, James Morgan. *The Apocalypse Unsealed: Being an Esoteric Interpretation of the Initiation of Iôannês Commonly Called the Revelation of St. John, with a New Translation*. Los Angeles: J. M. Pryse, 1910.

——. "An Important Statement by Mr. J. M. Pryse." *The Canadian Theosophist* 7, no. 6 (1926): 140–41.

——. "Memorabilia of H.P.B." *The Canadian Theosophist* 16, no. 1 (1935): 1–5.

Quijada, Danielle. "Ariz. Temple Leader Sentenced on Prostitution Charges." *USA Today*, May 19, 2016. https://www.usatoday.com/story/news/nation-now/2016/05/19/ariz-temple-leader-sentenced-prostitution-charges/84623744/.

Rajneesh, Bhagwan Shree. *Meditation: The Art of Ecstasy*. New York: Harper & Row, 1978.

——. *The Orange Book*. Rajneeshpuram, OR: Rajneesh Foundation International, 1983.

Rasimus, Tuomas. "Ophite Gnosticism, Sethianism and the Nag Hammadi Library." *Vigiliae Christianae* 59, no. 3 (January 2005): 235–63.

——. *Paradise Reconsidered in Gnostic Mythmaking: Rethinking Sethianism in Light of the Ophite Myth and Ritual*. Leiden, the Netherlands: Brill, 2009.

——. "The Serpent in Gnostic and Related Texts." In *L'Évangile selon Thomas et les textes de Nag Hammadi: Québec, 29–31 mai 2003*, ed. Louis Painchaud and

Paul-Hubert Poirier, 417–72. Québec, Canada: Presses de l'Université Laval, 2007.

Rele, Vasant G. *The Mysterious Kundalini.* Bombay, India: D. B. Taraporevala Sons & Co., 1931.

Riedweg, Christoph. *Pythagoras: His Life, Teaching, and Influence.* Trans. Steven Rendall and Andreas Schatzmann. Ithaca, NY: Cornell University Press, 2005.

Rist, John M. "On Greek Biology, Greek Cosmology and Some Sources of Theological Pneuma." In *Man, Soul, and Body: Essays in Ancient Thought from Plato to Dionysius*, ed. D. W. Dockrill and R. G. Tanner, 27–47. Auckland, New Zealand: University of Auckland, 1985.

Rosenman, Ellen Bayuk. *Unauthorized Pleasures: Accounts of Victorian Erotic Experience.* Ithaca, NY: Cornell University Press, 2003.

Rossman, Randi. "Lee Sherman Sannella." *The Press Democrat*, March 22, 2010. https://www.pressdemocrat.com/article/news/lee-sherman-sannella/.

Row, T. Subba. "The Twelve Signs of the Zodiac." In *Five Years of Theosophy*, 103–18. London: Reever and Turner, 1885.

Ruff, Jeffrey Clark. "Yoga in the Yoga Upaniṣads: Disciplines of the Mystical OṂ Sound." In *Yoga in Practice*, ed. David Gordon White, 97–116. Princeton, NJ: Princeton University Press, 2012.

Russell, Dick. *The Life and Ideas of James Hillman: Volume I; The Making of a Psychologist.* New York: Helios Press, 2013.

Sanches, Laura, and Michael Daniels. "Kundalini and Transpersonal Development: Development of a Kundalini Awakening Scale and a Comparison Between Groups." *Transpersonal Psychology Review* 12, no. 1 (January 2008): 73–83.

Sanderson, Alexis. "The Śaiva Age: The Rise and Dominance of Śaivism During the Early Medieval Period." In *Genesis and Development of Tantrism*, ed. Shingo Einoo, 41–350. Tokyo: Institute of Oriental Culture, University of Tokyo, 2009.

Sannella, Lee. *The Kundalini Experience: Psychosis or Transcendence?* Lower Lake, CA: Integral Publishing, 1987.

——. *Kundalini: Psychosis or Transcendence?* San Francisco: H. S. Dakin Company, 1976.

Satyeswarananda Giri, Swami. *Kriya: Finding the True Path.* San Diego, CA: Sanskrit Classics, 1991.

Schmidt, Leigh Eric. *Heaven's Bride: The Unprintable Life of Ida C. Craddock; American Mystic, Scholar, Sexologist, Martyr, and Madwoman*. New York: Basic Books, 2010.

Schwartz, Jason. "Parabrahman Among the Yogins." *International Journal of Hindu Studies* 21, no. 3 (December 2017): 345–89.

Scott, Mary. *The Kundalini Concept: Its Origin and Value* (Fremont, CA: Jain Publishing, 2006).

——. *Kundalini in the Physical World*. London: Routledge & Kegan Paul, 1983.

Shamdasani, Sonu. "Introduction: Jung's Journey to the East." In *The Psychology of Kundalini Yoga: Notes of the Seminar Given in 1932*, ed. Sonu Shamdasani, xvii–xlvi. Princeton, NJ: Princeton University Press, 1996.

Shaw, Gregory. "Theurgy and the Platonist's Luminous Body." In *Practicing Gnosis: Ritual, Magic, Theurgy and Liturgy in Nag Hammadi, Manichaean and Other Ancient Literature; Essays in Honor of Birger A. Pearson*, ed. April D. DeConick, Gregory Shaw, and John D. Turner, 537–58. Leiden, the Netherlands: Brill, 2013.

——. *Theurgy and the Soul: The Neoplatonism of Iamblichus*. University Park: Pennsylvania State University Press, 1995.

Silburn, Lilian. *Kuṇḍalinī: The Energy of the Depths; A Comprehensive Study Based on the Scriptures of Nondualistic Kashmir Shaivism*. Trans. Jacques Gontier. Albany: State University of New York Press, 1988.

Singleton, Mark. *Yoga Body: The Origins of Modern Posture Practice*. New York: Oxford University Press, 2010.

Singleton, Mark, and Tara Fraser. "T. Krishnamacharya, Father of Modern Yoga." In *Gurus of Modern Yoga*, ed. Mark Singleton and Ellen Goldberg, 83–106. New York: Oxford University Press, 2014.

Siorvanes, Lucas. *Proclus: Neo-Platonic Philosophy and Science*. Edinburgh: Edinburgh University Press, 1996.

Sivananda, Swami. *Kundalini Yoga*. Shivanandanagar, India: The Divine Life Society, 1994.

——. *Yogic Home Exercises: Easy Course of Physical Culture for Modern Men and Women*. Bombay, India: D. B. Taraporevala Son and Co., 1939.

Sivananda Radha, Swami. *Hatha Yoga: The Hidden Language; Symbols, Secrets, and Metaphor*. Boston: Shambhala, 1987.

——. "Kundalini: An Overview." In *Kundalini: Evolution and Enlightenment*, ed. John White, 49–60. New York: Paragon House, 1979.

——. *Kundalini Yoga*. Delhi: Motilal Banarsidass, 2011.

——. *Kundalini: Yoga for the West*. Spokane, WA: Timeless Books, 1978.

Sivananda Saraswathi, Swami. *Kundalini Yoga: Illustrated*. Madras, India: P. K. Vinayagam, 1935.

Smith, Frederick M., and Joan White. "Becoming an Icon: B. K. S. Iyengar as a Yoga Teacher and a Yoga Guru." In *Gurus of Modern Yoga*, ed. Mark Singleton and Ellen Goldberg, 122–46. New York: Oxford University Press, 2014.

Smith, Jonathan Z. "In Comparison a Magic Dwells." In *Imagining Religion: From Babylon to Jonestown*, ed. Jonathan Z. Smith, 19–35. Chicago: Chicago University Press, 1982.

Steiner, Rudolf. *Kundalini: Spiritual Perception and the Higher Element of Life*. Ed. Andreas Meyer. Forest Row, UK: Rudolf Steiner Press, 2019.

Strube, Julian. *Global Tantra: Religion, Science, and Nationalism in Colonial Modernity*. New York: Oxford University Press, 2022.

Taves, Ann, and Egil Asprem. "Experience as Event: Event Cognition and the Study of (Religious) Experiences." *Religion, Brain & Behavior* 7, no. 1 (2017): 43–62.

Taylor, Kathleen. *Sir John Woodroffe, Tantra and Bengal: "An Indian Soul in a European Body?"* London: Routledge, 2001.

Taylor, Steve. "Energy and Awakening: A Psycho-Sexual Interpretation of Kundalini Awakening." *The Journal of Transpersonal Psychology* 47, no. 2 (2015): 219–41.

Thaler, Marleen. "Approaching a Universal Pattern? Gopi Krishna's Transformational Kuṇḍalinī Experience Within the Frame of Universalism and Religious Scientism." In *Intentional Transformative Experiences*, ed. Sarah Perez, Jens Schlieter, and Bastiaan Vanrijn. Berlin: De Gruyter, forthcoming.

——. "Gaia's Energy Flows: The Interplay of Eco-Spirituality and Terrestrial Energy Healing." In *Subtle Energies in Therapy, Spirituality, Arts, and Politics, 1800–Present*, ed. Julian Strube, Marleen Thaler, and Dominic Zoehrer. Leiden, the Netherlands: Brill, forthcoming.

——. "The Rising Serpent at Esalen." Esalen, Esalen Institute and Esalen Theory & Research, May 24, 2023. https://www.esalen.org/post/the-rising-serpent-at-esalen-052323.

Thursby, Gene R. "Hindu Movements Since Mid-Century: Yogis in the States." In *America's Alternative Religions*, ed. Timothy Miller, 191–214. Albany: State University of New York Press, 1995.

Urban, Hugh B. "Osho, from Sex Guru to Guru of the Rich: The Spiritual Logic of Late Capitalism." In *Gurus in America*, ed. Thomas A. Forsthoefel and Cynthia Ann Humes, 169–92. Albany: State University of New York Press, 2005.

——. *Tantra: Sex, Secrecy, Politics, and Power in the Study of Religion*. Berkeley: University of California Press, 2003.

——. *Zorba the Buddha: Sex, Spirituality, and Capitalism in the Global Osho Movement*. Oakland: University of California Press, 2016.

Van den Broek, Roelof. "Gnosticism and Hermetism in Antiquity: Two Roads to Salvation." In *Gnosis and Hermeticism from Antiquity to Modern Times*, ed. Roelof Van den Broek and Wouter J. Hanegraaff, 1–20. Albany: State University of New York Press, 1998.

——. "Hermes Trismegistus I: Antiquity." In *Dictionary of Gnosis & Western Esotericism*, ed. Wouter J. Hanegraaff, Antoine Faivre, Roelof Van den Broek, and Jean-Pierre Brach, 474–78. Leiden, the Netherlands: Brill, 2006.

——. "Hermetic Literature I: Antiquity." In *Dictionary of Gnosis & Western Esotericism*, ed. Wouter J. Hanegraaff, Antoine Faivre, Roelof Van den Broek, and Jean-Pierre Brach, 487–99. Leiden, the Netherlands: Brill, 2006.

——. "Hermetism." In *Dictionary of Gnosis & Western Esotericism*, ed. Wouter J. Hanegraaff, Antoine Faivre, Roelof Van den Broek, and Jean-Pierre Brach, 558–70. Leiden, the Netherlands: Brill, 2006.

Vasudeva, Somadeva. *The Yoga of the Mālinīvijayottaratantra: Chapters 1–4, 7, 11–17*. Pondicherry, India: Institut français de Pondichéry, Ecole française d'Extrême-Orient, 2004.

Versluis, Arthur. *Wisdom's Children: A Christian Esoteric Tradition*. Albany: State University of New York Press, 1999.

Vivekananda, Swami. *The Complete Works of Swami Vivekananda*. Vol. 1. Calcutta, India: Advaita Ashrama, 1915.

Wallis, Christopher D. "The Descent of Power: Possession, Mysticism, and Initiation in the Śaiva Theology of Abhinavagupta." *Journal of Indian Philosophy* 36, no. 2 (April 2008): 247–95.

——. "The Real Story on Kundalini," January 31, 2021. https://hareesh.org/blog/2022/1/31/the-real-story-on-kundalini.

White, David Gordon. *The Alchemical Body: Siddha Traditions in Medieval India*. Chicago: Chicago University Press, 1996.

——. *Daemons Are Forever: Contacts and Exchanges in the Eurasian Pandemonium*. Chicago: Chicago University Press, 2021.

——. *The Kiss of the Yoginī: "Tantric Sex" in Its South Asian Contexts*. Chicago: University of Chicago Press, 2002.

——. *Sinister Yogis*. Chicago: University of Chicago Press, 2009.

——, ed. *Tantra in Practice*. Princeton, NJ: Princeton University Press, 2000.

——. *The Yoga Sutra of Patanjali: A Biography*. Princeton, NJ: Princeton University Press, 2014.

White, John, ed. *Kundalini: Evolution and Enlightenment*. New York: Paragon House, 1979.

Williamson, Lola. "The Perfectibility of Perfection: Siddha Yoga as a Global Movement." In *Gurus in America*, ed. Thomas A. Forsthoefel and Cynthia Ann Humes, 147–67. Albany: State University of New York Press, 2005.

Wood, Linda Sargent. *A More Perfect Union: Holistic Worldviews and the Transformation of American Culture After World War II*. New York: Oxford University Press, 2010.

Wrisberg, Heinrich August. *Observationum anatomicarum de nervis viscerum abdominalium*. Göttingen, Germany: Ioann Christian Dietrich, 1780.

Yogananda, Paramahansa. *Autobiography of a Yogi*. Nevada City, CA: Crystal Clarity Publishers, 1995.

——. "Awakening of Kundalini, or Serpent Force." *Yogoda Sat-Sanga Fortnightly Instructions*, n.d.

——. *The Second Coming of Christ: The Resurrection of the Christ Within You; A Revelatory Commentary on the Original Teachings of Jesus*. Los Angeles: Self-Realization Fellowship, 2008.

Zweig, Paul. "Shaktipat." In *Kundalini: Evolution and Enlightenment*, ed. John White, 172–83. New York: Paragon House, 1979.

INDEX

3HO (Healthy, Happy, Holy Organization), 216, 218, 220–21, 288, 295

Abhinavagupta, 47–48, 152, 233
Adam and Eve, 5, 59–60, 152, 270
Adi Da, 25, 253–55, 272, 282
Africa, 55–56
alchemy, 21, 97, 101, 339n19, 359n78; as symbolism, 10–11, 327n7; South Asian, 40, 44; European, 69–72; and Gichtel, 76; and Jung, 107; Hillman's use of, 198
amṛta, 33, 35, 46, 49, 133, 162, 261, 316
anima, 63, 78; in Aristotle, 62; as used by Jung, 107, 110, 198, 341n68
apāna, 51–52
Aristotle, 60, 61, 62–64, 333n12
Arundale, George Sydney, 89, 90, 91, 117, 281; on Kuṇḍalinī, 102–104; and danger of Kuṇḍalinī, 264–65; and sex, 271
āsana, 51, 136, 148, 229, 321; in Kuvalayananda, 137, 139–40; in Sivananda, 142; in Iyengar, 144–45; and Desai, 230, 231, 243
ascent, 56, 252; of the soul, 21–22, 61, 72, 80; in South Asian sources, 30–31, 36–37, 38, 39, 46; of Kuṇḍalinī, 47, 48–49, 125, 131, 191, 261, 327n5; theurgic, 56, 64–66, 70334n17; in Plato, 58; in Gichtel, 76; in Theosophy, 86, 89, 94, 96, 99–101, 106, 339n25; in Yogananda, 153, 155; in Aurobindo, 158–159, 16, in Bentov, 257; in Sannella, 260
asceticism, 47, 161, 190, 272, 342n83; and *tapas*, 35–36, 64, 146; and *haṭha* yoga 41, 49, 122–23, 139, 241n66
Asclepius, 21, 67–69, 72, 80
Assam, 13–14, 285, ethnography in, 301, 303–320

astral, 109, 116, 164; body, 63–64, 99, 135, 155, 156, 241; realm, 64, 74, 76, 91
astrology, 44, 62, 65, 69, 70, 78, 85, 164
ātman, 36, 38, 313, 317
Aurobindo, Sri. *See* Ghose, Aurobindo
authenticity, 5, 8–9, 11, 21, 22, 31, 168, 273, 299; and Avalon, 114, 115, 117, and Vivekananda, 124–25, and gurus, 207, 214; and Osho, 237, 240–42, 254
Avalon, Arthur, 22, 24, 47, 82, 94, 112–19, 191; referred to by others, 97, 110, 13, 144, 218, 248, 252, 280–81, 282, 341n66

Baier, Karl, 80, 87, 327n5
bandha, 41, 122, 133, 141, 145, 152, 229, 266, 321–23; *mūla-bandha*, 51, 52, 321–22; *jālaṅdhara-bandha*, 52, 265, 321–22
Bengal, 56, 112–13, 147, 150, 329n3, 343n83
Bentov, Itzhak, 256–60, 267, 281, 288, 290
Bernard, Pierre Arnold, 270–71, 272
Besant, Annie, 88, 102
Bhagavad Gītā, 50, 87
Bhajan, Yogi, 4, 24, 147, 210, 213–21, 224, 234, 243–44, 251, 265–66, 272, 280, 288, 295, 300
bindu. *See* semen
Blavatsky, Helena Petrova, 84–89, 264, 340n41; influence on others, 18, 91, 94, 98, 102, 255, 339n19
blockage, 56; Kuṇḍalinī as, 30, 46, 119, 143; Kuṇḍalinī clearing, 242, 243, 268
brain, 164, 202, 256, 275; abdominal, 1, 78, 79; as control center, 63; and Kuṇḍalinī, 96–97, 125, 139, 152, 220, 249, 254, 265; and collective unconscious, 106–107, and prāṇāyāma, 141, 145; Gopi Krishna's experience, 177, 179, 180, 181, 186–88, 193, 195, 196, 200
breath, 17, 59, 86, 202, 312; in Upaniṣads, 37; and *haṭha* yoga, 42; and Kuṇḍalinī, 45–46, 50, 51, 53, 259, 321–22; and pneumatic ascent, 63–65, 67, 88; in Swedenborg, 77, 78; in Vivekananda, 125–26, 128; in Gopi Krishna's experience, 173, 175, 184; in Yogi Bhajan, 217, 244; in Desai, 233, 234; in Osho, 238, 239, 244. *See also prāṇāyāma*
Buddhism, 7, 20, 30, 31, 86, 213, 275, 290–92; and *layayoga*, 48–49, 152

caduceus, 42, 299; and Hermes, 68, 69, 80; and alchemy, 70, 72; and Theosophy, 82, 101–102, 103, 107, 280
cakra, 11, 16, 22, 80, 121, 122, 145, 147, 236, 242, 252, 298, 299; Kuṇḍalinī rising through, 2, 48–49, 159, 248, 260, 268, 274, 316–17, 322; in pre-modern

sources, 39–40, 42, 45, 46–48, 51, 66, 115, 329n3, 337n6, 348n83; Theosophical models of, 92, 94, 99–100, 102, 338n16; in Jung, 110, 111; in Avalon, 115, 116–17, 118–19; as nerve plexuses, 127, 132–33, 118, 138, 344n13; in Gopi Krishna, 192–93, 194; *mūlādhāra*, 46–47, 50–51, 110, 117, 128, 152, 193, 236, 289, 313–14; *sahasrāra*, 115, 133, 314, 317
Campbell, Joseph, 218, 253, 277
caṇḍalī, 20, 30, 48, 49, 152
Chakras, The (1927), 73, 98–99, 101
Chaldean Oracles, 64, 334n17
Chaldea, 62, 84
channel. *See nāḍī*
Charlesworth, James H., 67
Chidvilasananda, Gurumayi, 210
Christ, Jesus, 59, 60, 76, 90, 108, 150
Christianity, 5, 58, 69, 90, 94, 98, 113, 249; mysticism, 21, 250, 262; and the serpent, 57; Yogananda and, 150, 151, 152
Chrysopoeia of Cleopatra, 71
coil: Kuṇḍalinī as 1, 2, 3, 20, 44, 45, 46, 48, 52, 93, 104, 128, 130, 132, 135, 139, 146, 153, 159, 190, 248, 249, 313; as *speirēma*, 92–93, 96; of hair in Yogi Bhajan, 219, 220; serpents and, 32, 67, 71, 73, 97, 99
colonialism, 3, 8, 56, 83–85, 123, 211, 271
Craddock, Ida C., 270, 272, 294
crisis: in Mesmerism, 78–79; in Gopi Krishna's experience, 176–79, 181, 187; in Osho, 239–40; as spiritual emergency, 263–69, 276
Comte de Gabalis, The, 97, 98

daimon, 65, 68, 72
De Michelis, Elizabeth, 144, 147
DeConick, April, 65
Degler, Teri, 166
Desai, Amrit, 208, 210, 218, 230–34, 243, 244, 251, 272
Deslippe, Philip, 214
Devi, Indra, 97
dhātu, 34, 49, 52
Dhirendra Brahmachari, Swami, 215
dhyana. See meditation
dīkṣā. See initiation
Divine Life Society, 141–42, 295
dragon, 1, 19, 72, 279
Dream of Ravan, The, 87–88
Dvivedi, Manilal N., 85
Dynamic Meditation, 236, 241, 244

earth, 1, 35, 37, 73, 96, 108, 160; as element, 49, 314; as planetary sphere, 58, 61; and serpents, 67, 68, 108; and Kuṇḍalinī as fire inside, 100–101, 102–103, 280, 340n41
Egypt, 65, 68–69, 71, 84, 101, 334n17
electricity, 299; in Theosophy, 85, 87–88, 89, 92, 337n6; in Vivekananda, 127, 128
energy-like somatic experiences (ELSEs), 290–93
Esalen Institute, 204, 269, 274–79

ether, 78, 88, 314; as ethereal body or realm, 63, 64, 74, 99, 135, 187; as etheric body in Osho, 241–43
evolution, 1, 3, 131, 220, 245, 248, 250, 254, 256, 269, 290; in Theosophy, 99, 100; in Vivekananda, 148–49; in Yogananda, 154–56; in Aurobindo, 160–62; in Gopi Krishna, 23, 164, 165, 170, 194–96, 199, 200, 201; at Esalen, 275, 276, 278, 282

feminine. *See* gender
fire, 3, 147, 217, 312, 314; as symbol, 21, 33, 34–37, 44, 48, 66, 109, 299; digestive, 11, 21, 34–35, 42, 45, 50; in the earth, 1, 98–105, 340n41; Kuṇḍalinī as, 45–64, 50, 52, 82, 86, 88, 97, 98–105, 116, 146, 280; and pneumatic body, 56, 63

Galen, 62–63
gender, 6, 10–11, 38, 42, 56, 59, 107, 152, 198, 202, 309, 319, 324, 341n68; as principles in tantra, 5, 6, 16, 44, 270, 315, 317, 341n66, 349n52; Kuṇḍalinī as feminine, 9, 10, 20, 41, 80, 304, 313; and sexed bodies, 7, 41, 51, 200, 272, 304, 308, 314–15, 317–19
Ghose, Aurobindo, 156–62, 218, 220, 250, 280, 281; and Gopi Krishna, 23, 162, 165–66, 167, 170–71, 175–80, 184, 187, 190, 194; and Michael Murphy, 274–75, 278
Ghosh, Atalbihari, 112–13
Gichtel, Johann Georg, 73–76, 78, 340n41
Gnosticism, 10, 18, 22, 73, 74, 80, 87, 119, 207, 270; in antiquity, 58–62, 64, 67, 71–72, 332n4, 333n7; and Theosophy, 84, 85, 90–92, 94–96, 101; and Jung, 107, 109–10
goddess, 10, 12, 42, 44, 146, 254, 294; in tantra, 6, 24, 38, 40–41, 47, 323; Kuṇḍalinī as, 30, 32, 47–50, 119, 135, 228, 233, 255, 287; as subject of practices in ethnography, 285, 302, 305, 309, 312, 315, 321
Gopi Krishna, 23, 74, 126, 206, 218, 220, 260, 261, 274, 190, 348n5; engagement with literature, 97, 98, 111, 167, 190, 342n69; early life, 166–68; and Aurobindo, 23, 162, 165–66, 167, 170–71, 175–80, 184, 187, 190, 194; experiential narrative of, 170–83; and analysis of narrative, 183–96, 349n52; collaborators and legacy of, 164–66; 168–69; 196–204, 248, 250, 256, 281–82, 359n78
Gorakṣa Śataka, 49
granthi, 46, 152
Grof, Christina and Stanislav, 263–69, 276–77, 279, 288, 292

Hanegraaff, Wouter, 18, 19
haṭha yoga. *See* yoga
harmonialism, 66, 89, 147, 220, 255, 270
heart, 12, 125, 131, 133, 134, 225, 257, 265; and central channel, 21, 256; and sun, 21, 37, 62, 63, 65, 102; and seat of self, 36, 37, 63, 77–78, 86; and Kuṇḍalinī, 44–45, 46, 51, 53, 86; and serpent in Gichtel, 73, 74, 76; in Gopi Krishna's experience, 173, 174, 175, 176, 177, 178, 187, 188
heat, 1, 35, 63, 64, 122, 337n6; in Kuṇḍalinī experience, 52, 105–6, 117, 176, 178, 203, 234, 268, 316
Hermes, 21, 61, 67–70, 72, 80, 82, 102. *See also* Mercury
Hermes Trismegistus, 68–69
Hermeticism, 18, 22, 61, 65, 69–72, 84, 90, 101, 102, 107, 109, 280, 333n7
Hevajra Tantra, 49
Hillman, James, 164, 183, 196–204, 350n52, 359n78
Holy Spirit, 59, 76, 92, 100, 249, 277
Hopman, Frederik Jan (Tontyn), 164, 183, 197, 203
Human Potential Movement, 24, 245, 250, 255, 269, 275–76, 278, 279, 282
Huxley, Aldous, 203, 204, 275

Ialdabaoth, 59–60
Iamblichus, 64
iḍā. *See* *nāḍī*
initiation, 92, 97, 126, 150, 230; in tantra, as *dīkṣā*, 41, 112, 114, 222, 313, 315, 317–18; and *śaktipāt*, 222, 232, 253
Integral Yoga, 158, 194, 274
internet: Kuṇḍalinī on, 295–301
Iyengar, B. K. S., 144–47

Jñāneśvarī, 40, 49, 50–54, 86, 87, 133, 264
Jois, K. Pattabhi, 144, 147
Jung, Carl, 10, 22, 106–12, 119, 204, 341n68, 342n69, 342n70; Jungian thought, 164, 194, 198, 199, 200, 253, 255, 298, 359n78

Kālī, 151, 321, 322, 323
Kāmākhyā, 13, 312–13, 317–18, 321, 324
karma, 35, 36, 148, 160, 217
Kaula, 20, 22, 46–47, 64, 115, 118, 150, 152, 194, 203, 228, 233
Kiehnle, Catharina, 50
Kripal, Jeffery J., 4, 9–10, 13, 25, 26, 213, 273
Kripalu Yoga, 230–31, 233–34, 244
Kripalvananda, Swami, 208, 230, 232–33, 243
Kriya Yoga, 32, 150, 152, 154–56, 215
kriyās, 152, 215, 228–29, 233–34, 244, 268
Krishnamacharya, Tirumalai, 143–44, 147
Kubjikāmata Tantra, 47

Kundalini: Evolution and Enlightenment (1979), 218, 248
Kundalini: Psychosis or Transcendence? (1976), 258
Kundalini: The Energy of the Depths (1983), 2, 273
Kundalini: The Evolutionary Energy in Man, 23, 164, 197, 206, 359n78
Kundalini Awakening Scale, 288, 324
Kundalini Concept: Its Origin and Value, The (2006), 281
Kundalini in the Physical World (1983), 280
Kundalini Yoga (1935), 141–42
Kuṇḍalinī yoga. *See* yoga
Kundalini Yoga as taught by Yogi Bhajan, 4, 24, 147, 213–21, 234, 244, 266, 288, 300
Kundalini Yoga for the West (1978), 252
Kuvalayananda, Swami, 137–41, 143, 145, 255

Leadbeater, Charles Webster, 73, 86, 89, 90, 91, 98–102, 103, 104, 193, 281, 338n8, 240n40; and Avalon, 116, 117; and danger of Kuṇḍalinī, 264–65; and sex, 271
Leland, Kurt, 89, 99
Life Divine, The (1919), 275
Living with Kundalini. *See Kundalini: The Evolutionary Energy in Man*
Logos, 90, 92, 99–100
lotus, 33, 44, 126, 132, 153, 172, 184, 232; heart as, 36, 45; *cakras* as, 46, 115, 118, 121, 126, 192, 329n3
Lucia, Amanda, 212
Majercik, Ruth, 64
Mallinson, James, 30, 41, 49, 122, 123, 324n83
Maslow, Abraham, 253
māyā, 38, 86, 146, 152, 153, 160
Mead, G. R. S., 107, 110
meditation, 35, 76, 126, 129, 139, 157, 256, 262, 277, 290–92; in Gopi Krishna's account, 167, 168, 172, 173, 175, 181, 184, 185; Yogi Bhajan on, 217, 218; Muktananda on, 223, 228, 353n50; Desai and, 230, 232, 233–34, Osho and, 236, 238, 239, 240, 241, 244
mental illness, 146, 258, 259, 262–66, 272–73, 283
Mercury: as god, 21, 82, 101, 102; as planet, 61, 74, 76; as substance, 10–11, 44, 70
Mesmer, Franz Anton, 78–80
Mithras Liturgy, 65, 334n17
moon, 34, 61, 68, 74; as symbol, 10, 35, 70, 198; in *haṭha* yoga, 42, 44, 49, 132, 198
Mukhopadhyay, Pramathanath, 113, 114
Muktananda, Swami, 24, 207, 210–11, 218, 221–29, 234, 243, 244, 245, 251, 253, 255, 260, 262, 265–66, 272, 274, 280
mūlādhāra. *See cakra*
Murphy, Michael, 27, 274–79, 282
Mysterious Kundalini, The (1927), 130–35

nāda. *See* sound
nāḍī, 16, 37, 43, 46, 65, 129, 138, 144, 145, 154, 268; *iḍā* and *piṅgalā*, 42, 94, 101, 103, 116, 127, 133, 176–78, 187, 198; *suṣumnā* or central channel, 20–21, 30, 42, 44, 46, 94, 96, 101, 103, 116, 118, 125, 127, 129, 133, 135, 188, 289
Nāga. *See* serpent
navel, 21, 45, 46, 48, 49, 51, 74, 76, 174, 176
Neoplatonism. *See* Platonism
Neo-Tantra, 4–5, 235, 273, 293–94, 320
nerve plexuses, 78, 79–80, 99, 118, 119, 122, 126–27, 132–34, 138, 154, 193, 236, 265, 344n13
Nityananda, Swami, 222–24, 228
nonduality, 38, 123, 144, 147, 262; in Śaiva and Śākta tantra, 2, 5, 6, 20, 40, 45, 47, 115, 222, 233, 269; and Yogananda, 152, 153, 154; and Adi Da, 251, 255, 282

Ophites, 59–60, 80, 332n4
Osho, 211, 235–44, 253–54, 255, 266, 272, 279, 294, 295, 354n65
ouroboros, 16, 67, 70–72, 86

Pādma Saṃhitā, 30, 45, 337n4
Patañjani. *See Yoga Sūtras*
penis, 46, 48, 51, 320, 321, 322, 323
physio-kundalini, 256, 259, 282, 288
piṅgalā. *See nāḍī*
planetary spheres, 21, 59, 61–62, 64–67, 72, 74–76, 89, 92, 337n6
Platonism, 57–58, 61, 62, 63, 109, 236, 333n12; Neoplatonism, 60–61, 64, 66, 84, 109, 202
Play of Consciousness (1974), 223–25
pneuma, 59, 60, 62–64, 88, 92, 333n12
prāṇa, 17, 30, 155, 233–34, 243, 249, 265; as *prāṇakuṇḍalinī*, 47, 118, 152, 233
prāṇāyāma, 35, 126, 128, 129, 130, 133, 136, 137, 140–41, 142, 145, 148, 152, 172, 229, 233, 262, 321
Price, Richard, 274–75, 277, 279
Pryse, James Morgan, 89, 90, 91–98, 101, 116, 117, 339n19
psychology, 79, 128, 141, 146, 165, 204, 244, 270, 275, 276, 291, 298; Jungian, 22, 106–12, 141, 194, 198–99; transpersonal, 253, 255, 288–89, 292; and physio-kundalini, 259, 260; and spiritual emergency, 267–68, 283

Ramakrishna Paramahansa, 125, 126, 151, 167
Raja Yoga (1896), 22, 125–30, 135, 136, 165
Rajneesh, Bhagwan Shree. *See* Osho
Rele, Vasant G., 130–35, 218, 248, 256
Row, Tallapragada Subba, 85, 337n6
Rudrananda, Swami, 253

Sabhapati Swami, 94, 338n16, 339n25
sahasrāra. *See cakra*

Śaiva. *See* tantra
Śākta. *See* tantra
śakti: as goddess, 1, 32, 44–45, 48, 50, 52, 53, 114, 153, 3350n52; as energy, 10, 20, 24, 38, 41, 44, 46, 47, 85, 132, 145, 152, 157, 178, 209, 312, 316
śaktipāt, 24, 41, 210, 218–19, 242; and Muktananda, 221–25, 228–29, 243, 244, 253, 266; and Desai, 230–34, 243
Saṃgīta Ratnākara, 46
Sanderson, Alexis, 39
Sannella, Lee, 255, 258–63, 266–67, 268, 277, 280, 281–83, 288, 289–90
Sārdhatriśatikālottara Tantra, 44
Ṣaṭcakra Nirūpaṇa, 22, 47, 114–15, 117, 192, 343n83
Scott, Mary, 280–81, 359n78
Self-Realization Fellowship, 151, 152, 215, 346n66
semen, 10, 34, 35, 36, 44, 200, 321, 322; as *bindu*, 30, 35, 42, 44–45, 49, 122, 193, 198, 199, 313
serpent, 9, 21, 24, 30, 34, 48, 250, 255, 274, 289, 298, 299, 325, 327n5; Kuṇḍalinī described as, 2–3, 9–10, 12, 24, 31, 44–46, 48, 52, 83, 248, 249, 267, 276, 280, 313–14; in Western sources, 5, 56–57, 59–60, 67–68, 70–74, 76, 80, 96–97, 270, 3332n5; as Nāga, 31–32, 86, 329n5, 329n6; in Theosophy, 84–88, 89, 91–93, 97–98, 99, 100, 102; in Jung, 106, 107, 108–9, 110, 342n68; in Yogananda, 152; in Aurobindo, 159; in Gopi Krishna, 188, 189, 190; in discourse of modern gurus, 207; in Yogi Bhajan, 220; in Osho, 237
Śeṣa, 31–33, 86, 249
Siddha Yoga, 207, 218, 221, 228–29, 353n50
Siddhasiddhānta Paddhati, 47, 50
siddhi, 53, 129, 135, 155, 191, 278, 304, 305, 309, 310, 311, 316–17, 361n15
Silburn, Lilian, 2, 273–74
Singh, Maharaj Virsa, 214
Śiva, 10, 32, 33, 34, 40–41, 44, 48, 49, 54, 114, 153, 162, 323
Śiva Saṃhitā, 44, 46, 136
Sivananda Saraswati, Swami, 141–42, 143, 144, 145, 218, 295
Sivananda Radha, Swami, 251–53, 255, 272, 273, 280
Serpent Power, The (1919), 22, 47, 97, 110, 112, 114–19, 132, 144, 191, 281, 341n66, 359n78. *See also* Avalon, Arthur
Sikhism, 137, 214, 216, 219–20
Singleton, Mark, 30, 215, 342n83
snake. *See* serpent
social media. *See* internet
solar body, 92, 96, 97
solar plexus, 78–80, 265
Sophia, 59–60, 76, 80
soul, 68, 69, 73, 76, 96, 108, 135, 202, 295, 316; ascent of, 21, 30, 34, 56, 58–61, 63–67, 70, 72, 75–76, 80, 339n25; Kuṇḍalinī as, 47, 228; nature and capacities of, 62–64,

109, 333n12; World Soul, 58, 60, 86–87; and Mesmerism, 78–80
sound, 44–45, 53, 153, 223, 256, 259, 268; *nāda*, 48, 122, 152; in Gopi Krishna's experience, 173, 175, 188, 189, 191
speirēma, 92–93, 96–97
Spiegelberg, Frederic, 168–69, 189, 201, 204, 275, 282
spine, 33, 98, 102, 107, 139–41, 176, 195; and subtle channels and *cakras*, 44, 94, 118, 127, 133, 135, 153, 154, 192; Kuṇḍalinī at base of, 2, 20, 103, 104, 126, 146, 172, 193, 248, 260, 280, 289; Kuṇḍalinī rising along, 12, 97, 105, 187–88, 190, 203, 219, 249, 250, 256–57, 260, 262, 268, 289; sensation in, 79, 105, 159, 173, 177, 178, 181, 186–88, 190, 203, 234, 257, 268, 289
Spiritual Emergency (1989), 267–69
Spiritual Emergency/e Network (SEN), 263, 266–67, 269
Steiner, Rudolf, 82
Stoicism, 60, 63
stress, 256–57, 260
Strube, Julian, 83, 112–13, 114, 342n83, 344n13
sun, 34, 61, 187, 193, 258, 299, 324; as symbol, 1, 10–11, 21, 35, 42, 44, 52, 62, 63, 70, 74, 76, 108; and path of the soul, 34, 36–37, 62, 64–65, 334n17; black sun, 76, 101; in Theosophical models, 90, 92, 100–101, 102–6, 340n40, 240n41
sunthemata, 65
suṣumnā. *See nāḍī*
Swedenborg, Emanuel, 76–78
sympathetic nervous system, 94, 97, 106–7, 132–33

tantra, 2, 4–5, 12, 15–16, 21, 24, 83, 85, 113, 123, 152, 203, 219, 250, 273, 277, 285, 287, 292; non-dual Śaiva and Śakta, 6, 13–14, 20, 22, 46–47, 40, 54, 115, 135, 152; textual sources on Kuṇḍalinī, 44–49; and Yogananda, 150, 152; and Aurobindo, 157–58, 161, 162; and Muktananda, 228; and Kripalu yoga, 233; and sex, 270–71, 273–74, 294; ethnographic accounts of, 302, 304–24. *See also* Neo-Tantra
Tantra Sadbhāva, 44–45
tapas, 35, 41, 49, 64, 122, 146. *See also* asceticism
tattvas, 39, 53, 131, 252, 314, 317
Taylor, Kathleen, 112–13
Taylor, Steve, 289
Theosophy, 21–22, 73, 82–83, 122, 135, 138, 147, 148; early engagement with Kuṇḍalinī, 84–90, 337n6, 338n14; hybrid Kuṇḍalinī models, 90–106; influence on Jung, 107, 109; and Avalon, 114, 115–19; and Gopi Krishna, 165, 167, 193; and danger of Kuṇḍalinī, 264, 271–72; and Mary Scott, 280–81
theurgy, 64–67, 69, 88, 89, 334n15, 334n17

Thoth, 68–69
Transcendental Meditation (TM), 217, 262

Upaniṣads, 34, 36–37, 42, 65, 92–93, 123, 154, 157
Urban, Hugh B., 4, 236, 244, 273

vagina, 320–21, 322
vagus nerve, 131–35
Vaiṣṇava, 45–46, 50, 143, 144, 147, 208, 329n3
Varieties of Contemplative Experience (VCE) project, 290–92, 298
Vasiṣṭha Saṃhitā, 46
Vedānta, 38, 92, 123, 144, 147, 167, 262, 271; Yogananda and, 150, 152, Aurobindo and, 157–8, 160, 161
Versluis, Arthur, 73
Vivekananda, Swami, 22, 123, 135, 136, 138, 142, 165, 207, 220, 245, 251; on Kuṇḍalinī, 124–30; on evolution, 148–49; references to, 130, 131, 135, 138, 218, 248; and Yogananda, 151; and Aurobindo, 156, 157
Voice of the Silence, The (1889), 86–87, 98

Weizsäcker, Carl Friedrich Freiherr von, 199–201
West Bengal, 8, 24; fieldwork in, 320–24
White, David Gordon, 36, 40, 41
White, John, 218, 248–49, 250, 280
Woodroffe, John. *See* Avalon, Arthur
Wrisberg, Heinrich August, 78

yoga, 2, 16–18, 22, 36–37, 40, 46, 64, 90, 107, 115, 116, 253, 260, 270, 271, 276, 279, 288, 294, 295, 337n6; *haṭha* yoga, 30, 41–42, 49, 122–24, 133, 134, 136, 150, 152, 167, 168, 215, 217, 229, 241, 271, 321; *laya* yoga, 41, 48; Kuṇḍalinī yoga, 4, 13, 111, 141–42, 144, 156, 190–91, 195, 206, 214, 215, 216, 233, 234, 252, 253, 287, 300, 302, 308, 310, 311, 313–15, 320; and modernization of yogic physiology, 121, 127–48; and Vivekananda, 124–30; postural yoga, 136–48, 214, 215, 233, 288; modern metaphysical yoga, 148–62; Gopi Krishna and, 167, 168, 169, 170, 172, 190–91, 194; as brand, 206–7; Yogi Bhajan and, 213–21, 265, 288, 300; Muktananda and, 221, 228–29, 265–66, 353n50; Desai and, 230–34; Osho and, 241, 244
Yoga Sūtras, 17, 32, 125, 129, 136, 140, 145–49, 233
Yoga Vāsiṣṭha, 7
Yogananda, Paramahansa, 22, 126, 150–56, 160, 162, 165, 211, 215, 245, 251, 246n66
Yoginī, 40–41

zodiac, 66, 85, 88, 92–93, 94, 119, 154
Zweig, Paul, 226–27

GPSR Authorized Representative: Easy Access System Europe, Mustamäe tee 50, 10621 Tallinn, Estonia, gpsr.requests@easproject.com

www.ingramcontent.com/pod-product-compliance
Lightning Source LLC
Chambersburg PA
CBHW022025290426
44109CB00014B/757
* 9 7 8 0 2 3 1 2 1 2 5 3 3 *